Taking SIDES

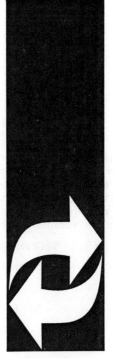

Clashing Views on Controversial Issues in Health and Society

Third Edition

Edited, Selected, and with Introductions by

Eileen L. Daniel

State University of New York College at Brockport

Dushkin/McGraw-Hill
A Division of The McGraw-Hill Companies

To Ann

Cover Art Acknowledgment

Charles Vitelli

Library of Congress Cataloging-in-Publication Data

Main entry under title:
    Taking sides: clashing views on controversial issues in health and society/edited, selected, and with introductions by Eileen L. Daniel.—3rd ed.
    Includes bibliographical references and index.
    1. Health. 2. Medical care—United States. 3. Medical ethics. 4. Social medicine—United States. I. Daniel, Eileen L., *comp.*

362.1

0-697-39111-6   ISSN: 1094-7531

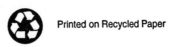 Printed on Recycled Paper

Taking SIDES

Clashing Views on
Controversial Issues in
Health and Society

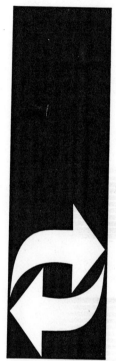

Third Edition

PREFACE

This book contains 38 articles arranged in 19 *pro* and *con* pairs. Each pair addresses a controversial issue in health and society, expressed in terms of a question in order to draw the lines of debate more clearly.

Most of the questions that are included here relate to health topics of modern concern, such as AIDS, managed health care, environmental health, and drug use and abuse. The authors of these articles take strong stands on specific issues and provide support for their positions. Although we may not agree with a particular point of view, each author clearly defines his or her stand on the issues.

This book is divided into six parts, each containing related issues. Each part opener provides a brief overview of the issues and offers several related sites on the World Wide Web, including Web addresses. Each issue is preceded by an *introduction*, which sets the stage for the debate, gives the historical background of the subject, and provides a context for the controversy. Each issue concludes with a *postscript*, which offers a summary of the debate and some concluding observations and suggests further readings on the subject. The postscript also raises further points, since most of the issues have more than two sides. At the back of the book is a listing of all the *contributors to this volume*, which gives information on the physicians, professors, journalists, and scientists whose views are debated here.

Taking Sides: Clashing Views on Controversial Issues in Health and Society is a tool to encourage critical thought on important health issues. Readers should not feel confined to the views expressed in the articles. Some readers may see important points on both sides of an issue and may construct for themselves a new and creative approach, which may incorporate the best of both sides or provide an entirely new vantage point for understanding.

Changes to this edition   The third edition of *Taking Sides: Clashing Views on Controversial Issues in Health and Society* includes some important changes from the second edition. Seven completely new issues have been added: *Will Managed Care Improve Health Care in the United States?* (Issue 1); *Can Spirituality Overcome Disease?* (Issue 6); *Should Moderate Use of Alcohol Be Recommended?* (Issue 8); *Is Marijuana Dangerous and Addictive?* (Issue 9); *Are Silicone Breast Implants a Health Risk to Women?* (Issue 10); *Public Policy and Health: Is Global Warming a Real Threat?* (Issue 16); and *Are Homeopathic Remedies Legitimate?* (Issue 19). For eight of the issues, I have retained the topic from the second edition but have replaced one or both of the selections in order to bring the debate up-to-date or to focus more clearly on the controversy: Issue 2 on physician-assisted suicide; Issue 4 on gun control as a public health issue; Issue 5 on mandating healthy behavior; Issue 12 on AIDS; Issue 14 on the Gulf War Syndrome; Issue 15 on pesticide exposure; Issue 17 on yo-yo dieting; and Issue 18 on immunization. As a result, there is a total of 24 new readings. The issue introductions and postscripts have all been revised and updated.

In addition to changes in topics and selections, a new feature, *On the Internet*, has been added to each part opener. Several relevant sites on the World Wide Web have been identified and annotated.

A word to the instructor An *Instructor's Manual With Test Questions* (both multiple-choice and essay) is available through the publisher for instructors using *Taking Sides* in the classroom. Also available is a general guidebook, *Using Taking Sides in the Classroom*, which discusses teaching techniques and methods for integrating the pro-con approach of *Taking Sides* into any classroom setting.

An online version of *Using Taking Sides in the Classroom* and a correspondence service for Taking Sides adopters can be found at www.cybsol.com/usingtakingsides/.

Taking Sides: Clashing Views on Controversial Issues in Health and Society is only one title in the Taking Sides series. If you are interested in seeing the table of contents for any of the other titles, please visit the Taking Sides Web site at http://www.dushkin.com/takingsides/.

Acknowledgments Special thanks again to John, Diana, and Jordan. Also, thanks to my colleagues at the State University of New York College at Brockport for all their helpful contributions. I was also assisted in preparing this edition by the valuable suggestions from the adopters of *Taking Sides* who filled out comment cards and questionnaires:

Catherine Cardina
SUNY College at
   Brockport

Patricia Goodson
University of Texas–
   San Antonio

Cindy Groh
Chicago State University

Carol Johnson
University of Richmond

Kathryn Schneider
Pacific Union College

Marsha Schreiber
Biola University

Michael Stahly
Olivet College

Many of your recommendations were incorporated into this edition. Finally, I appreciate the assistance of David Dean, list manager of the Taking Sides series at Dushkin/McGraw-Hill.

Eileen L. Daniel
State University of New York
College at Brockport

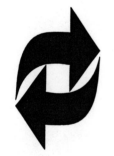

CONTENTS IN BRIEF

CONTENTS

Surgeon David Jacobsen makes the claim that health maintenance organizations (HMOs) offer quality care and that high-quality medical care at an affordable price is not only possible under managed care; it is a reality. Journalism professor A. Kent MacDougall contends that joining a managed care program was the most painful mistake in his life.

Marcia Angell, M.D., executive editor of *The New England Journal of Medicine*, believes that physician-assisted suicide should be permitted under some circumstances and that not all of the pain of the dying can be controlled. Physician Kathleen M. Foley believes that doctors do not know enough about their patients, themselves, or suffering, to provide assistance with dying as a medical treatment for the relief of suffering.

Hastings Center director Daniel Callahan believes that medical care for elderly people should not involve expensive health care services that serve only to forestall death. Physicians Ezekiel J. Emanuel and Linda L. Emanuel argue that cost savings due to limitations in medical care at the end of life are not likely to be substantial.

Josh Sugarmann, executive director of the Violence Policy Center, an education foundation that researches firearm violence and advocates gun control, argues that guns increase the costs of hospitalization, rehabilitation, and lost wages, making them a serious public health issue. Attorney Don B. Kates, Professor Henry E. Schaffer and William C. Waters IV, a physician, counter that most gun-related violence is caused by aberrants, not ordinary gun owners.

Michael F. Jacobson, a microbiologist and the director of the Center for Science in the Public Interest, claims that federal policies emphasizing healthy behavior would not only improve public health but reduce health care spending. Journalist and author Jacob Sullum argues that, by treating risky behavior like a communicable disease, the public health establishment invites the government to meddle in our private lives.

Herbert Benson, associate professor of medicine at Harvard Medical School, and journalist Marg Stark contend that faith and spirituality will enhance and prolong life. William B. Lindley, associate editor of *Truth Seeker*, counters that there is no scientific way to determine that spirituality can heal.

The editors of *Consumer Reports* argue that there is sound scientific data proving that secondhand smoke causes lung cancer and other illnesses. Editor and journalist Jacob Sullum argues that there is no evidence that secondhand smoking carries the dangers associated with actually smoking.

Writer Dave Shiflett claims that for years the antidrinking establishment has insisted that even moderate drinking is bad for health despite the fact that science indicates otherwise. Physicians Meir J. Stampfer and Eric B. Rimm and professor Diana Chapman Walsh argue that encouraging the use of alcohol, even in moderation, could lead to an increase in its consumption, with potentially dangerous results.

Eric A. Voth, medical director of Chemical Dependency Services at St. Francis Hospital in Topeka, Kansas, argues that marijuana produces many adverse effects and that its effectiveness as a medicine is supported only by anecdotes. Ethan A. Nadelmann, director of the Lindesmith Center, a New York drug policy research institute, claims that government officials continue to promote the myth that marijuana is harmful and leads to the use of hard drugs; he states that the war on marijuana is being fought for purely political, not health, reasons.

Reporter Jennifer Washburn challenges two studies that claim silicone gel implants do no harm and finds over 10 percent of the women who received implants are ill. Journalist Michael Fumento claims that special interests and the press have conspired to ban implants despite the fact that no scientific study has linked them to cancer or other diseases.

Health and medical reporters Leslie Laurence and Beth Weinhouse claim that women have been excluded from most research on new drugs and medical treatments. Physician Andrew G. Kadar argues that women actually receive more medical care and benefit more from medical research than do men.

William B. Johnston, a senior research fellow and the vice president of the Hudson Institute, and Kevin R. Hopkins, an adjunct senior fellow of the

Hudson Institute, describe the rise of AIDS cases among heterosexuals and warn that unless people make a serious attempt to alter behaviors that put them at risk for the disease, this population will be facing an AIDS epidemic. Columnist for the *Philadelphia Inquirer* David R. Boldt claims that public health officials with the help of the media have exaggerated the risk of heterosexual AIDS.

Author Mary Gordon believes that abortion is an acceptable means to end an unwanted pregnancy. Editor Jason DeParle argues that the 3 out of 10 pregnancies that currently end in abortion raise many moral questions.

Journalists Dennis Bernstein and Thea Kelley claim that disabling, sometimes life-threatening medical problems related to environmental and chemical exposure are currently affecting thousands of soldiers who fought in the Persian Gulf War. Michael Fumento, a science and economics reporter, argues that medical experts have not found any evidence to support the existence of a syndrome related to the war.

Martha Honey, research fellow at the Institute for Policy Studies, claims that pesticides in the food chain are building up in animals and humans and are disrupting the immune system, causing cancers, and birth defects. Professor of biochemistry and molecular biology Bruce Ames argues that any risks from pesticides in foods are minimal and that fears are greatly exaggerated.

Journalist Ross Gelbspan contends that we need to act now to prevent future catastrophic climatic changes that may result from global warming. Atmospheric physicist S. Fred Singer argues that 18 years of weather-satellite data actually show a global cooling trend.

Nutritionist Frances M. Berg contends that yo-yo dieting, or weight cycling, is associated with an elevated risk of physical and mental health problems and that it increases the risk of regaining lost weight. The editors of the *Harvard Heart Letter* claim that there is no convincing evidence that weight cycling has any major effects on heart disease risk, the effectiveness of future diets, increased percentage of body fat, or metabolism.

Physicians Gary L. Freed and Samuel L. Katz and epidemiologist Sarah J. Clark maintain that the benefits of vaccination substantially outweigh the risks and that childhood vaccination has significantly reduced the incidence of many common childhood infections. Health journalist Richard Leviton maintains that many vaccines are neither safe nor effective and that parents should have a say in whether or not their children receive them.

Author Nancy Bruning claims that neither skeptics nor believers can exactly
explain how homeopathy works, but it can successfully treat a wide range
of health problems. Physician and health consumer advocate Stephen Barrett
argues that homeopathic remedies are so dilute that they are useless.

INTRODUCTION

Dimensions and Approaches to the Study of Health and Society

Eileen L. Daniel

WHAT IS HEALTH?

Traditionally, being healthy meant being absent of illness. If someone did not have a disease, then he or she was considered to be healthy. The overall health of a nation or specific population was determined by numbers measuring illness, disease, and death rates. Today, this rather negative view of assessing individual health and health in general is changing. A healthy person is one who is not only free from disease but also fully well.

Being well, or wellness, involves the interrelationship of many dimensions of health: physical, emotional, social, mental, and spiritual. This multifaceted view of health reflects a holistic approach, which includes individuals taking responsibility for their own well-being.

Our health and longevity are affected by the many choices we make every day: Medical reports tell us that if we abstain from smoking, drugs, excessive alcohol consumption, fat, and cholesterol, and if we get regular exercise, our rate of disease and disability will significantly decrease. These reports, although not totally conclusive, have encouraged many people to make positive lifestyle changes. Millions of people have quit smoking, alcohol consumption is down, and more and more individuals are exercising regularly and eating low-fat diets. These changes are encouraging, but many people have been unable or unwilling to make them and are left feeling worried and/or guilty over continuing their negative health behaviors.

Additionally, experts disagree about the exact nature of positive health behaviors, and this causes confusion. For example, some scientists claim that Americans should make efforts to reduce their serum cholesterol in order to lower their risk of heart disease. Other researchers claim that lowering serum cholesterol has no significant effect on heart health. Whom do you believe? Experts also disagree on the risks of global warming, whether or not sex education prevents unwanted pregnancy, and the role of exercise in increasing longevity.

Health status is also affected by society and government. Societal pressures have helped pass smoking restrictions in public places, mandatory safety belt legislation, and laws permitting condom distribution in public schools. The government plays a role in the health of individuals as well, although it has failed to provide minimal health care for many low-income Americans.

Unfortunately, there are no absolute answers to many questions regarding health and wellness issues. Moral questions, controversial concerns, and individual perceptions of health matters all can create opposing views. As you evaluate the issues in this book, you should keep an open mind toward both sides. You may not change your mind regarding the morality of abortion or the limitation of health care for the elderly, but you will still be able to learn from the opposing viewpoint.

WELLNESS, BEHAVIOR, AND SOCIETY

The issues in this book are divided into six parts. The first deals with health care and society. The topics addressed in Part 1 include a debate on whether or not managed health care offers consumers an improvement over traditional care. In the United States, approximately 35 to 40 million Americans have no health insurance. There has been a resurgence in diseases such as tuberculosis and antibiotic-resistant strains of bacterial infections, which threaten thousands of Americans and strain the current system. Those enrolled in government programs such as Medicaid often find few, if any, physicians who will accept them as patients since reimbursements are low and the paperwork is cumbersome. On the other hand, Americans continue to live longer and longer, and for most of us, the health care available is among the best in the world.

Issue 2 deals with whether or not physicians should intervene in hastening death for hopelessly ill persons. Many Americans agree that we cannot and should not prolong the lives of terminally ill patients, although others believe that physicians should not hasten the process of dying but rather should offer these persons relief from pain and quality of life management strategies. In Issue 3, Daniel Callahan, the director of the Hastings Center, believes that the increasing proportion of health care dollars that is going to the elderly cannot be allowed to continue. Physicians Ezekiel and Linda Emanuel disagree with Callahan. The fourth controversy in this section is about the epidemic of homicide and the potential benefits of more stringent gun control. Doctors and public health officials claim that homicides involving guns are increasing and that owning a gun is dangerous. They maintain that gun control would help slow down the shootings and deaths. Opponents of gun control argue that only criminals—not law-abiding citizens—would have access to guns. They also contend that doctors should leave the gun control issue to criminologists.

MIND/BODY RELATIONSHIP

Part 2 discusses two important issues related to the relationship between mind and body. Should the government mandate healthy behaviors, and can spirituality overcome disease? Over the past 10 years, both laypeople and the medical profession have placed an emphasis on the prevention of illness as a way to improve health. Not smoking, for instance, certainly reduces the risk of developing lung cancer. Unfortunately, the current U.S. health care system places an emphasis on treatment rather than on prevention, even though prevention is less expensive, less painful, and more humane. Michael Jacobson, director of the Center for Science in the Public Interest, states that the emphasis on treatment has neglected prevention. Jacob Sullum claims that by treating risky behavior like a communicable disease, the medical establishment invites the government to meddle in our personal lives.

SUBSTANCE USE AND ABUSE

Part 3 introduces current issues related to drug use and abuse in the United States. Millions of Americans use and abuse drugs that alter their minds and affect their bodies. These drugs range from illegal substances, such as crack cocaine and marijuana, to the widely used legal drugs, alcohol and tobacco. Use of these substances can lead to physical and psychological addiction and the related problems of family dysfunction, reduced worker productivity, and crime. Because of drug-related crime, many experts have argued for the legalization of drugs, particularly marijuana. The legalization of marijuana for medicinal purposes is another relevant issue concerning the drug.

The American drug crisis is often related to changes in or a breakdown of traditional values. The collapse of strong family and religious influences may affect drug usage, especially among young people. Illicit drugs remain a problem in this country, and alcohol also continues to be a major concern. Alcohol is a factor in car crashes, violence, and health problems. Heavy drinkers are at risk for cirrhosis, cancer, hypertension, malnutrition, and other illnesses. Although these risks are well known, some experts maintain that moderate drinking can actually improve health by reducing stress and heart attacks. They believe that moderate drinking should be promoted as a means of reducing heart disease. Also in this section is a debate on passive smoking. The individual's right to smoke in public is set against the nonsmoker's health risks when forced to breathe tobacco smoke. There is also debate over the research used to link passive smoking and health concerns.

SEXUALITY AND GENDER ISSUES

For years, women in North America have had the option of augmenting the size of their breasts by having silicone implants placed under their skin. Some women have the operation to reconstruct their breasts following a mastectomy, but most opt for the surgery for cosmetic reasons. Recently, some women with breast implants have claimed that the silicone has caused health problems ranging from headaches to autoimmune diseases. Several successful lawsuits were based on the premise that silicone caused these health problems. Jennifer Washburn holds this opinion, but Michael Fumento in "A Confederacy of Boobs" argues that there is no conclusive evidence that silicone causes disease.

Other issues discussed in this section include the debate over whether or not our health care system favors men at the expense of women. Although they live longer than men, many women claim that they have been excluded from drug tests and other medical research and receive inferior care when they see doctors. Physician Andrew Kadar disagrees with this premise. He claims that women see their doctors more frequently than men, are hospitalized more often, and continue to outlive men by several years.

Issue 12 focuses on whether or not AIDS is a serious risk to the heterosexual, non-drug-abusing population. Author David Boldt believes that the AIDS epidemic has peaked and heterosexual transmission has actually decreased. The general population was never at a high risk for contracting the disease, he claims. Researchers William B. Johnston and Kevin R. Hopkins have an opposing viewpoint. They feel that as heterosexuals become more sexually active, their risk of contracting AIDS increases.

The United States has one of the highest teenage pregnancy rates. Is abortion an acceptable means to end an unwanted pregnancy? Mary Gordon believes that abortion is acceptable and argues in Issue 13 that it is not an immoral choice for women. Jason DeParle, in opposition, discusses why liberals and feminists do not like to talk about the morality of abortion. The abortion issue continues to cause major controversy. More restrictions have been placed on the right to abortion as a result of the political power wielded by the pro-life faction. Pro-choice followers, however, argue that making abortion illegal again will force many women to obtain dangerous, back alley abortions.

ENVIRONMENTAL ISSUES

Debate continues over the two fundamental issues surrounding the environment: human needs and the future of the environment. The debate becomes more heated as the environmental issues move closer to human concerns such as health, economic interests, and politics. In Issue 14, for example, the debate focuses on whether or not troops stationed overseas during the Persian Gulf War were exposed to harmful environmental or chemical substances that caused their present health problems. Issue 15 discusses the safety of pesticide usage on fruits and vegetables. The Alar (a chemical growth regulator for apples) scare convinced many Americans that the apple supply was not safe and that an apple a day could cause cancer. At the same time, nutritionists as well as the Department of Agriculture were urging people to eat more fruits and vegetables to help *prevent* cancer.

The question of whether or not environmental changes are having a serious impact on the average global temperature is debated in Issue 16. Global warming has many implications, including political, health, economic, and environmental. Due to increased levels of greenhouse gases in the atmosphere, global temperatures appear to be rising. Rising temperatures could cause major catastrophes such as loss of plant and animal species, a reduction of the food supply, drought, disease, and flooding of low-lying coastal areas.

NUTRITION, EXERCISE, AND CONSUMER HEALTH

Is yo-yo dieting harmful to health? Should children be immunized? Are homeopathic remedies legitimate? These questions are discussed in Part 6, which deals with consumer health and nutrition.

Millions of Americans are dieting, many going on one diet after another, in an effort to achieve a lean figure. Does constant dieting increase one's risk of heart disease and other medical problems? And does it become harder to lose weight the more frequently one diets? These questions are explored in Issue 17.

This section also introduces questions about particular issues related to choices about health care services: (1) Should all children be immunized against childhood diseases? and (2) Are homeopathic remedies legitimate?

At the turn of the century, millions of American children developed childhood diseases such as tetanus, polio, measles, and pertussis (whooping cough). Many of these children died or became permanently disabled because of these illnesses. Today, vaccines can prevent all of these conditions; however, not all children receive their recommended immunizations. Some do not get vaccinated until the schools require them, and others are allowed exemptions. More and more, parents are requesting exemptions for some or all vaccinations based on fears over their safety and/or their effectiveness. The pertussis vaccination seems to generate the biggest fears. Reports of serious injury to children following the pertussis vaccination (usually given in a combination of diphtheria, pertussis, and tetanus, or DPT) have convinced many parents to forgo immunization. As a result, the incidence rates of measles and pertussis have been climbing after decades of decline. Is it safer to be vaccinated than to risk getting pertussis? Most medical societies and physicians believe so, but Richard Leviton argues that many vaccines are neither safe nor effective.

Current views of homeopathy and the use of homeopathic remedies are discussed in Issue 19. Due to demand by the public, homeopathy is achieving new legitimacy, despite the efforts of traditional medicine to discredit the practice. As more consumers turn their backs on traditional medicine, the use of homeopathic remedies has increased.

Will the many debates presented in this book ever be resolved? Some issues may resolve themselves because of the availability of resources. For instance, funding for health care for the elderly may become restricted in the United States, as it is in the United Kingdom, simply because there are increasingly limited resources to go around. As health costs continue to rise, an overhaul of the health care system to provide managed care for all while keeping costs down seems inevitable. Other controversies may require the test of time for resolution. Several more years may be required before it can be determined whether or not global warming is really a serious environmental hazard.

Other controversies may never resolve themselves. There may never be a consensus over the abortion issue, gun control, or the dangers of secondhand smoke. This book will introduce you to many ongoing controversies on a variety of sensitive and complex health-related topics. In order to have a good grasp of one's own viewpoint, it is necessary to be familiar with and understand the points made by the opposition.

On the Internet . . .

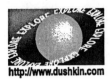

National Committee for Quality Assurance

The National Committee for Quality Assurance's World Wide Web page features an HMO accreditation status list, updated monthly; accreditation summary reports on a number of HMO plans, and other consumer information on managed care plans. *http://www.ncqa.org*

Euthanasia World Directory

This site deals with euthanasia and contains a newsletter and a main page featuring Dr. Jack Kevorkian. There is also a discussion on the book *Final Exit* and numerous citations about different laws regarding assisted suicide. *http://www.efn.org/~ergo/*

Huffington Center on Aging

The Huffington Center on Aging, Baylor College of Medicine's home page, offers great links to related sites on aging, Alzheimer's disease, and other material related to aging. *http://www.bcm.tmc.edu/hcoa/*

National Institutes of Health

The National Institutes of Health supports and conducts health and medical research. There is also information here about the history of medicine. *http://www.nih.gov*

PART 1

Health and Society

The United States currently faces many challenging health problems, including an aging population and lack of health care insurance for millions. Society must confront the enormous financial burden of providing health care to the elderly. At the same time, millions of Americans have enrolled in health maintenance organizations, which attempt to control health care costs through managing care. Although many people are happy with managed care, others claim it restricts access to the health care they need. To further complicate the problem, public policy and medical ethics have not always kept pace with rapidly growing technology and scientific advances. This section discusses some of the major controversies concerning the role of society in health concerns.

■ Will Managed Care Improve Health Care in the United States?

■ Should Doctors Ever Assist Terminally Ill Patients to Commit Suicide?

■ Should Health Care for the Elderly Be Limited?

■ Is Gun Control a Public Health Issue?

ISSUE 1

Will Managed Care Improve Health Care in the United States?

YES: David Jacobsen, from "Cost-Conscious Care," *Reason* (June 1996)

NO: A. Kent MacDougall, from "Health-Care Hell: One Man's Descent into the Abyss," *The Progressive* (March 1995)

ISSUE SUMMARY

YES: Surgeon David Jacobsen makes the claim that health maintenance organizations (HMOs) offer quality care and that high-quality medical care at an affordable price is not only possible under managed care; it is a reality.

NO: Journalism professor A. Kent MacDougall contends that joining a managed care program was the most painful mistake in his life.

Many Americans have perceived serious wrongs with the current health care system. In general, these concerns are (1) increasing health care access to the 35–40 million uninsured, (2) gaining the ability to keep one's health insurance when one changes or loses a job, and (3) controlling the escalating costs of health care.

Health care in this country is handled by various unrelated agencies and organizations and through a number of programs, including private insurance, government-supported Medicaid for the needy, and Medicare for the elderly. Currently there are between 35 and 40 million people, about 16 percent of the population, who do not have any health insurance and who do not qualify for government-sponsored programs. These people must often do without any medical care or suffer financial catastrophe if illness occurs. A *New York Times* article in 1992 claimed that 50 percent of personal bankruptcies in the United States have been attributed to medical costs.

In addition to the number of uninsured Americans, our health care is the most expensive in the world. The United States spends more on health care than any other nation, about $2,600 per capita. The share of the national output of wealth, the gross domestic product (GDP), expended by the United States on health is 14 percent and rising. Yet the United States has a lower life expectancy, higher infant mortality, and a higher percentage of low birth weight infants than Canada, Japan, or most western European nations. Ironically, the United States is the only industrialized nation other than South Africa that does not provide government-sponsored health care to all its citizens.

One solution to our health care problems has been the shift to managing care through various plans such as health maintenance organizations (HMOs). HMOs are organizations that provide health care in return for pre-fixed payments. Most HMOs provide care through a network of doctors and hospitals that their members must use in order to be covered. Currently, more than 50 million workers, 70 percent of the nation's eligible employees, now have health care through some type of managed care. The rise in managed care is related to employer efforts to reduce health care benefit costs. There are cost savings, but consumer groups and physicians worry that managed care will move medical decisions from doctors to accountants. The managed care industry argues that health care will actually improve under its care. They claim that it makes good financial sense for them to intervene early before patients get more sick. Unfortunately, seriously ill patients, who are the most expensive to treat, may lose out under managed care.

The underlying principle of managed health care is to maintain the health of a community by offering early detection tests and preventive care such as cholesterol screenings, vaccinations, physical exams, and smoking cessation programs. These services are usually provided at a modest fee or co-pay. In exchange for these reduced fees, the consumer agrees to see a limited group of doctors and providers selected by the managed care plan. The plan keeps rates down by limiting the patient's access to costly specialists and procedures, using less expensive and lesser trained providers, and by reducing hospital stays. Some health care workers have complained that pressure has been put on them to discharge patients as quickly as possible. Managed care plans have also increasingly demanded that certain medical procedures that were once done only in a hospital now be done in a less costly outpatient setting.

Does managed care compromise quality? Studies comparing traditional fee-for-service and managed care have found that the quality of care is similar. Consumer satisfaction surveys do not necessarily agree. Managed care patients are less likely to be satisfied with their care than those in a traditional practice. The more seriously ill they are, the more dissatisfaction they report. A recent survey by the Harvard School of Public Health found that managed care patients reported longer waits to see a specialist. They were also more likely to report incorrect care by their primary care physician. Most experts believe there is a wide range in quality among managed care plans. In cities where managed care is relatively new, managed care plans tend to offer the lowest possible premiums in order to attract new subscribers. Quality is often sacrificed. In communities where managed care has been well established, the quality tends to be higher.

In the following selections, physician and surgeon David Jacobsen argues that HMOs offer quality care that is comparable with the traditional fee-for-service. Journalism professor A. Kent MacDougall enrolled in an HMO and claims that it was the most painful decision of his life.

YES
David Jacobsen

COST-CONSCIOUS CARE

"Torture by HMO" is the title of a March 18 [1996] column by Bob Herbert in *The New York Times*. Herbert tells the story of a North Carolina family with a baby suffering from leukemia. Their health maintenance organization insisted that the child undergo treatment in another state, at great cost and inconvenience. Herbert condemns the HMO's "inflexible and thoroughly inhumane" policies, adding that "humanitarian concerns are not what corporate care is about. In the competition with profits, patients must always lose."

This portrait of HMOs as soulless money-making machines has become increasingly popular in recent years, as skyrocketing health care costs have driven a shift from fee-for-service medicine to managed care. Critics such as Harvard Medical School professor David Himmelstein contend that HMOs reward doctors for providing less care, trapping them in a conflict between their incomes and their patients' welfare, and impose "gag clauses" that forbid them to discuss this conflict with patients. "The bottom line is superseding the Hippocratic oath," write Jeff Cohen and Norman Solomon in their syndicated column. "Cost-cutting edicts from HMO managements put doctors in a box. . . . Faced with directives to help maximize profits, many physicians are under constant pressure to shift their allegiance from patients to company stockholders."

From my perspective as both a physician and a patient in the same HMO, these charges do not ring true. I do not doubt that HMOs, like any other business, sometimes serve their customers poorly. But there is no reason to believe that managed care systematically undermines patient welfare because of the imperative to cut costs. To the contrary, I have found that efficiency is perfectly compatible with compassionate, effective health care. (Since this article was written, I have myself become a cancer patient. Thus far, my care has been unsurpassed. I have the option of being treated outside my HMO, but would not think of going anywhere else. I expect from my plan the same level of care as a patient that I have provided as a physician.)

My plan delivers care at several neighborhood health centers. Each member chooses a "home" center and a primary care physician at that center. Surgical,

From David Jacobsen, "Cost-Conscious Care," *Reason* (June 1996). Copyright © 1996 by The Reason Foundation, 3415 S. Sepulveda Boulevard, Suite 400, Los Angeles, CA 90034. Reprinted by permission.

pediatric, obstetrical, and mental health services, as well as radiology, laboratory, pharmacy, and physical therapy, are all provided under one roof. While our "staff model" HMO does not offer as extensive a choice of physicians as many "network" HMOs, our arrangement does offer economies of scale and strict control of physician quality. Surveys consistently show that patients rate quality of care above greater choice of providers.

I am paid a straight salary and modest bonuses tied to both the plan's profitability and a patient satisfaction index. Frequent advisory audits help me and my patients sort out health care they *need* from health care they *want*. My goal is healthy, satisfied patients and a financially sound business. Every day, I put my professional reputation on the line. So does my HMO. Our challenge is to cut costs without cutting quality. Fortunately, there are many ways to do this.

* * *

Changing the venue of medical care from hospital to out-patient center, office, or home is the most important factor driving health care costs down and quality up. Hospitals are very expensive pieces of architecture. They are also complex places and therefore potentially hazardous to your health. Despite rigorous safeguards, medication and treatment errors can and do occur. As many as 15 percent of hospitalized patients go home with a hospital-acquired infection, often caused by antibiotic-resistant organisms. Furthermore, most patients do not wish to be in a hospital. In the last three years, my HMO has reduced hospital use by 25 percent.

Inguinal hernia repair is one of the most frequently performed operations.

Just a few years ago, the cost of this operation included a preoperative night in the hospital, one to two hours in the operating room under general anesthesia, and up to five postoperative days in the hospital. The patient had to take four to six weeks off work, and the recurrence rate was 10 percent. In 1996, at my HMO, this operation requires 40 minutes of surgery in a free-standing, outpatient surgical center under local anesthesia using a $100 plastic-mesh plug. Patients have less discomfort, return to unrestricted work in one week, and enjoy a recurrence rate of less than 1 per 1,000. This approach to hernia repair has been technically feasible for several years but was usually employed sporadically, at the discretion of the surgeon or the patient. In the era of cost containment, it has rapidly become the standard in the profession, regardless of reimbursement mode.

Thanks to the innovation of laparoscopic surgery, 80 percent of my patients who need their gallbladder removed can undergo the operation as outpatients and return to work in a week. The original inspiration for this procedure was the development of miniature video cameras, and the early reports were dismissed as mere technical wizardry. But as it became clear that laparoscopic gallbladder removal was not only safe but much less expensive than conventional surgery, surgeons quickly adopted the procedure as the standard approach, and patients demanded it.

* * *

The challenge of providing better care at lower cost has spurred not only the development of new procedures but the resurrection of old ones. Pilonidal abscess, a chronic and painful anorectal condition, used to be treated with radical surgery in the hospital. Recovery was frequently prolonged and painful. I now treat this problem with a 20-minute office procedure. Patients can return to work in two days, and the recurrence rate is less than 2 percent. This procedure was first described 15 years ago but languished until managed care created the incentive to implement it on a wider scale.

Open-heart surgery is expensive. Traditionally, the payer is billed separately by the hospital, the surgeon, and the anesthesiologist. My HMO recently negotiated a contract in which we pay a flat fee per operation that is about half our previous cost. As for concerns that surgeons might offer less surgery for less money, our studies show no change in mortality or morbidity since this contract went into effect. Beyond the question of ethics, no reputable provider group would risk a lucrative contract with a large HMO by delivering less than first-class care. Based on this experience, we are exploring package pricing for other high-cost procedures, such as organ transplantations.

Childhood asthma is a distressing and sometimes frightening problem for parents and children. Our studies showed that repeated visits to the emergency room were not only unnerving for families but accounted for a substantial portion of the cost of treating asthma. Through an aggressive program of family education, we are teaching our patients how to handle most asthma attacks at home, even how to give adrenaline injections. A nurse practitioner is available by telephone 24 hours a day to advise families whether a visit to the hospital may be necessary. Emergency room visits are down 40 percent in the last two years. So far, we have noted no adverse effects on patient care, and the response from families has been almost entirely positive.

Treatment of minor lacerations used to involve a trip to the hospital emergency room and frequently entailed a long wait. On nights and weekends our health centers are now staffed with specially trained physician assistants who repair 90 percent of all minor lacerations. In the first year this program has saved more than $100,000 in hospital emergency room charges while taking care of our patients better and more quickly.

For many of our patients with chronic wounds, such as bedsores and diabetic ulcers, treatment has often involved lengthy stays in rehabilitation hospitals or prolonged, expensive home visits by nurses. Under our wound-care program, most patients with chronic wounds can be treated directly at our health centers under the supervision of a physician. In most cases, patients and their families can be trained to do the daily wound care at home. In the first year, this program saved more than $70,000 in outside utilization costs.

Patients needing hip replacement surgery are often elderly and suffering from other medical problems. We now begin physical therapy evaluation in the patient's home *prior* to surgery. By knowing the level of family support and the location of stairs and bathrooms, we can much better prepare the patient for recuperation and rehabilitation. The new approach has cut the average hospital stay in half, eliminated the need for intermediate rehab hospital care in many cases, and accelerated recuperation.

For the past three years, my HMO has followed a policy of early discharge after childbirth. The childbirth program includes comprehensive prenatal education, post-partum home visits, and individual screening. A 16-year-old first-time mother with no family support and no telephone at home is not sent home in 24 hours. But 70 percent of women with uncomplicated vaginal deliveries are discharged in 24 to 36 hours. And despite the recent brouhaha over "drive-thru" deliveries, a recent survey documents that 90 percent of our patients are satisfied with their care—the same percentage as before the early discharge policy was adopted. There is no evidence that the health of mother or infant has been compromised. Most mothers and their babies belong at home with an attentive family, rather than in a potentially dangerous hospital.

Unnecessary diagnostic tests are probably the most familiar example of American medicine's spendthrift ways. Our computers are now set up so that every time a physician orders a laboratory test or X-ray procedure, a window on the screen displays the cost. Before managed care we neither knew nor asked. Preliminary analysis shows that this minor innovation has significantly reduced the ordering of routine laboratory and X-ray tests, especially among medical residents (physicians in training).

* * *

Much criticism of HMO care focuses not on common procedures such as these but on rare, emotionally charged illnesses. The cover story in the January 22 [1996] issue of *Time*, for example, chronicles the experience of a woman with advanced breast cancer whose HMO refused to pay for bone marrow transplantation. In such desperate cases, everyone understandably feels that something ought to be done. But the truth is that bone marrow transplantation for advanced breast cancer is a dangerous and expensive treatment of *no* proven benefit. This kind of case must be handled on an individual basis with consummate compassion and understanding, but it should not divert our attention from the myriad ways in which good medical care can be delivered for less money.

The significance of the potential conflict between physician income and patient welfare has also been exaggerated. First of all, it is offensive to me and the overwhelming majority of my colleagues to suggest that we would pad our bank accounts by obstructing or denying *necessary* medical care to our patients. I hew to an ethical standard of care, and so does my HMO. I am first and foremost the advocate of my patients, but always within the constraints of appropriate care and limited resources. More care is not always better care, and wishing that medicine could be exempt from the laws of economics does not make it so.

While there are various arrangements by which physicians are compensated under managed care, the incentives are to provide neither too little care nor too much care but *optimal* care. Under managed care, the worst course I could follow is to provide less than optimal care. Delay in diagnosis or treatment would only invite more expensive diagnosis and treatment down the line (and probably a lawsuit as well). Denying needed care is not only bad ethics; it is bad business.

As for the highly publicized "gag clauses," which have been outlawed in Massachusetts and a number of other states, my HMO does not have one. HMOs are entitled to insist on the confidentiality of proprietary information, but my HMO and most others encourage physicians to discuss financial incentives, covered benefits, and care options with patients. Many physicians are understandably dispirited by what they view as the demise of traditional health care and by projections of a 150,000-physician glut by the year 2000. But grievances and frustrations should be discussed with management and peers. Discussing them with patients can only erode an already embattled doctor–patient relationship.

* * *

Despite the charges of conflict and carnage, the evidence suggests that most physicians and patients are adjusting remarkably well to the managed care revolution and that the quality of care remains high. Studies have consistently shown that HMO patients are at least as satisfied with their care as patients receiving traditional fee-for-service care. A recent survey by CareData Reports, a New York health care information firm, revealed that, among members of 33 HMOs nationwide, nearly 80 percent were satisfied with their care. (The lowest ratings were not for quality of care but for administration and communication.) A 1994 study of 25,000 employees conducted by Xerox showed that HMO patients were significantly more satisfied with their overall care than were fee-for-service patients. In a 1994 Federal Employee Health Benefits Program survey of 90,000 federal employees, 86 percent of HMO members said they were satisfied with their plans, compared with 82 percent in fee-for-service plans. Interestingly, a 1994 survey by Towers Perrin revealed that patient satisfaction with HMO care rose with years of membership.

The results of research using objective measures have been similar. A 1996 study by KPMG Peat Marwick found that, in cities where most health care was provided by HMOs, costs were 11 percent lower, hospital stays 6 percent shorter, and death rates 5 percent lower than in cities where most care was provided under fee-for-service arrangements. A study recently published in the *Journal of the American Medical Association* looked at costs and outcomes of treatment for several chronic illnesses. Compared with fee-for-service specialists, HMO primary care physicians used 40 percent fewer hospital days and 12 percent less drugs. At four- and seven-year follow-ups, patient outcomes were the same.

A 1995 North Carolina study looked at the cost and outcome of treatment for lower-back pain. Costs for a single episode ranged from $169 in an HMO to $545 at a fee-for-service chiropractor, while outcomes were identical. As David Nash, an HMO expert at Jefferson Medical College in Philadelphia, told the *Chicago Sun-Times* last year [1995], "Overwhelmingly, the published evidence supports the notion that quality of care in the managed care arena equals, if not surpasses, the care in the private, fee-for-service sector."

The shift to managed care unquestionably imposes greater responsibility on patients. More information is becoming available to enable them to compare costs and benefits and make intelligent choices. We ought to disabuse ourselves of the notion that we can have a perfect health care system in which no one is ever misdiagnosed, mismanaged, or missed altogether. But high-quality medical care at an affordable price is not only possible under managed care; it is a reality.

NO

A. Kent MacDougall

HEALTH-CARE HELL: ONE MAN'S DESCENT INTO THE ABYSS

I got a sinking feeling about my decision to entrust my health to Kaiser Permanente the moment I arrived at the big health maintenance organization's medical center in Oakland. My wife let me off at the entrance to the center's parking garage and I hobbled on painful feet into the garage-attendants' office. We had been told it lent wheelchairs to Kaiser patients who needed assistance getting to their appointments.

I took a seat in the last wheelchair available, only to find it lacked foot rests. Without this standard equipment, the only way I could avoid dragging my feet along the sidewalk and possibly injuring them further was to keep my knees raised. After a few yards I realized I wouldn't be able to sustain the muscular effort this required. So my wife returned the damaged wheelchair to the garage and I hobbled on my damaged feet the rest of the way.

It was Monday, January 3, 1994, two days after my membership in the Kaiser Foundation Health Plan took effect, and I was getting my first painful lesson in how things work—and don't work—at Kaiser. Before the morning was over, it was clear that in spite of Kaiser's reputation for delivering quality care at a reasonable cost, there are a lot of things in the Kaiser system besides wheelchairs that need fixing.

My personal misadventures at Kaiser last year included misdiagnoses of my foot condition, inappropriate treatments that worsened it, an unsupervised, uncoordinated, scattershot approach to my case, waits of two to three months to see doctors, and the passage of a full six months for an accurate diagnosis.

Can my own unhappy experience be laid to bad luck, inexperience in "working" the Kaiser system, or some other personal aberration? Unfortunately not. Kaiser's own membership surveys show widespread dissatisfaction with access and service, and its self-confessed "poor performance in this area" is costing it business. A 1994 survey conducted for ten major California employers ranked Kaiser near the bottom among fifty-two health plans in two categories: member satisfaction with doctors, and waiting time for appointments.

My Kafkaesque struggle to break through Kaiser's all-but-impermeable institutional detachment, to get someone—anyone—to take my problem seriously, is a cautionary case study of the haphazard care all too commonly dispensed by prepaid medical plans. These plans have a financial interest in delaying and denying service because they receive the same fee no matter how much or how little care they provide.

Kaiser has grown from the World War II health service for Henry J. Kaiser's California shipyard and steel-mill workers into the world's largest nongovernmental health-care system. It couldn't have expanded so impressively if it didn't do a lot of things well. But Kaiser has been slipping. And Kaiser's performance in meeting—or not meeting—its 6.6 million members' expectations is significant because Kaiser sets the "cost-effective" standard of medicine that both nonprofit and for-profit health-maintenance organizations (HMOs) and other "managed-care" health plans across the nation are scrambling to emulate. This standard includes restricting patient choice of caregivers and access to specialists, inserting a layer of gatekeepers between patients and physicians, giving short shrift to emotional health problems, and basing doctors' compensation partly on the amount of treatment they avoid and deny.

As employers shift the financial burden of providing health-care benefits to their workers and retirees by making them pay more for traditional fee-for-service reimbursement insurance, HMOs and other managed-care plans are fast taking over the medical delivery system. Only one in eight medically insured Americans is still covered by traditional fee-for-service insurance. Membership in HMOs is past the 50 million mark, and industry experts predict HMOs will account for nearly half of the health-care market by the year 2000.

Solo and small-group practitioners are joining managed-care networks in order to survive. Hospitals are setting up managed-care networks of their own in order to compete. Others are merging or selling out to national chains. Some hospitals, along with insurers such as Blue Cross of California, are converting from nonprofit to for-profit status.

This oligopolization is not improving health care. Typically, patients are denied care they formerly received without question, and the care they do receive is down-sized, with doctors, physical therapists, and other caregivers spending less time with patients. Meanwhile, cost savings are dissipated on "utilization reviewers," who micro-manage each request for treatment. Savings are also drained by stepped-up advertising and sales promotion, lavish executive salaries, and generous shareholder benefits.

* * *

"You'll love Kaiser," a number of Berkeley friends told my wife, Kathleen, and me before we signed up with it. Our friends, who were already Kaiser members, promised we would get one-stop, all-inclusive care. No need to go elsewhere for an x-ray or blood test; it was all available under one roof, or at least in the cluster of buildings at Kaiser's medical center on Oakland's north side. No insurance forms to fill out; just a nominal $5 co-payment when visiting a doctor or picking up a prescription. We could pick our primary-care doctor and he or she would take care of the rest, referring us to specialists as needed. What could be simpler? And, in any case, how much did it matter? Kathleen and I figured on continuing to coast along in good health, seeing doctors infrequently, and needing Kaiser mainly as insurance against an unlikely catastrophic illness or injury.

How wrong we were. For between the time we authorized the switch to Kaiser in November 1993 and when it took effect January 1, 1994, my feet started hurting —bad. I attributed the pain to having done too much flutter kicking in the swimming pool one day. A specialist our family doctor referred me to diagnosed my foot condition as possible tendinitis and prescribed rest, ice, and physical therapy. By now it was late December, time for only two whirlpool, ultrasound, and massage treatments at a physical-therapy center in Berkeley before it was Kaiser's turn to take over.

On January 3, a Monday, I presented myself at Kaiser's physical therapy department in Oakland with my painful feet and a photocopy of a letter my private-care specialist had sent to my family doctor describing my condition and prescribing physical therapy two or three times a week for four to six weeks. A Kaiser physical therapist assessed my condition and requested an urgent-care appointment within a week, explaining that patients with less urgent problems routinely wait two months before starting physical therapy.

Kaiser defines "an urgent medical problem [as] one that requires attention within twenty-four to forty-eight hours," and it includes "mild to moderate pain" as such an urgent problem. Despite this, the first available appointment with a Kaiser physical therapist was in two and a half weeks. As I was to learn, Kaiser just doesn't have enough physical therapists to meet the demand. It copes by rationing

therapy sessions to thirty minutes, half the time I got in private care, and by limiting the number of sessions—in my case, to six. Six sessions might have sufficed if complications had not set in. But they did. Doing one of the home exercises prescribed by my therapist, an exercise designed to stretch the calf muscles and thereby to loosen up the feet, instead inflamed the heels of both feet and set my lower back to aching.

The heel pain was so severe I couldn't walk, much less leave home. For the first time in thirteen years of university teaching, I canceled a class because of illness. Desperate for help, I tried to get an appointment with a Kaiser sports-injury expert who had treated two of my friends, only to learn that seeing a specialist requires a referral from one's primary-care physician. Since my primary-care physician had yet to be assigned, I was out of luck.

I had to settle for an appointment with one of the part-time, fill-in general practitioners whom Kaiser is increasingly relying on in lieu of taking on more full-time physician "partners." The G.P. made an off-the-cuff diagnosis that proved grievously off the mark. He misdiagnosed my foot condition as plantar fasciitis. Plantar fasciitis is inflammation of the thick sheet of dense fibrous tissue that connects the heel bone to the toes on the underside of the foot. Plantar fasciitis pain usually comes on gradually over months or years and is most intense when first getting out of bed and walking in the morning, diminishing as the foot stretches out. My symptoms didn't fit, inasmuch as my heel pain came on suddenly, and was least bothersome when getting out of bed in the morning, increasing as the feet stretched out. Nonetheless, the G.P. said I had plantar fasciitis in both feet. He wrote out a referral to Kaiser's podiatry department that entitled me to attend a "heel pain class" with a dozen plantar fasciitis sufferers five weeks later.

Classes, I soon learned, are one of the ways Kaiser holds down the workload on its doctors so it can avoid hiring more of them. There are classes for patients with arthritis, asthma, back pain, cataracts, diabetes, and a dozen other maladies. The nurses who typically run these classes dispense useful advice that in many cases adequately substitutes for an appointment with a doctor. In other cases, including mine, classes merely delay diagnosis and treatment.

The primary-care doctor I was finally assigned and given an appointment with two months after my arrival at Kaiser was plainly at a loss to explain either my painful feet or my aching back. But he was friendly and accommodating. He guessed that the trouble with my feet was peripheral neuropathy, a localized nerve disorder, and referred me to Neurology. He ordered x-rays of my back and referred me to a "back-care class" for instruction in home exercises and ways to avoid aggravating my condition.

He also loaded me down with drugs. Substituting drugs for time and attention pervades U.S. medical practice, of course, but seems especially pervasive at Kaiser. At one point I was taking no fewer than four drugs: an anti-inflammatory (Clinoril), an analgesic (Darvocet), an antidepressant (Nortriptyline), and an anticonvulsant (Tegretol). The anticonvulsant was a bizarre choice since it matched none of my symptoms. But my primary-care doctor added it to the drugs already sloshing around in my system after I asked him to lean on Neurology for an earlier appointment. He said the neurologist I had an appointment with in two

and a half months couldn't see me sooner, but had suggested I take the anticonvulsant in the meantime. However, when I finally got in to see the neurologist, he disclaimed knowledge of or responsibility for the prescription, and I concluded it was just my primary-care doctor's well-intentioned sop to soothe my disappointment over not getting an earlier appointment with the specialist.

A wait of two to three months for an appointment with a specialist is par for the course at Kaiser. The presumption throughout the system is that care must be strictly rationed lest it be abused. If Kaiser made it too easy to see doctors, hypochondriacs with nothing better to do would clutter up waiting rooms and impose trivial complaints on busy doctors.

* * *

I had a burning sensation in both heels even when I was off my feet. I seemed in a downward spiral of pain, fatigue, weakness, and depression. The ten pounds I had lost from an already lean frame had reduced my weight to 145, the lowest since I was fifteen years old. My blood pressure, normally 140/72, had shot up to 170/86. I couldn't stand, much less walk, without pain. Neither could I drive because just resting my heel on the floorboard next to the accelerator was excruciating. Kathleen became my lifeline to the public pool in Berkeley where I swam and to Kaiser in Oakland. She also drove me to the University of California campus several times. But hobbling around the Graduate School of Journalism there was more than I was up for. I reneged on my office hours, and my students agreed to attend seminars at my home a mile from campus. Even then, conducting an eighty-minute class around my dining-room table invariably left me exhausted and sent me to bed.

My mysterious foot affliction was also hard to take psychologically. Kaiser's indifference to it was especially disturbing. Nearly three months into the system, and here I was, still bouncing around, begging for attention. My primary-care doctor was willing, but he just wasn't able to figure out what was wrong, much less what to do about it. And he wasn't getting any help.

I started having nightmares of being lost and endangered in scary settings —a rundown underground shopping arcade, a midnight warehouse, an empty cafeteria—that were stand-ins for the labyrinthine basement complex at Kaiser where I went for x-rays, blood tests, and podiatry. Childhood feelings of being ignored and uncared for that I thought I had resolved came roaring back. I felt trapped in a medical maze without a guide to help me find the way out.

"You've got to work the system," my friends who were loyal Kaiser members reminded me. "Unless you scream, nothing happens at Kaiser," one advised. "Tell them you can't walk and you can't wait," a second said.

What no friend told me, however, is that insisting on seeing a doctor sooner rather than later typically results in an appointment with the least experienced, least qualified doctor on the staff. The part-time G.P. who misdiagnosed my foot condition as plantar fasciitis was my first lesson. My second came courtesy of a recent podiatry school graduate serving a residency at Kaiser. This young woman didn't attempt to diagnose my foot condition other than to say, "It could be a tendon. It could be the transverse fascia." But she knew what to do with the more painful foot: she put it in a cast.

The cast came with a sandal, permitting me to walk. But limping about did nothing for the pain in the casted foot, while the additional stress it placed on the uncasted foot caused it to flare up. Worse, the cast prevented me from swimming, which I considered essential for easing both my backache and the emotional ache of being reduced to semi-invalidism.

After four days I wanted out. The apprentice podiatrist agreed the cast probably was doing more harm than good. As a substitute I was given a pair of strap-on plastic splints to wear in bed at night and while sitting or lying around the house during the day. Like the cast, the splints kept the foot at a right angle to the leg. This is useful in cases of plantar fasciitis. But I didn't have plantar fasciitis, according to the full-fledged podiatrist I eventually got to see, but rather inflammation of a tendon on the outside edge of the heel. He said the splints kept this tendon stretched, preventing it from healing, and so was counterindicated in my case. That was nice to know, but it came seven weeks after I had used the splints day and night, only to have them aggravate my heels. Only after I stopped using the splints did the inflammation in my heels begin to subside.

By now it was time to see the neurologist. He gave my feet a good going-over only to conclude, "I don't see neuropathy." So my primary-care doctor's hunch had been off. More likely your problem is rheumatological, the neurologist said, writing out a referral.

It was now mid-May, four months since my heels had flared up. And still no diagnosis. Would Rheumatology have one? I eagerly awaited the postcard in the mail that would notify me of my appointment with a rheumatologist. One day it came. July 21, it announced. Another two months to find out. Was there no way to speed up the process? I tried working the system once again. I phoned the rheumatologist's appointment/advice nurse and told her I still couldn't walk and was in too much pain to wait another two months. "Well, if you don't like July 21," she said, "I have an opening on July 27."

* * *

Working the system clearly wasn't working. Helping me regain my health seemed low on this HMO's list of priorities. So what if I couldn't walk, only hobble in pain? There were lots of other members in even worse shape. Hundreds of them, some on crutches, others in wheelchairs, filled Kaiser-Oakland's waiting rooms on any given day, while hundreds of others occupied its hospital beds. These folks needed help even more than I did. Some of them would die if they didn't get it. I seemed in no danger of that. Kaiser had just so many doctors—and way too many patients. Some would have to wait. It was logical, even defensible, for this "cost-effective" HMO to decide that the waitees should include me. Get in line, No. 8456513, and be grateful for whatever crumbs of care fall your way.

But they weren't falling my way. Stressed out by the professional demands placed on him at Kaiser, and with personal problems of his own, my primary-care doctor went off on an indefinite leave of absence and was still out five months later. An appointment I had with him was canceled. I was told that if and when he returned, he would no longer be anyone's primary-care doctor. I could choose a new primary-care doctor. But few were accepting new patients and getting an appointment with those

who were would take—predictably—two months.

It was time to give up on Kaiser, to admit the system had me beat. I decided to go outside for help even though it would mean paying for it out of my own pocket. I returned to the specialist who had examined my feet the preceding December just before I joined Kaiser. This rheumatologist had not suspected a systemic condition at that time. Now he did. He ordered a blood test that came back positive. The test was for a genetic marker, known as HLA-B27, associated with a family of arthritis, one type of which inflames the ligaments and tendons where they attach to the heels. Fairly common among white men, attachment arthritis when mild sometimes goes undiagnosed for decades.

Diagnosing my condition was no snap, then. But it shouldn't have taken Kaiser more than six months. The Kaiser rheumatologist I finally got to see in late July conceded as much. He pointed to the clues: the unlikelihood that either plantar fasciitis or peripheral neuropathy would afflict both feet simultaneously, the fact that my heel pain lay behind and along the sides of the heels, that x-rays showed pitting of the heel bones from chronic inflammation, and that back x-rays revealed moderate osteoarthritis of the lower spine. Had a single doctor, even a G.P., been coordinating my case and providing continuity, he or she might have put the clues together and suspected attachment arthritis. But both coordination and continuity easily get lost in the shuffle at Kaiser.

My visit with the rheumatologist was no exception. When we met in his examining room, he had no idea who I was or what other doctors had found.

My medical-records file was checked out to another doctor I had never heard of —why, neither of us knew. On the basis of what I told him and a hurried look at my x-rays, the Kaiser rheumatologist confirmed my outside rheumatologist's diagnosis. He seconded the course of treatment my outside rheumatologist had prescribed, assured me that "we can carry on here," and gave me a return appointment in two months.

Should I have been content at this point to drop my outside rheumatologist and let Kaiser carry on alone? The prospect was scary, given what had preceded my visit with the Kaiser rheumatologist. The day before my scheduled July 21 appointment, I had gotten a phone call that the rheumatologist was sick and would be unable to see me, and that the next available appointment would be in another two months. I replied that a two-month delay was unacceptable, given the two and a half months I had already waited and the pain and disability I was still in. And lo and behold, Kaiser found a way to squeeze me in with the rheumatologist the following week. I had won a skirmish in what I continued to consider an unevenly matched battle against the Kaiser system.

When my heel pain flared up and both feet swelled up a week after I saw the Kaiser rheumatologist, I had no hesitancy in making my choice. Instead of trying Kaiser again, I pulled out my checkbook and went back to my private-care rheumatologist.

Joining Kaiser has turned out to be the most painful mistake of my life. In retrospect, my old fee-for-service, small-practice family doctor looks better than ever. Alone among half a dozen doctors, he suspected an inflammatory systemic condition from the start. He was right. Dropping him for Kaiser may not have been a sin, but it added to my suffering. Repentant, I returned to his care last September following complications caused by all the anti-inflammatory drugs I had been taking.

But I noticed a new name, Alta Bates Medical Associates, on the door of the suite of offices he shares with several other family practitioners. In the nine months I had been away, he and his colleagues had become affiliated, along with several hundred other formerly independent physicians, with a 500-bed Berkeley hospital in a managed-care network designed to keep patients, cut costs, and stay competitive in an increasingly "get big or get out" industry.

"You realize, of course," my doctor explained after welcoming me back, "everyone's going Kaiser."

POSTSCRIPT

Will Managed Care Improve Health Care in the United States?

Should managed care scare the typical health care consumer? Will our access to necessary care be denied in favor of the bottom line? Many experts think that is the case since managed care plans reward physicians for providing less care. In some plans, gag orders have been imposed on member doctors. The doctors are forbidden, or "gagged," from disclosing expensive treatment options not covered by the plan. As more and more workers are enrolled in managed care programs by their employers, can we assume that companies can make better health care choices than their employees would individually? On the other hand, can we as a nation cope with rising health costs, especially as our population ages? While there is evidence that managed care offers service that is similar in quality to fee-for-service care, many consumers have expressed dissatisfaction with their HMO. The people most likely to be unhappy with managed care are those who are the most sick.

An overview of managed care is provided by "Managed-Care Plan Performance Since 1980: A Literature Analysis," *Journal of the American Medical Association* (May 18, 1994) and "Managed Care: Do Health-Care Firms Sacrifice Quality to Cut Costs?" *CQ Researcher* (April 12, 1996).

Although there are dissatisfied consumers, several articles claim that the quality of care through managed care is comparable to fee-for-service care. These include the following: "A Report Card on HMOs," *Fortune* (June 28, 1993); "The Effectiveness of Health Care Cost Management Strategies: A Review of the Evidence," *Employee Benefit Research Institute Issue Brief* (October 1994); "Good Managed Care Means Good Health Care," *Boston Globe* (November 21, 1995); "Managed Care Can Help Curb Medicare Costs," *USA Today* (February 8, 1995); "Managed Care Means Shared Responsibilities," *St.Louis Post-Dispatch* (January 29, 1996); and "Learning to Accentuate the Positive in Managed Care," *The New England Journal of Medicine* (February 13, 1997).

Many articles, books, and reports, however, claim that patients suffer under managed care. These include "On the Examining Table," *Harper's Magazine* (May 1994); "The Case Against Managed Care and for a Single-Payer System," *JAMA* (January 4, 1995); "Do HMOs Ration Their Health Care?" *Los Angeles Times* (August 27, 1995); "Managed Care Is Not Health Care," *Boston Globe* (September 5, 1995); "U.S. Health Reform: Unkindest Cuts," *The Nation* (January 1996); "How Your HMO Could Hurt You," *U.S. News and World Report* (January 15, 1996); "Humanistic Economics," *The Humanist* (September/October 1996); "Can HMOs Help Solve the Health-Care Crisis?" *Consumer Reports on Health* (October 1996); "Quality and the Medical Marketplace," *The New England Journal of Medicine* (September 19, 1996); and "Bedside Mania: Medicine Turned Upside Down," *The American Prospect* (March/April 1997).

If managed care is not the solution for reforming medical services in the United States, are there alternatives? The Canadian system has often been considered the solution to rising health care costs in the United States. The Canadian medicare program, however, has been under attack for not providing necessary services for its patients, especially in regard to making referrals to specialists. Although a Gallup poll found that 96 percent of Canadians prefer their health care system to that of the United States, the system is becoming a frequent target for a government interested in cost cutting. For information on the Canadian system, read "Canada's Health Care System Faces Its Problems," *The New England Journal of Medicine* (February 22, 1990) and "Bitter Medicine: Canada Is Taking an Ax to Its Popular Health Care System," *In These Times* (January 20, 1997).

ISSUE 2

Should Doctors Ever Assist Terminally Ill Patients to Commit Suicide?

YES: Marcia Angell, from "The Supreme Court and Physician-Assisted Suicide: The Ultimate Right," *The New England Journal of Medicine* (January 2, 1997)

NO: Kathleen M. Foley, from "Competent Care for the Dying Instead of Physician-Assisted Suicide," *The New England Journal of Medicine* (January 2, 1997)

ISSUE SUMMARY

YES: Marcia Angell, M.D., executive editor of *The New England Journal of Medicine*, believes that physician-assisted suicide should be permitted under some circumstances and that not all of the pain of the dying can be controlled.

NO: Physician Kathleen M. Foley believes that doctors do not know enough about their patients, themselves, or suffering, to provide assistance with dying as a medical treatment for the relief of suffering.

Should doctors ever help their patients die? Whereas doctors should provide every support possible to their dying patients, do they have the right or obligation to actually hasten the process of death even if a patient requests it? This topic has been the subject of numerous debates over the past few years.

The debate over aided suicide has reached a new plateau. In June 1997 the Supreme Court justices unanimously rejected a plea to declare physician-assisted suicide a constitutional right. The justices did leave the way open for states to legalize the practice. Although most states make aided suicide a crime, legislators in nine states want to repeal the laws. In Oregon, voters narrowly approved the legalization of assisted suicide in 1994; the bill comes up again in November of 1997.

Some of the practices that were controversial a short time ago in the care of terminally ill patients have become accepted and routine. Many doctors now believe that it is ethical to use "do-not-resuscitate" orders on dying patients, while others feel that it is also acceptable to withhold food and water from patients who are hopelessly ill and dying. The word *euthanasia*, which comes from Greek roots—the prefix *eu*, meaning good, fortunate, or easy, and the word *thanatos*, meaning death—describes a good or easy death. Withdrawing care or treatment (referred to as *passive euthanasia*) may be acceptable to many doctors, but *active euthanasia*, or playing an active role in a patient's death, may not. One form of active euthanasia, physician-assisted suicide, has been the subject of numerous debates in recent years.

In early 1988, the *Journal of the American Medical Association* published a short article entitled "It's Over, Debbie" (January 8, 1988), which was written by an anonymous physician who described administering a lethal dose of morphine to a young woman with terminal cancer. The doctor claimed her suffering was extreme and that there was absolutely no hope of recovery. The morphine was requested by the patient, who said, "Let's get this over with." The patient died within minutes of receiving the drug, while the doctor looked on. This article generated a great deal of criticism because the doctor had met the patient for the first time that evening and had not consulted with colleagues or family members before making his decision. The doctor did, however, believe he was correctly responding to the patient's request.

Soon after this incident, Dr. Jack Kevorkian assisted in the suicide of an Oregon woman who suffered from Alzheimer's disease. Dr. Kevorkian supplied the woman with a device that he developed—a "suicide machine"—that allowed her to give herself a lethal dose of drugs. Intense criticism followed regarding the ability of Dr. Kevorkian to diagnose the patient's illness (which was not immediately terminal) and whether or not the patient was able to make an informed decision to end her life.

In March 1991, Dr. Timothy E. Quill published an editorial in the *New England Journal of Medicine* that described an assisted suicide. A woman, Quill's patient for eight years, was suffering from leukemia. She had decided not to undergo chemotherapy, which would have offered her only a 25 percent chance of long-term survival with considerable side effects. In addition to refusing treatment, the patient requested that Quill help her commit suicide. She later killed herself with sleeping pills that Quill had prescribed. Quill is an outspoken advocate of physician-assisted suicide under certain conditions.

Other physicians believe that many hopelessly ill patients contemplate taking their own lives because their doctors do not help them manage their pain. Pain is one of the principal reasons the sick ask their doctors to help them to die. Many doctors believe that the best antidote to the appeal of doctor-assisted suicide would be better treatment of pain. In "The Quality of Mercy: Effective Pain Treatments Already Exist. Why Aren't Doctors Using Them?" *U.S. News and World Report* (March 17, 1997), the authors claim that health providers are unwilling to treat pain adequately out of fear of litigation, fear their patients will become addicted, or because they lack adequate knowledge in pain management.

In the following articles, Dr. Marcia Angell supports a patient's right to assisted suicide and cites personal reasons for her decision. Dr. Kathleen Foley argues that physicians should provide competent care for the dying, including adequate pain management, and should not offer physician-assisted suicide.

YES

Marcia Angell

THE SUPREME COURT AND PHYSICIAN-ASSISTED SUICIDE— THE ULTIMATE RIGHT

The U.S. Supreme Court will decide later this year whether to let stand decisions by two appeals courts permitting doctors to help terminally ill patients commit suicide.[1] The Ninth and Second Circuit Courts of Appeals last spring held that state laws in Washington and New York that ban assistance in suicide were unconstitutional as applied to doctors and their dying patients.[2,3] If the Supreme Court lets the decisions stand, physicians in 12 states, which include about half the population of the United States, would be allowed to provide the means for terminally ill patients to take their own lives, and the remaining states would rapidly follow suit. Not since *Roe* v. *Wade* has a Supreme Court decision been so fateful.

The decision will culminate several years of intense national debate, fueled by a number of highly publicized events. Perhaps most important among them is Dr. Jack Kevorkian's defiant assistance in some 44 suicides since 1990, to the dismay of many in the medical and legal establishments, but with substantial public support, as evidenced by the fact that three juries refused to convict him even in the face of a Michigan statute enacted for that purpose. Also since 1990, voters in three states have considered ballot initiatives that would legalize some form of physician-assisted dying, and in 1994 Oregon became the first state to approve such a measure.[4] (The Oregon law was stayed pending a court challenge.) Several surveys indicate that roughly two thirds of the American public now support physician-assisted suicide,[5,6] as do more than half the doctors in the United States,[6,7] despite the fact that influential physicians' organizations are opposed. It seems clear that many Americans are now so concerned about the possibility of a lingering, high-technology death that they are receptive to the idea of doctors' being allowed to help them die.

In this editorial I will explain why I believe the appeals courts were right and why I hope the Supreme Court will uphold their decisions. I am aware that this is a highly contentious issue, with good people and strong argu-

From Marcia Angell, "The Supreme Court and Physician-Assisted Suicide: The Ultimate Right," *The New England Journal of Medicine*, vol. 336, no. 1 (January 2, 1997), pp. 50–53. Copyright © 1997 by The Massachusetts Medical Society. Reprinted by permission. All rights reserved.

ments on both sides. The American Medical Association (AMA) filed an amicus brief opposing the legalization of physician-assisted suicide,[8] and the Massachusetts Medical Society, which owns the *Journal* was a signatory to it. But here I speak for myself not the *Journal* or the Massachusetts Medical Society. The legal aspects of the case have been well discussed elsewhere, to me most compellingly in Ronald Dworkin's essay in the *New York Review of Books*.[9] I will focus primarily on the medical and ethical aspects.

I begin with the generally accepted premise that one of the most important ethical principles in medicine is respect for each patient's autonomy, and that when this principle conflicts with others, it should almost always take precedence. This premise is incorporated into our laws governing medical practice and research, including the requirement of informed consent to any treatment. In medicine, patients exercise their self-determination most dramatically when they ask that life-sustaining treatment be withdrawn. Although others may sometimes consider the request ill-founded, we are bound to honor it if the patient is mentally competent—that is, if the patient can understand the nature of the decision and its consequences.

A second starting point is the recognition that death is not fair and is often cruel. Some people die quickly, and others die slowly but peacefully. Some find personal or religious meaning in the process, as well as an opportunity for a final reconciliation with loved ones. But others, especially those with cancer, AIDS, or progressive neurologic disorders, may die by inches and in great anguish, despite every effort of their doctors and nurses. Although nearly all pain

can be relieved, some cannot, and other symptoms, such as dyspnea, nausea, and weakness, are even more difficult to control. In addition, dying sometimes holds great indignities and existential suffering. Patients who happen to require some treatment to sustain their lives, such as assisted ventilation or dialysis, can hasten death by having the life-sustaining treatment withdrawn, but those who are not receiving life-sustaining treatment may desperately need help they cannot now get.

If the decisions of the appeals courts are upheld, states will not be able to prohibit doctors from helping such patients to die by prescribing a lethal dose of a drug and advising them on its use for suicide. State laws barring euthanasia (the administration of a lethal drug by a doctor) and assisted suicide for patients who are not terminally ill would not be affected. Furthermore, doctors would not be *required* to assist in suicide; they would simply have that option. Both appeals courts based their decisions on constitutional questions. This is important, because it shifted the focus of the debate from what the majority would approve through the political process, as exemplified by the Oregon initiative, to a matter of fundamental rights, which are largely immune from the political process. Indeed, the Ninth Circuit Court drew an explicit analogy between suicide and abortion, saying that both were personal choices protected by the Constitution and that forbidding doctors to assist would in effect nullify these rights. Although states could regulate assisted suicide, as they do abortion, they would not be permitted to regulate it out of existence.

It is hard to quarrel with the desire of a greatly suffering, dying patient for a quicker, more humane death or to disagree that it may be merciful to help bring that about. In those circumstances, loved ones are often relieved when death finally comes, as are the attending doctors and nurses. As the Second Circuit Court said, the state has no interest in prolonging such a life. Why, then, do so many people oppose legalizing physician-assisted suicide in these cases? There are a number of arguments against it, some stronger than others, but I believe none of them can offset the overriding duties of doctors to relieve suffering and to respect their patients' autonomy. Below I list several of the more important arguments against physician-assisted suicide and discuss why I believe they are in the last analysis unpersuasive.

Assisted suicide is a form of killing, which is always wrong. In contrast, withdrawing life-sustaining treatment simply allows the disease to take its course. There are three methods of hastening the death of a dying patient: withdrawing life-sustaining treatment, assisting suicide, and euthanasia. The right to stop treatment has been recognized repeatedly since the 1976 case of Karen Ann Quinlan[10] and was affirmed by the U.S. Supreme Court in the 1990 *Cruzan* decision[11] and the U.S. Congress in its 1990 Patient Self-Determination Act.[12] Although the legal underpinning is the right to be free of unwanted bodily invasion, the purpose of hastening death was explicitly acknowledged. In contrast, assisted suicide and euthanasia have not been accepted; euthanasia is illegal in all states, and assisted suicide is illegal in most of them.

Why the distinctions? Most would say they turn on the doctor's role: whether it is passive or active. When life-sustaining treatment is withdrawn, the doctor's role is considered passive and the cause of death is the underlying disease, despite the fact that switching off the ventilator of a patient dependent on it looks anything but passive and would be considered homicide if done without the consent of the patient or a proxy. In contrast, euthanasia by the injection of a lethal drug is active and directly causes the patient's death. Assisting suicide by supplying the necessary drugs is considered somewhere in between, more active than switching off a ventilator but less active than injecting drugs, hence morally and legally more ambiguous.

I believe, however, that these distinctions are too doctor-centered and not sufficiently patient-centered. We should ask ourselves not so much whether the doctor's role is passive or active but whether the *patient's* role is passive or active. From that perspective, the three methods of hastening death line up quite differently. When life-sustaining treatment is withdrawn from an incompetent patient at the request of a proxy or when euthanasia is performed, the patient may be utterly passive. Indeed, either act can be performed even if the patient is unaware of the decision. In sharp contrast, assisted suicide, by definition, cannot occur without the patient's knowledge and participation. Therefore, it must be active— that is to say, voluntary. That is a crucial distinction, because it provides an inherent safeguard against abuse that is not present with the other two methods of hastening death. If the loaded term "kill" is to be used, it is not the doctor who kills, but the patient. Primarily because euthanasia can be performed without the patient's participation, I oppose its legalization in this country.

Assisted suicide is not necessary. All suffering can be relieved if care givers are sufficiently skillful and compassionate, as illustrated by the hospice movement. I have no doubt that if expert palliative care were available to everyone who needed it, there would be few requests for assisted suicide. Even under the best of circumstances, however, there will always be a few patients whose suffering simply cannot be adequately alleviated. And there will be some who would prefer suicide to any other measures available, including the withdrawal of life-sustaining treatment or the use of heavy sedation. Surely, every effort should be made to improve palliative care, as I argued 15 years ago,[13] but when those efforts are unavailing and suffering patients desperately long to end their lives, physician-assisted suicide should be allowed. The argument that permitting it would divert us from redoubling our commitment to comfort care asks these patients to pay the penalty for our failings. It is also illogical. Good comfort care and the availability of physician-assisted suicide are no more mutually exclusive than good cardiologic care and the availability of heart transplantation.

Permitting assisted suicide would put us on a moral "slippery slope." Although in itself assisted suicide might be acceptable, it would lead inexorably to involuntary euthanasia. It is impossible to avoid slippery slopes in medicine (or in any aspect of life). The issue is how and where to find a purchase. For example, we accept the right of proxies to terminate life-sustaining treatment, despite the obvious potential for abuse, because the reasons for doing so outweigh the risks. We hope our procedures will safeguard patients. In the case of assisted suicide, its voluntary nature is the best protection against sliding down a slippery slope, but we also need to ensure that the request is thoughtful and freely made. Although it

is possible that we may someday decide to legalize voluntary euthanasia under certain circumstances or assisted suicide for patients who are not terminally ill, legalizing assisted suicide for the dying does not in itself make these other decisions inevitable. Interestingly, recent reports from the Netherlands, where both euthanasia and physician-assisted suicide are permitted, indicate that fears about a slippery slope there have not been borne out.[14–16]

Assisted suicide would be a threat to the economically and socially vulnerable. The poor disabled, and elderly might be coerced to request it. Admittedly, overburdened families or cost-conscious doctors might pressure vulnerable patients to request suicide, but similar wrongdoing is at least as likely in the case of withdrawing life-sustaining treatment, since that decision can be made by proxy. Yet, there is no evidence of widespread abuse. The Ninth Circuit Court recalled that it was feared *Roe* v. *Wade* would lead to coercion of poor and uneducated women to request abortions, but that did not happen. The concern that coercion is more likely in this era of managed care, although understandable, would hold suffering patients hostage to the deficiencies of our health care system. Unfortunately, no human endeavor is immune to abuses. The question is not whether a perfect system can be devised, but whether abuses are likely to be sufficiently rare to be offset by the benefits to patients who otherwise would be condemned to face the end of their lives in protracted agony.

Depressed patients would seek physician-assisted suicide rather than help for their depression. Even in the terminally ill, a request for assisted suicide might signify treatable depression, not irreversible suffering. Patients suffering greatly at the end of life may also be depressed, but the depression does not necessarily explain their decision to commit suicide or make it irrational. Nor is it simple to diagnose depression in terminally ill patients. Sadness is to be expected, and some of the vegetative symptoms of depression are similar to the symptoms of terminal illness. The success of antidepressant treatment in these circumstances is also not ensured. Although there are anecdotes about patients who changed their minds about suicide after treatment,[17] we do not have good studies of how often that happens or the relation to antidepressant treatment. Dying patients who request assisted suicide and seem depressed should certainly be strongly encouraged to accept psychiatric treatment, but I do not believe that competent patients should be *required* to accept it as a condition of receiving assistance with suicide. On the other hand, doctors would not be required to comply with all requests; they would be expected to use their judgment, just as they do in so many other types of life-and-death decisions in medical practice.

Doctors should never participate in taking life. If there is to be assisted suicide, doctor must not be involved. Although most doctors favor permitting assisted suicide under certain circumstances, many who favor it believe that doctors should not provide the assistance.[6,7] To them, doctors should be unambiguously committed to life (although most doctors who hold this view would readily honor a patient's decision to have life-sustaining treatment withdrawn). The AMA, too, seems to object to physician-assisted suicide primarily because it violates the profession's mission. Like others, I find that position too abstract.[18] The highest ethical imperative of doctors should be to provide care in whatever way best serves patients' interests, in accord with each patient's wishes, not with a theoretical commitment to preserve life no matter what the cost in suffering.[19] If a patient requests help with suicide and the doctor believes the request is appropriate, requiring someone else to provide the assistance would be a form of abandonment. Doctors who are opposed in principle need not assist, but they should make their patients aware of their position early in the relationship so that a patient who chooses to select another doctor can do so. The greatest harm we can do is to consign a desperate patient to unbearable suffering —or force the patient to seek out a stranger like Dr. Kevorkian. Contrary to the frequent assertion that permitting physician-assisted suicide would lead patients to distrust their doctors, I believe distrust is more likely to arise from uncertainty about whether a doctor will honor a patient's wishes.

Physician-assisted suicide may occasionally be warranted, but it should remain illegal. If doctors risk prosecution, they will think twice before assisting with suicide. This argument wrongly shifts the focus from the patient to the doctor. Instead of reflecting the condition and wishes of patients, assisted suicide would reflect the courage and compassion of their doctors. Thus, patients with doctors like Timothy Quill, who described in a 1991 *Journal* article how he helped a patient take her life,[20] would get the help they need and want, but similar patients with less steadfast doctors would not. That makes no sense.

People do not need assistance to commit suicide. With enough determination, they can do it themselves. This is perhaps the cruelest of the arguments against physician-assisted suicide. Many patients at the end of life are, in fact, physically unable to commit suicide on their own. Others lack the resources to do so. It has sometimes been suggested that they can simply stop eating and drinking and kill themselves that way. Although this method has been described as peaceful under certain conditions,[21] no one should count on that. The fact is that this argument leaves most patients to their suffering. Some, usually men, manage to commit suicide using violent methods. Percy Bridgman, a Nobel laureate in physics who in 1961 shot himself rather than die of metastatic cancer, said in his suicide note, "It is not decent for Society to make a man do this to himself."[22]

My father, who knew nothing of Percy Bridgman, committed suicide under similar circumstances. He was 81 and had metastatic prostate cancer. The night before he was scheduled to be admitted to the hospital, he shot himself. Like Bridgman, he thought it might be his last chance. At the time, he was not in extreme pain, nor was he close to death (his life expectancy was probably longer than six months). But he was suffering nonetheless—from nausea and the side effects of antiemetic agents, weakness, incontinence, and hopelessness. Was he depressed? He would probably have freely admitted that he was, but he would have thought it beside the point. In any case, he was an intensely private man who would have refused psychiatric care. Was he overly concerned with maintaining control of the circumstances of his life and death? Many people would say so, but that was the way he was. It is the job of medicine to deal with patients as they are, not as we would like them to be.

I tell my father's story here because it makes an abstract issue very concrete. If physician-assisted suicide had been available, I have no doubt my father would have chosen it. He was protective of his family, and if he had felt he had the choice, he would have spared my mother the shock of finding his body. He did not tell her what he planned to do, because he knew she would stop him. I also believe my father would have waited if physician-assisted suicide had been available. If patients have access to drugs they can take when they choose, they will not feel they must commit suicide early, while they are still able to do it on their own. They would probably live longer and certainly more peacefully, and they might not even use the drugs.

Long before my father's death, I believed that physician-assisted suicide ought to be permissible under some circumstances, but his death strengthened my conviction that it is simply a part of good medical care—something to be done reluctantly and sadly, as a last resort, but done nonetheless. There should be safeguards to ensure that the decision is well considered and consistent, but they should not be so daunting or violative of privacy that they become obstacles instead of protections. In particular, they should be directed not toward reviewing the reasons for an autonomous decision, but only toward ensuring that the decision is indeed autonomous. If the Supreme Court upholds the decisions of the appeals courts, assisted suicide will not be forced on either patients or doctors, but it will be a choice for those patients who need it and those doctors willing to help. If, on the other hand, the Supreme Court overturns the lower courts' decisions, the issue will continue to be grappled with state by state, through the political process. But sooner or later, given the need and the widespread public support, physician-assisted suicide will be demanded of a compassionate profession.

REFERENCES

1. Greenhouse L. High court to say if the dying have a right to suicide help. New York Times. October 2, 1996:A1.
2. Compassion in Dying v. Washington, 79 F.3d 790 (9th Cir. 1996).
3. Quill v. Vacco, 80 F.3d 716 (2d Cir. 1996).
4. Annas GJ. Death by prescription—the Oregon initiative. N Engl J Med 1994;331:1240-3.
5. Blendon RJ, Szalay US, Knox RA. Should physicians aid their patients in dying? The public perspective. JAMA 1992; 267:2658-62.
6. Bachman JG, Alcser KH, Doukas DJ, Lichtenstein RL, Corning AD, Brody H. Attitudes of Michigan physicians and the public toward legalizing physician-assisted suicide and voluntary euthanasia. N Engl J Med 1996;334:303-9.
7. Lee MA, Nelson HD, Tilden VP, Ganzini L, Schmidt TA, Tolle SW. Legalizing assisted suicide —views of physicians in Oregon. N Engl J Med 1996;334:310-5.
8. Gianelli DM. AMA to court: no suicide aid. American Medical News. November 25, 1996:1, 27, 28.
9. Dworkin R. Sex, death, and the courts. New York Review of Books. August 8, 1996.
10. In re: Quinlan, 70 N.J. 10, 355 A.2d 647 (1976).
11. Cruzan v. Director, Missouri Department of Health, 497 U.S. 261, 110 S.Ct. 2841 (1990).
12. Omnibus Budget Reconciliation Act of 1990, P.L. 101-508, sec. 4206 and 4751, 104 Stat. 1388, 1388-115, and 1388-204 (classified respectively at 42 U.S.C. 1395cc(f) (Medicare) and 1396a(w) (Medicaid) (1994).
13. Angell M. The quality of mercy. N Engl J Med 1982;306:98-9.
14. van der Maas PJ, van der Wal G, Haverkate I, et al. Euthanasia, physician-assisted suicide, and other medical practices involving the end of life in the Netherlands, 1990–1995. N Engl J Med 1996;335:1699-705.
15. van der Wal G, van der Maas PJ, Bosma JM, et al. Evaluation of the notification procedure for physician-assisted death in the Netherlands. N Engl J Med 1996;335:1706-11.
16. Angell M. Euthanasia in the Netherlands—good news or bad? N Engl J Med 1996;335:1676-8.
17. Chochinov HM, Wilson KG, Enns M, et al. Desire for death in the terminally ill. Am J Psychiatry 1995;152:1185-91.
18. Cassel CK, Meier DE. Morals and moralism in the debate over euthanasia and assisted suicide. N Engl J Med 1990;323:750-2.
19. Angell M. Doctors and assisted suicide. Ann R Coll Physicians Surg Can 1991;24:493-4.
20. Quill TE. Death and dignity—a case of individualized decision making. N Engl J Med 1991;324:691-4.
21. Lynn J, Childress JF. Must patients always be given food and water? Hastings Cent Rep 1983;13(5):17-21.
22. Nuland SB. How we die. New York: Alfred A. Knopf, 1994:152.

NO

Kathleen M. Foley

COMPETENT CARE FOR THE DYING INSTEAD OF PHYSICIAN-ASSISTED SUICIDE

While the Supreme Court is reviewing the decisions by the Second and Ninth Circuit Courts of Appeals to reverse state bans on assisted suicide, there is a unique opportunity to engage the public, health care professionals, and the government in a national discussion of how American medicine and society should address the needs of dying patients and their families. Such a discussion is critical if we are to understand the process of dying from the point of view of patients and their families and to identify existing barriers to appropriate, humane compassionate care at the end of life. Rational discourse must replace the polarized debate over physician-assisted suicide and euthanasia. Facts, not anecdotes, are necessary to establish a common ground and frame a system of health care for the terminally ill that provides the best possible quality of living while dying.

The biased language of the appeals courts evinces little respect for the vulnerability and dependency of the dying. Judge Stephen Reinhardt, writing for the Ninth Circuit Court, applied the liberty-interest clause of the Fourteenth Amendment, advocating a constitutional right to assisted suicide. He stated, "The competent terminally ill adult, having lived nearly the full measure of his life, has a strong interest in choosing a dignified and humane death, rather than being reduced to a state of helplessness, diapered, sedated, incompetent."[1] Judge Roger J. Miner, writing for the Second Circuit Court of Appeals, applied the equal-rights clause of the Fourteenth Amendment and went on to emphasize that the state "has no interest in prolonging a life that is ending."[2] This statement is more than legal jargon. It serves as a chilling reminder of the low priority given to the dying when it comes to state resources and protection.

The appeals courts' assertion of a constitutional right to assisted suicide is narrowly restricted to the terminally ill. The courts have decided that it is the patient's condition that justifies killing and that the terminally ill are special—so special that they deserve assistance in dying. This group alone can receive

From Kathleen M. Foley, "Competent Care for the Dying Instead of Physician-Assisted Suicide," *The New England Journal of Medicine*, vol. 336, no. 1 (January 2, 1997), pp. 54–58. Copyright © 1997 by The Massachusetts Medical Society. Reprinted by permission. All rights reserved.

such assistance. The courts' response to the New York and Washington cases they reviewed is the dangerous form of affirmative action in the name of compassion. It runs the risk of further devaluing the lives of terminally ill patients and may provide the excuse for society to abrogate its responsibility for their care.

Both circuit courts went even farther in asserting that physicians are already assisting in patients' deaths when they withdraw life-sustaining treatments such as respirators or administer high doses of pain medication that hasten death. The appeals courts argued that providing a lethal prescription to allow a terminally ill patient to commit suicide is essentially the same as withdrawing life-sustaining treatment or aggressively treating pain. Judicial reasoning that eliminates the distinction between letting a person die and killing runs counter to physicians' standards of palliative care.[3] The courts' purported goal in blurring these distinctions was to bring society's legal rules more closely in line with the moral value it places on the relief of suffering.[4]

In the real world in which physicians care for dying patients, withdrawing treatment and aggressively treating pain are acts that respect patients' autonomous decisions not to be battered by medical technology and to be relieved of their suffering. The physician's intent is to provide care, not death. Physicians do struggle with doubts about their own intentions.[5] The courts' arguments fuel their ambivalence about withdrawing life-sustaining treatments or using opioid or sedative infusions to treat intractable symptoms in dying patients. Physicians are trained and socialized to preserve life. Yet saying that physicians struggle with doubts about their inten-

tions in performing these acts is not the same as saying that their intention is to kill. In palliative care, the goal is to relieve suffering, and the quality of life, not the quantity, is of utmost importance.

Whatever the courts say, specialists in palliative care do not think that they practice physician-assisted suicide or euthanasia.[6] Palliative medicine has developed guidelines for aggressive pharmacologic management of intractable symptoms in dying patients, including sedation for those near death.[3,7,8] The World Health Organization has endorsed palliative care as an integral component of a national-health care policy and has strongly recommended to its member countries that they not consider legalizing physician-assisted suicide and euthanasia until they have addressed the needs of their citizens for pain relief and palliative care.[9] The courts have disregarded this formidable recommendation and, in fact, are indirectly suggesting that the World Health Organization supports assisted suicide.

Yet the courts' support of assisted suicide reflects the requests of the physicians who initiated the suits and parallels the numerous surveys demonstrating that a large proportion of physicians support the legalization of physician-assisted suicide.[10-15] A smaller proportion of physicians are willing to provide such assistance, and an even smaller proportion are willing to inject a lethal dose of medication with the intent of killing a patient (active voluntary euthanasia). These survey data reveal a gap between the attitudes and behavior of physicians; 20 to 70 percent of physicians favor the legalization of physician-assisted suicide, but only 2 to 4 percent favor active voluntary euthanasia, and only approximately 2 to 13 percent have actually aided patients in dying, by either providing a prescription or administering a lethal injection. The limitations of these surveys, which are legion, include inconsistent definitions of physician-assisted suicide and euthanasia, lack of information about nonrespondents, and provisions for maintaining confidentiality that have led to inaccurate reporting.[13,16] Since physicians' attitudes toward alternatives to assisted suicide have not been studied, there is a void in our knowledge about the priority that physicians place on physician-assisted suicide.

The willingness of physicians to assist patients in dying appears to be determined by numerous complex factors, including religious beliefs, personal values, medical specialty, age, practice setting, and perspective on the use of financial resources.[13,16-19] Studies of patients' preferences for care at the end of life demonstrate that physicians' preferences strongly influence those of their patients.[13] Making physician-assisted suicide a medical treatment when it is so strongly dependent on these physician-related variables would result in a regulatory impossibility.[19] Physicians would have to disclose their values and attitudes to patients to avoid potential conflict.[13] A survey by Ganzini et al. demonstrated that psychiatrists' responses to requests to evaluate patients were highly determined by their attitudes.[13] In a study by Emanuel et al., depressed patients with cancer said they would view positively those physicians who acknowledged their willingness to assist in suicide. In contrast, patients with cancer who were suffering from pain would be suspicious of such physicians.[11]

In this controversy, physicians fail into one of three groups. Those who support physician-assisted suicide see it as a compassionate response to a medical need, a symbol of nonabandonment, and a means to reestablish patients' trust in doctors who have used technology excessively.[20] They argue that regulation of physician-assisted suicide is possible and, in fact, necessary to control the actions of physicians who are currently providing assistance surreptitiously.[21] The two remaining groups of physicians oppose legalization.[19,22-24] One group is morally opposed to physician-assisted suicide and emphasizes the need to preserve the professionalism of medicine and the commitment to "do no harm." These physicians view aiding a patient in dying as a form of abandonment, because a physician needs to walk the last mile with the patient, as a witness, not as an executioner. Legalization would endorse justified killing, according to these physicians, and guidelines would not be followed, even if they could be developed. Furthermore, these physicians are concerned that the conflation of assisted suicide with the withdrawal of life support or adequate treatment of pain would make it even harder for dying patients because there would be a backlash against existing policies. The other group is not ethically opposed to physician-assisted suicide and, in fact, sees it as acceptable in exceptional cases, but these physicians believe that one cannot regulate the unregulatable.[19] On this basis, the New York State Task Force on Life and the Law, a 24-member committee with broad public and professional representation, voted unanimously against the legalization of physician-assisted suicide.[24] All three groups of physicians agree that a national effort is needed to improve the care of the dying. Yet it does seem that those in favor of legalizing physician-assisted suicide are disingenuous in their use of this issue as a wedge. If this form of assistance with dying is legalized, the courts will be forced to broaden the assistance to include active voluntary euthanasia and, eventually, assistance in response to requests from proxies.

One cannot easily categorize the patients who request physician-assisted suicide or euthanasia. Some surveys of physicians have attempted to determine retrospectively the prevalence and nature of these requests.[10] Pain, AIDS, and neurodegenerative disorders are the most common conditions in patients requesting assistance in dying. There is a wide range in the age of such patients, but many are younger persons with AIDS.[10] From the limited data available, the factors most commonly involved in requests for assistance are concern about future loss of control, being or becoming a burden to others, or being unable to care for oneself and fear of severe pain.[10] A small number of recent studies have directly asked terminally ill patients with cancer or AIDS about their desire for death.[25-27] All these studies show that the desire for death is closely associated with depression and that pain and lack of social support are contributing factors.

Do we know enough, on the basis of several legal cases, to develop a public policy that will profoundly change medicine's role in society?[1,2] Approximately 2.4 million Americans die each year. We have almost no information on how they die and only general information on where they die. Sixty-one percent die in hospitals, 17 percent in nursing homes, and the remainder at home, with approximately 10 to 14 percent of those at home receiving hospice care.

The available data suggest that physicians are inadequately trained to assess and manage the multifactorial symptoms commonly associated with patients' requests for physician-assisted suicide. According to the American Medical Association's report on medical education, only 5 of 126 medical schools in the United States require a separate course in the care of the dying.[28] Of 7048 residency programs, only 26 percent offer a course on the medical and legal aspects of care at the end of life as a regular part of the curriculum. According to a survey of 1068 accredited residency programs in family medicine, internal medicine, and pediatrics and fellowship programs in geriatrics, each resident or fellow coordinates the care of 10 or fewer dying patients annually.[28] Almost 15 percent of the programs offer no formal training in terminal care. Despite the availability of hospice programs, only 17 percent of the training programs offer a hospice rotation, and the rotation is required in only half of those programs; 9 percent of the programs have residents or fellows serving as members of hospice teams. In a recent survey of 55 residency programs and over 1400 residents, conducted by the American Board of Internal Medicine, the residents were asked to rate their perception of adequate training in care at the end of life. Seventy-two percent reported that they had received adequate training in managing pain and other symptoms; 62 percent, that they had received adequate training in telling patients that they are dying; 38 percent, in describing what the process will be like; and 32 percent, in talking to patients who request assistance in dying or a hastened death (Blank L: personal communication).

The lack of training in the care of the dying is evident in practice. Several studies have concluded that poor communication between physicians and patients, physicians' lack of knowledge about national guidelines for such care, and their lack of knowledge about the control of symptoms are barriers to the provision of good care at the end of life.[23,29,30]

Yet there is now a large body of data on the components of suffering in patients with advanced terminal disease, and these data provide the basis for treatment algorithms.[3] There are three major factors in suffering: pain and other physical symptoms, psychological distress, and existential distress (described as the experience of life without meaning). It is not only the patients who suffer but also their families and the health care professionals attending them. These experiences of suffering are often closely and inextricably related. Perceived distress in any one of the three groups amplifies distress in the others.[31,32]

Pain is the most common symptom in dying patients, and according to recent data from U.S. studies, 56 percent of outpatients with cancer, 82 percent of outpatients with AIDS, 50 percent of hospitalized patients with various diagnoses, and 36 percent of nursing home residents have inadequate management of pain during the course of their terminal illness.[33-36] Members of minority groups and women, both those with cancer and those with AIDS, as well as the elderly, receive less pain treatment than other groups of patients. In a survey of 1177 physicians who had treated a total of more than 70,000 patients with cancer in the previous six months, 76 percent of the respondents cited lack of knowledge as a barrier to their ability to control pain.[37] Severe pain that is not adequately controlled interferes with the quality of life, including the activities of daily living, sleep, and social interactions.[33,38]

Other physical symptoms are also prevalent among the dying. Studies of patients with advanced cancer and of the elderly in the year before death show that they have numerous symptoms that worsen the quality of life, such as fatigue, dyspnea, delirium, nausea, and vomiting.[36,38]

Along with these physical symptoms, dying patients have a variety of well-described psychological symptoms, with a high prevalence of anxiety and depression in patients with cancer or AIDS and the elderly.[27,39] For example, more than 60 percent of patients with advanced cancer have psychiatric problems, with adjustment disorders, depression, anxiety, and delirium reported most frequently. Various factors that contribute to the prevalence and severity of psychological distress in the terminally ill have been identified.[39] The diagnosis of depression is difficult to make in medically ill patients[3,26,40]; 94 percent of the Oregon psychiatrists surveyed by Ganzini et al. were not confident that they could determine, in a single evaluation, whether a psychiatric disorder was impairing the judgment of a patient who requested assistance with suicide.[13]

Attention has recently been focused on the interaction between uncontrolled symptoms and vulnerability to suicide in patients with cancer or AIDS.[41] Data from studies of both groups of patients suggest that uncontrolled pain contributes to depression and that persistent pain interferes with patients' ability to receive support from their families and others. Patients with AIDS have a high risk of suicide that is independent of physical symptoms. Among New York City residents with AIDS, the relative risk of suicide in men between the ages of 20 and 59 years was 36 times higher than the risk among men without AIDS in the same age group and 66 times higher than the risk in the general population.[41] Patients with AIDS who committed suicide generally did so within nine months after receiving the diagnosis; 25 percent had made a previous suicide attempt, 50 percent had reported severe depression, and 40 percent had seen a psychiatrist within four days before committing suicide. As previously noted, the desire to die is most closely associated with the diagnosis of depression.[26,27] Suicide is the eighth leading cause of death in the United States, and the incidence of suicide is higher in patients with cancer or AIDS and in elderly men than in the general population. Conwell and Caine reported that depression was under-diagnosed by primary care physicians in a cohort of elderly patients who subsequently committed suicide; 75 percent of the patients had seen a primary care physician during the last month of life but had not received a diagnosis of depression.[22]

The relation between depression and the desire to hasten death may vary among subgroups of dying patients. We have no data, except for studies of a small number of patients with cancer or AIDS. The effect of treatment for depression on the desire to hasten death and on requests for assistance in doing so has not been examined in the medically ill population, except for a small study in which four of six patients who initially wished to hasten death changed their minds within two weeks.[26]

There is also the concern that certain patients, particularly members of minority groups that are estranged from the health care system, may be reluctant to receive treatment for their physical or psychological symptoms because of the fear that their physicians will, in fact, has-

ten death. There is now some evidence that the legalization of assisted suicide in the Northern Territory of Australia has undermined the Aborigines' trust in the medical care system[42]; this experience may serve as an example for the United States, with its multicultural population.

The multiple physical and psychological symptoms in the terminally ill and elderly are compounded by a substantial degree of existential distress. Reporting on their interviews with Washington State physicians whose patients had requested assistance in dying, Back et al. noted the physicians' lack of sophistication in assessing such nonphysical suffering.[10]

In summary, there are fundamental physician-related barriers to appropriate, humane, and compassionate care for the dying. These range from attitudinal and behavioral barriers to educational and economic barriers. Physicians do not know enough about their patients, themselves, or suffering to provide assistance with dying as a medical treatment for the relief of suffering. Physicians need to explore their own perspectives on the meaning of suffering in order to develop their own approaches to the care of the dying. They need insight into how the nature of the doctor-patient relationship influences their own decision making. If legalized, physician-assisted suicide will be a substitute for rational therapeutic, psychological, and social interventions that might otherwise enhance the quality of life for patients who are dying. The medical profession needs to take the lead in developing guidelines for good care of dying patients. Identifying the factors related to physicians, patients, and the health care system that pose barriers to appropriate care at the end of life should be the first step in a national dialogue to educate health care professionals and the public on the topic of death and dying. Death is an issue that society as a whole faces, and it requires a compassionate response. But we should not confuse compassion with competence in the care of terminally ill patients.

REFERENCES

1. Reinhardt, Compassion in Dying v. State of Washington, 79 F. 3d 790 9th Cir. 1996.
2. Miner, Quill v Vacco 80 F. 3d 716 2nd Cir. 1996.
3. Doyle D, Hanks GWC, MacDonald N. The Oxford textbook of palliative medicine. New York: Oxford University Press, 1993.
4. Orentlicher D. The legalization of physician-assisted suicide. N Engl J Med 1996;335:663-7.
5. Wilson WC, Smedira NG, Fink C, McDowell JA, Luce JM. Ordering and administration of sedatives and analgesics during the withholding and withdrawal of life support from critically ill patients. JAMA 1992;267:949-53.
6. Foley KM. The relationship of pain and symptom management to patient requests for physician-assisted suicide. J Pain Symptom Manage 1991;6:289-97.
7. Cherny NI, Coyle N, Foley KM. Guidelines in the care of the dying patient. Hematol Oncol Clin North Am 1996;10:261-86.
8. Cherny NI, Portenoy RK. Sedation in the management of refractory symptoms: guidelines for evaluation and treatment. J Palliat Care 1994;10(2):31-8.
9. Cancer pain relief and palliative care. Geneva: World Health Organization, 1989.
10. Back AL, Wallace JI, Starks, HE, Pearlman RA. Physician-assisted suicide and euthanasia in Washington State: patient requests and physician responses. JAMA 1996;275:919-25.
11. Emanual EJ, Fairclough DL, Daniels ER, Clarridge BR. Euthanasia and physician-assisted suicide: attitudes and experiences of oncology patients, oncologists, and the public. Lancet 1996;347:1805-10.
12. Lee MA, Nelson HD, Tilden VP, Ganzini L, Schmidt TA, Tolle SW. Legalizing assisted suicide —views of physicians in Oregon. N Engl J Med 1996;334:310-5.
13. Ganzini L, Fenn DS, Lee MA, Heintz RT, Bloom JD. Attitudes of Oregon psychiatrists toward physician-assisted suicide. Am J Psychiatry 1996;153:1469-75.
14. Cohen JS, Fihn SD, Boyko EJ, Jonsen AR, Wood RW. Attitudes toward assisted suicide and euthanasia among physicians in Washington State. N Engl J Med 1994;331:89-94.
15. Doukas DJ, Waterhouse D, Gorenflo DW, Seid J. Attitudes and behaviors on physician-assisted death: a study of Michigan oncologists. J Clin Oncol 1995;13:1055-61.
16. Morrison S, Meier D. Physician-assisted dying: fashioning public policy with an absence of data. Generations. Winter 1994:48-53.
17. Portenoy RK, Coyle N, Kash K, et al. Determinants of the willingness to endorse assisted suicide: a survey of physicians, nurses, and social workers. Psychosomatics (in press).
18. Fins J. Physician-assisted suicide and the right to care. Cancer Control 1996;3:272-8.
19. Callahan, D, White M. The legalization of physician-assisted suicide: creating a regulatory Potemkin Village. U Richmond Law Rev 1996;30:1-83.
20. Quill TE. Death and dignity—a case of individualized decision making. N Engl J Med 1991;324:691-4.
21. Quill TE, Cassel CK, Meier DE. Care of the hopelessly ill—proposed clinical criteria for physician-assisted suicide. N Engl J Med 1992;327:1380-4.
22. Conwell Y. Caine ED. Rational suicide and the right to die—reality and myth. N Engl J Med 1991;325:1100-3.
23. Foley KM. Pain, physician assisted suicide and euthanasia. Pain Forum 1995;4:163-78.
24. When death is sought: assisted suicide and euthanasia in the medical context. New York: New York State Task Force on Life and the Law, May 1994.
25. Brown JH, Henteleff P, Barakat S, Towe CJ. Is it normal for terminally ill patients to desire death? Am J Psychiatry 1986;143:208-11.
26. Chochinov HM, Wilson KG, Enns M, et al. Desire for death in the terminally ill. Am J Psychiatry 1995;152:1185-91.
27. Breitbart W. Rosenfeld BD, Passik SD. Interest in physician-assisted suicide among ambulatory HIV-infected patients, Am J Psychiatry 1996;153:238-42.
28. Hill TP. Treating the dying patient: the challenge for medical education. Arch Intern Med 1995;155:1265-9.
29. Callahan, D. Once again reality: now where do we go. Hastings Cent Rep 1995;25(6):Suppl:S33-S36.
30. Solomon MZ, O'Donnell L, Jennings B, et al. Decisions near the end of life: professional views on life-sustaining treatments. Am J Public Health 1993;83:14–23.
31. Cherny NI, Coyle, N. Foley KM. Suffering in the advanced cancer patient: definition and taxonomy. J. Palliat Care 1994;10(2):57-70.

32. Cassel EJ. The nature of suffering and the goals of medicine. N Engl J Med 1982;306:639-45.

33. Cleeland CS, Gonin R, Hatfield AK, et al. Pain and its treatment in outpatients with metastatic cancer. N Engl J Med 1994;330:592-6.

34. Breitbart W, Rosenfeld BD, Passik SD, McDonald NV, Thaler H, Portenoy RK. The undertreatment of pain in ambulatory AIDS patients. Pain 1996;65:243-9.

35. The SUPPORT Principal Investigators. A controlled trial to improve care for seriously ill hospitalized patients. JAMA 1995;274:1591-8.

36. Seale C, Cartwright A. The year before death. Hants, England: Avebury, 1994.

37. Von Roenn JH, Cleeland CS, Gonin R, Hatfield AK, Pandya KJ. Physician attitudes and practice in cancer pain management: a survey from the Eastern Cooperative Oncology Group. Ann Intern Med 1993;119:121-6.

38. Portenoy RK. Pain and quality of life: clinical issues and implications for research. Oncology 1990;4:172-8.

39. Breitbart W. Suicide risk and pain in cancer and AIDS patients. In: Chapman CR, Foley KM, eds. Current and emerging issues in cancer pain. New York: Raven Press, 1993.

40. Chochinov H, Wilson KG, Enns M, Lander S. Prevalence of depression in the terminally ill: effects of diagnostic criteria and symptom threshold judgments. Am J Psychiatry 1994;151:537-40.

41. Passik S, McDonald M. Rosenfeld B, Breitbart W. End of life issues in patients with AIDS: clinical and research considerations. J Pharm Care Pain Symptom Control 1995;3:91-111.

42. NT "success" in easing rural fear of euthanasia. The Age. August 31,1996:A7.

POSTSCRIPT

Should Doctors Ever Assist Terminally Ill Patients to Commit Suicide?

As our population ages and the incidence of certain diseases, such as cancer and AIDS, continues to increase, it appears that the ranks of the dying and suffering will grow. In the past, there were limited means of prolonging life; however, due to advances in modern medicine and technology, the dying can be kept alive sometimes for lengthy time periods. Although some doctors are beginning to speak more often of euthanasia, in the United States the American Medical Association has unequivocally reaffirmed its opposition to the practice.

In the Netherlands the Dutch have taken a different viewpoint: Although Dutch law still refers to euthanasia as a crime, the highest courts there have determined that doctors may practice it if they follow specific guidelines set up by the Royal Dutch Medical Association [see "Euthanasia in the Netherlands," *The New England Journal of Medicine*, (vol. 335, 1996)].

Articles that support euthanasia include "The Physician's Responsibility Toward Hopelessly Ill Patients," *The New England Journal of Medicine* (March 30, 1989); "Suicide: Should the Doctor Ever Help?" *Harvard Health Letter* (August 1991); and "What Quinlan Can Tell Kevorkian About the Right to Die," *The Humanist* (March/April 1997).

Opponents of euthanasia and physician-assisted suicide argue that all life has value and that doctors do not have the right to end it. These include Leon R. Kass, in "Neither for Love Nor Money: Why Doctors Must Not Kill," *The Public Interest* (December 1989), and philosophy professor Richard Momeyer of Miami University, in "Does Physician Assisted Suicide Violate the Integrity of Medicine?" *Journal of Medicine and Philosophy* (vol. 20, 1995). Other articles that discuss the issue include "Coming Soon: Your Neighborhood T.S.C.," *America* (April 30, 1994); "Should Physicians Aid Their Patients in Dying?" *Journal of the American Medical Association* (May 20, 1992); "Assisted Suicide: Should Doctors Help Hopelessly Ill Patients Take Their Lives?" *CQ Researcher* (February 21, 1992); "Are Laws Against Assisted Suicide Unconstitutional?" *Hastings Center Report* (May/June 1993); "The Euthanasia Follies," *Commonweal* (June 3, 1994); "Attitudes Toward Assisted Suicide and Euthanasia Among Physicians in Washington State," *The New England Journal of Medicine* (July 14, 1994); "Assisted Suicide Controversy: Should Physicians Help the Dying to End Their Lives?" *CQ Researcher* (May 5, 1995); and "Whose Right to Die?" *The Atlantic Monthly* (March 1997).

ISSUE 3

Should Health Care for the Elderly Be Limited?

YES: Daniel Callahan, from "Setting Limits: A Response," *The Gerontologist* (June 1994)

NO: Ezekiel J. Emanuel and Linda L. Emanuel, from "The Economics of Dying: The Illusion of Cost Savings at the End of Life," *The New England Journal of Medicine* (February 24, 1994)

ISSUE SUMMARY

YES: Hastings Center director Daniel Callahan contends that medical care for elderly people who have lived their natural life expectancy should consist only of pain relief rather than expensive health care services that serve only to forestall death.

NO: Physicians Ezekiel J. Emanuel and Linda L. Emanuel argue that cost savings accrued by restricting medical care at the end of life are not likely to be substantial and that health care costs would be reduced if changes were made in the overall delivery of health care.

In 1980, 11 percent of the U.S. population was over age 65, but they utilized about 29 percent ($219 billion) of the total American health care expenditures. By the end of the decade, the percentage of the population over 65 had risen to 12 percent, which consumed 31 percent of total health care expenditures, or $450 billion. The costs of Medicare, the government insurance for the elderly, is expected to increase to $114 billion by the year 2000. It has been projected that by the year 2040, people over 65 will represent 21 percent of the population and consume 45 percent of all health care expenditures.

Medical expenses at the end of life appear to be extremely high in relation to other health care costs. Studies have shown that nearly one-third of annual Medicare costs are for the 5–6 percent of beneficiaries who die that year. Expenses for dying patients increase significantly as death nears, and payments for health care during the last weeks of life make up 40 percent of the medical costs for the entire last year of life. Some studies have shown that up to 50 percent of the medical costs incurred during a person's entire life are spent during their last year!

Many surveys have indicated that most Americans do not want to be kept alive if their illness is incurable and irreversible, for both economic and humanitarian reasons. Many experts believe that if physicians stopped using high technology at the end of life to prevent death, then we would save billions of dollars, which could be used to insure the uninsured and provide basic health care to millions.

In England the emphasis of health care is on improving the quality of life through primary care medicine, well-subsidized home care, and institutional programs for the elderly and those with incurable illnesses, rather than through life-extending acute care medicine. The British seem to value basic medical care for all rather than expensive technology for the few who might benefit from it. As a result, the British spend a much smaller proportion of their gross national product (6.2 percent) on health services than do Americans (10.8 percent) for a nearly identical health status and life expectancy.

In the following selection, Daniel Callahan argues that using medical technologies to extend the lives of the terminally ill and/or individuals who have lived out their natural life spans is an expensive and inappropriate use of modern medicine. Technology, he feels, should be used to avoid premature death and to relieve suffering, not to prolong full and complete lives. He believes that most elderly and hopelessly ill people agree with these principles: they indicate a wish that their lives not be aggressively extended beyond a point at which they still possess a good level of physical and mental functioning and a certain degree of value and meaning. Callahan also states that the attempt to indefinitely extend life can be an economic disaster. This goal also fails to put health in its proper place as only one among many human values, and it discourages the acceptance of aging and death as part of life.

Ezekiel J. Emanuel and Linda L. Emanuel counter that the actual savings from withholding treatment at the end of life would be minimal. The amount that may be saved by reducing the use of aggressive life-sustaining interventions for dying patients is at most 3.3 percent of total national health care costs. They claim that high-quality care, such as providing pain medications and helping in the activities of daily living, requires skilled and expensive personnel. Even low-technology medical care is costly. They also argue that since death is often unpredictable, it is not always possible to say accurately which patients will benefit from high-technology treatment and which ones will not.

YES

Daniel Callahan

SETTING LIMITS: A RESPONSE

Some six years ago, in the fall of 1987, I published *Setting Limits: Medical Goals in an Aging Society* (Callahan, 1987). I argued that we would have to rethink once again the place of aging in the life cycle and that, in the future, scarcity of resources could force an age limit on medical entitlements for the elderly. That was not a popular thesis. I expected controversy and I got it, ranging from scholarly debates conducted with academic decorum to nasty public and media exchanges. Some six books of commentary and criticism, and an issue of a law review, were directly or indirectly inspired by *Setting Limits* (St. Louis University Law Journal, 1989; Homer & Holstein, 1990; Binstock & Post, 1991; Jecker, 1991; Barry & Bradley, 1991; Winslow & Walters, 1993; Hackler, in press).

The birth of *Setting Limits* came about because, beginning in the mid-1980s, I became aware of the striking demographic trends being reported, often accompanied by worries about their economic and social impact in the decades ahead (Preston, 1984). I saw us moving—through no one's fault, and surely not the elderly—toward a potential tragic dilemma of the first order. Something would have to give somewhere. We could not possibly guarantee indefinitely to the growing number and proportion of the elderly all of the potentially limitless fruits of medical progress at public expense without seriously distorting sensible social priorities. Where and how could we set some sensible and fair limits?

WHAT I TRIED TO SAY

Setting Limits was the result of my effort to think through that problem. I argued that we should begin now, *before* the crisis is fully upon us, to change our expectations about elderly care in the future. I stressed in the book the *trend* in the development of expensive technologies, not their present costs, and the likely need for *future* change in entitlement policies, not at present. As a way into these likely changes, I said that we need to rethink two deeply imbedded ideas, widely if not universally held. The first is the cherished notion that we should try endlessly through medical progress to modernize

From Daniel Callahan, "Setting Limits: A Response," *The Gerontologist*, vol. 34, no. 3 (June 1994), pp. 373–398. Copyright © 1994 by The Gerontological Society of America. Reprinted by permission.

old age, to turn it into a more or less permanent middle age. We should instead accept aging as a part of life, not just another medical obstacle to be overcome. The valuable and necessary campaign against ageism, highly individualistic in its premises, runs the risk of emptying age as a stage in life of meaningful content and, with the help of science, trying to turn it into a kind of repairable biological accident. The second idea I criticized was the view that there should be no limits to the claims of the elderly as a group to expensive life-extending medicine under *public* entitlement programs, that only their individual needs should count, and count in an age-blind way.

After criticizing those two ideas, I offered a different picture of what a future health care policy for the elderly might look like, one designed to balance the new limits with some enriched entitlements. I was seeking a public policy that: (1) would guarantee the elderly, along with everyone else, access to universal health care; (2) would help everyone to avoid an early, premature death; (3) would achieve a better balance of caring and curing to overcome the powerful bias toward the latter (whose effect is to undermine the former), and in particular to greatly strengthen long-term and home care support; and (4) would use age as a categorical standard to cut off life-extending technologies under the Medicare entitlement program—but using it as a standard *if and only if the* other reforms were put in place first.

I proposed the idea of a "natural life span" as a rough way of determining such a cut-off point. I would have been wise to have chosen a different word than "natural," since I meant by that concept a biographical not a biological standard,

that is, a notion of when it might be said that most people will have lived an adequately full, if not necessarily totally full, life. I drew that notion from my own experience, and the traditions of most cultures, which perceives an important moral and social distinction between the sadness but fittingness of death in old age and the tragedy or outrage of an avoidable early, particularly, childhood death. I did not specify an exact age but suggested that the "late 70s or early 80s" would be an appropriate age range in which to look for it.

The great need is to find a type of limit that would dampen the potent trend to apply ever more expensive technologies to saving and extending the life of the elderly. That trend has seen a steady rise in the age of various surgical and other medical procedures, and in particular a rise often marked by successful results (Hosking, Warner, Lobdell, Offord, & Melton, 1989; Latta & Keene, 1989; Breidenbaugh, Sarsitis, & Milam, 1990). But it is the success, I argued, that was creating the problem for us, not the failures, and I did not foresee us going backwards in care for the elderly, but radically slowing up and eventually plateauing the forward march of expensive medical progress.

I held, finally, that the needed changes should be effected, not by compulsion —the young imposing it by force on the unwilling old—but democratically, preceded by a decades-long period of changing our thinking, attitudes, and expectations about elderly health care. Those of us still reasonably young should be prepared in the future to impose an age limit on ourselves. As I noted in the Preface to my book, in a passage often overlooked, "what I am looking for is not any quick change but the beginning of a long-term discussion, one that will lead people to change their thinking and, most important, their expectations, about old age and death" (Callahan, 1987, p. 10).

RESPONSES TO CRITICS

Let me take up, in turn, the major objections leveled at my argument. Since there were well over 100 papers written about the book, and I was given the back of someone's hand in at least that many more, I will consolidate here the criticisms.

The Use of Age as a Standard for Limiting Health Care Would Be Ageist and Unjust. There are two discordant ways of thinking about the place and relevance of age from an individual and from a policy perspective. From an individual perspective, it is said, age as such should have no place in resource allocation. It is not a good predictor of health, mental or physical. True. Yet the difficulty here is obvious from a policy perspective: Age *is* a relevant and conspicuous variable in health care costs, and the elderly are more costly as a group than people of younger ages. The fact that many elderly people remain healthy most of their final years—and that there is a heterogeneous pattern of health care usage—does not change the fact that the average per capita costs of the elderly are significantly higher than for younger people. Public policy must take account of, and work with, those averages. They are what count in devising programs, in projecting future costs, and in estimating different health care needs. Age matters.

If age matters, how does it matter? It matters when, as we can now see, meeting the health care costs of the elderly as a group begins to threaten the possibility of meeting the needs of other age groups. In the nature of the case, moreover, there are no fixed boundaries to the amount of money that can be spent combating the effects of biological aging and attempting to forestall death in old age. It is an unlimited frontier. One could say exactly the same thing about trying to save the life of low birthweight infants. We can go from the present 450–500 grams and 24–25 weeks gestation to 400 to 300 grams, and 20–21 weeks gestation, and so on. There are no end of possibilities there as well, and thus some very good reasons to set limits to those efforts, using either weight or gestational age as a categorical standard (Callahan, 1990). It is no more an anti-aging act than it is an anti-baby act to set limits (for instance, on neonatal care) in order to avoid pursuing unlimited, potentially ruinous possibilities.

Aging and death in old age are inevitable, and there should be no unlimited claim on public resources to combat them. But premature death, and bad schools, and blighted urban areas of great poverty, are not inevitable. The first health task of a society is that the young should have the chance to become old. That should always take priority over helping, at great cost, those who are already old from becoming still older. That is exactly what we can look forward to, as we throw more and more money into the fight to cure the chronic and degenerative diseases of aging, but not to care well for those who cannot be saved.

But if we set a limit on public entitlement for the elderly would this not be unfair and ageist? I believe we cannot achieve perfect equality in this world, much less in a health care system, without some harmful consequences. No country in the world, save the communist countries, has achieved any such goal, and the price they paid was rampant corruption and bribery; the wealthy and powerful still got better care. An age limit on entitlement benefits would of course perpetuate a two-tier system, with the rich able to buy health benefits not available to the poor, but that need not be the disaster many fear. The test should not be whether everyone receives exactly the same level of care. It should instead be whether the poorest and worst off receive decent health care. I believe the system I propose, guaranteeing universal care, a powerful effort to beat back premature death, a full range of health services through the late 70s or early 80s, a good range of social and caring services thereafter for one's entire life, and then (and only then) an age limit on expensive life-extending therapies, would be decent. If combined, moreover, with other kinds of limits in the health care systems for all groups, it would not be ageist even if it used age as a standard. It would use age as a standard simply because, as argued above, age does matter from a policy perspective.

It Is Unduly Pessimistic to Take Seriously the Projections That Show a Steadily Increasing Burden of Elderly Health Care Costs. "Callahan," one commentator said, "is overly alarmist about the relative burden of older persons..." (Lawlor, 1992, p. 132). I have never known quite what to make of that charge. I have used the standard research available on demographic trends and projected health care costs. I have never been able to find *any* optimistic projections based on historical and current demographic and economic projections. Even the critic who said I was "alarmist" concluded that paragraph by

criticizing the optimists for failing to note that "the arithmetic of compound growth is at work in the increase of health expenditures (prices, demographic change, and increasing intensity of care)" (Lawlor, 1992, p. 132). Since I wrote *Setting Limits,* moreover, the "pessimistic" data have continued to pour forth, even from those who are my critics on other grounds (Schneider & Guralnik, 1990).

Since I have been unable to locate *any* optimistic data and reassuring projections, nor have any been cited in rebuttal, I can only observe that those who find me pessimistic rely on hopeful, but essentially still imaginary, scenarios about the future. One scenario is that in the future there will be a "compression of morbidity" and thus a decrease in the costs of elderly morbidity. That is a most invigorating hope, but the present evidence has moved in exactly the opposite direction, to greater not lesser morbidity, even if there is at least one recent report suggesting a slight amelioration of that trend (Manton, Corder, & Stallard, 1993). The second scenario is that advances in medical research will find cures or inexpensive treatments for the degenerative diseases of aging (Schneider & Guralnik, 1990). I hope that is true, but there is no evidence so far to support that hope as a likely outcome. The third scenario is that the elderly in the future will retire later and work longer, thus contributing more and much later to their health care costs. That could surely happen, and may by force happen, but it will as such not do a great deal about the disproportion of resources that could go to the elderly, although it surely might help. It is not likely to be helpful with the large number of people who live beyond 85, a rapidly growing group.

It Is Only Because Our Health Care System Is Wasteful, Capitalistic, and Paternalistic That We Are Even Thinking of Rationing and Limits on Care for the Elderly. There is no doubt that ours is a wasteful, fragmented, and excessively costly system, and that we could spend more on the elderly if we reduced waste elsewhere (Estes, 1988). The amount of money we spend in comparison with other developed countries, which get as good and often better outcomes for considerably less money, establishes that point well enough (though it does not establish that the money saved should go to the elderly as distinguished, say, from improving the schools). There are two points to consider here. The first is that, after more than 20 years of trying, we have not discovered in this country how, short of the universal health care and global budgeting we have been slow to embrace, to significantly control our costs; they just keep rising.

The second point is that, even if we can achieve those needed reforms, the problem will still not go away. The experience of other developed countries is already showing how an aging population can continue to push costs and demand up even in efficient, cost-effective, non-market health care systems (Hollander & Becker, 1987; Loriaux, 1990; Jouvenel, 1989). Those countries, controlling the fees of health care workers, rationing technology, keeping a lid on drug and equipment costs, still have a growing age-related problem even so. Better health care systems can delay the problem, or ameliorate it; but they are not going to be a solution to it.

A popular proposal to reduce elderly costs is the promotion of "advance directives" to allow the elderly to voluntarily forgo expensive, useless, and un-desired care at the end of life. Could that make a difference? The evidence is mixed on that point and still scanty. One study found that advance directives made no difference in the medical treatment or in the medical costs (Schneiderman, Kronick, Kaplan, Anderson, & Langer, 1992), while another found evidence of dramatic savings (Chambers, Diamond, Perkel, & Lasch, 1994). My own guess is that advance directives will in the long run make some economic difference in relatively clear-cut cases of terminal illness for some classes of patients. There are two problems, however, which will make the greatest difference over time. One of them is the number of people who will execute advance directives, now still a significant minority. The other is the extent of expensive medical treatments that successfully avert the need to invoke advance directives, putting them off to another day; that's where the real bill is likely to add up, even if money can be saved in the last illness. To save money in the last days of life is not identical with saving money in the last years of life.

Even If It Becomes Necessary to Set Limits on Public Expenditures for Elderly Health Care, That Should Be Done on a Case-by-Case Basis Rather Than Categorically by Age. Should rationing or limits be necessary, almost everyone's ideal would be a system that was simultaneously individualized, fair, and effective. Each patient would be considered on his or her medical merits, not on the basis of some categorical standard. Rejecting categorical standards, "the impersonal application of a rule to a faceless group," Dr. Norman G. Levinsky has written that "society must not insulate itself from the agony of each decision to forgo beneficial treatment as it is experienced by patients, families, and care givers" (Levinsky, 1990, p. 1815).

I can well understand the sentiment behind Dr. Levinsky's thinking, but I have simply never been able to understand how it would be possible to limit health care in general while individualizing it in particular. If the assumption is that people should receive care on the basis of its individual efficacy for them, then we will run afoul of what I would call the "efficacy fallacy," that is, the notion that those treatments that are individually efficacious are therefore socially affordable. But precisely the problem we are likely to face is this: It will be the efficacious, not wasteful, treatments that will cause us the most financial grief, simply because it will be all the harder to deny people such treatment. There is a related fallacy, what I will dub the "hidden hand fallacy," that is, the view that the aggregate impact of meeting individual needs will turn out to be identical with the available common resources. Why should that be the case?

My assumption, by contrast—using the available projections—is that we will be forced to limit some proven, efficacious treatments, of a kind that people will want and that would extend their lives. The choices we will have to make will then be genuinely tragic choices. The pain of such choices is that they allow us no happy way out. It is an easy exercise to measure age-limit proposals against the standard of unlimited resources and no hard choices; and, naturally, an age limit looks terrible by that standard. But if we understand that we may one day be faced only with nasty options, then our task will be to compare those options with each other, not compare them against a world where no unpleasant choices are needed.

The Idea of Using a "Natural Life Span" as a Basis for Setting an Age Limit is Too Vague, and Too Controverted, to Be Useful.

With great frequency I felt my proposal ran up against the individualism of our culture, not only in the repeated assertion about the heterogeneity of the elderly, but also in the rejection of a use of the life cycle as a place to look for an age limit. Yet I find it hard to know where else we might fruitfully look. If our standard is simply individual benefit, regardless of age, then there is no possible way we could effectively limit elderly health care costs; they will inexorably rise as technology improves. My alternative approach is to ask: How can we design a health care and entitlement system that would allow each of us to live a long and full life, but would not entail unlimited public support for whatever technology turned up at whatever cost?

I turned to the idea of a "natural life span" in order to capitalize on a common culture sentiment, still alive in the United States. It is that, while all death is a cause for sadness, a death in old age after a long and full life is, given the inevitability of death, the most acceptable kind of death. Unlike the death of a child, or a young adult, death in old age is part of our biology and part of the life cycle. It is no accident, think, that there is less weeping at the death of a very old person than at the death of a child. Although the idea of a "natural life span" as a biographical notion was thoroughly assaulted by many of my critics, a recent survey indicates that the idea is still strong in our society, even if most people would at present probably resist using it for rationing purposes (Zweibel, Cassel, & Karvison, 1993). Increased financial pressure, certain in the years ahead, may perhaps change the public bias against an age-based rationing standard.

I come back to a fundamental question. Do the elderly have an unlimited medical claim on public resources? No, they have only a reasonable and thus limited claim. What is a "reasonable" claim? I take it to be a claim to live a long life with public support, but not indefinitely long, and not at the price of potential harm to others. If we can agree with that proposition, then a "natural life span" is one that is highly useful—though admittedly not precise —allowing us a way of talking about what should count as a premature death, and as the basis for a claim on the public purse. It will surely work better than, say, "individual need," which is subject to technological escalation and intractable subjective desires. If we agree, for instance, that the preservation of life is a basic medical need, then in the nature of the case with the aging person there are no necessary limits at all, scientific or economic, to what can be done to achieve that goal. To be sure, any specific age to invoke as a limit will be arbitrary, but not necessarily capricious. That was true of age 65 when Medicare was established. It could have been 66 or 64. The point is that it was within a generally acceptable range of choices, and that is sufficient for fair public policy.

SOME TELLING POINTS

My response so far might indicate that I have been unwilling to give way to my critics or to admit any validity to what they say. Up to a point that is true. Nonetheless, on the old principle that much of life and policy lies in the details, some telling points have been made against me. They are worth further thought.

The most powerful criticism is political: Whatever the rational arguments in its favor, neither the public nor legislators would ever accept an open, explicit use of age as a criterion for cutting off life-extending medical care. One critic called this assumption on my part a "blunder," and (in some sympathy with my general argument about the need for limits) said that we might be forced to covertly have an age standard (Moody, 1991). I have no doubt that an age limit would, politically, be obnoxious to politicians, at least at present. Even those countries known for using age as a norm (such as England and Switzerland) have done so tacitly and quietly, out of the public eye. Yet, if it is true that an explicit age standard is now and will remain for some time politically unacceptable as public policy, then we will be left with another dilemma. We will either have to come up with some other standard, bound to be unwanted also if it has any bite, or resign ourselves to euphemism and evasion, using age privately but never admitting it publicly.

There is a telling scientific criticism also. One of my goals with an age limit is to discourage the kind of scientific "progress" that endlessly generates new, almost always expensive, ways of extending the lives of elderly people. If those modalities were not going to be reimbursed, that would be a powerful disincentive to developing them in the first place. The problem here, as many noted, is that most of the technologies now used with the elderly were first developed with younger people in mind; few life-extending technologies are created for the elderly as such.

I cannot deny the force of those contentions. But that leaves us with another dilemma: If scientific progress moves along in an unchecked fashion, generating still more expensive ways of saving life, our tragic dilemma will become all the more painful. The gap between what we know we can or could do to save life will all the more harshly and conspicuously clash with our economic limitations. My own preference would be for a sharp increase in research designed to decrease morbidity and disability, discouraging when possible explicit efforts to develop more life-extending technologies.

Still another criticism might, for lack of a better name, be called the repugnance argument. It takes a number of forms. One of them is that we would find it repugnant to deny reimbursement to someone for a form of care that would clearly save that person's life; we could not just stand by and let the person die for lack of money. Another form is that, however nice my theory of justice between age groups, it would *look* like we were devaluing the worth of the elderly if we used age as an exclusive standard for denying care; we would find that hard to stand.

I agree that most people would find these consequences of an age limit repugnant. But again we are left with a dilemma, indeed more than one. What will we do about the repugnance that could well result from seeing a larger and larger, and even more disproportionate, share of resources going to the elderly while the needs of younger groups are going unmet? Or placing heavier and heavier economic burdens on the young to sustain the old? If we leave all choices about resource allocation to doctors and families at the bedside, what will we do about the repugnance regarding the variations in treatment that method will

bring, with some getting too much treatment and others getting too little? If we find the open use of an age limit repugnant, will we feel any better about a covert use, one that could be forced by a shortage of money?

Another telling point, in some ways the most fundamental, leaves me with a deep and unresolved problem. In an unpublished paper Per Anderson suggests that the "high quality aging that Callahan wants medicine and society to support will serve to make the idea of the life cycle increasingly implausible ... one can wonder whether Callahan would have us adopt an ethic of limits because it is the human good or because it is the grim necessity to which we must be resigned" (Anderson, 1991, p. 3). On this point, a profound one for medicine in general and not just for care of the aged, I am deeply ambivalent.

My own reading of history is that those people and cultures who live with some sense of intrinsic limits, whether natural or culturally inspired, better adapt to the human situation, and to aging and mortality, than do those who want to carry out endless warfare against human finitude. Yet I cannot ignore the other side of that coin, which is that we have enormously benefited from many efforts to transcend what earlier generations took to be fixed limits. I might not now be alive but for those efforts. How do we find the right balance here, between acceptance and acquiescence and the desire to struggle against our human condition? It is open to my critics to make a good case for fighting the ravages of age and to seek to further postpone death. I will respond by asking: Why should we believe that will necessarily increase our human satisfaction and sense of well-being? We will, I am sure, go back and forth on that point—and no doubt so will future generations.

WHAT ABOUT THE FUTURE?

There were three reasons why I was drawn to the use of an age limit as a likely way to eventually control health care allocation to the elderly. One reason was that it seems to me better in general for human beings to live with a strong sense of their mortality and to be willing to understand that their lives must come to an end. A second reason is that it seems to me merely the prejudice of an affluent, hyper-individualistic, technologically driven society to think that a denial of reimbursement for life-extending care beyond a certain point is tantamount to a denial of value and dignity to the elderly. The third reason for being drawn to age was that I simply could not imagine—and still cannot imagine—any other way of decisively and effectively and uniformly drawing a clear policy line than the use of age. It is precisely because it cuts through, and transcends, our individual differences that it is attractive for policy purposes.

That of course is precisely its greatest liability in the eyes of my critics, and I am more persuaded than I was initially that, for both symbolic and practical reasons, an age-based policy will appear, and well could be, obnoxious. Yet, having conceded that, I must then add: Show me an equally decisive alternative, one that will work to hold down costs, that does not depend upon variable bedside judgments, and that takes with full seriousness the need to find a solution —and a solution that does not depend on evading the problem altogether by invoking some yet-to-be-seen hopeful scientific or economic miracle.

If we agree on the eventual need for limits, does it follow that only an age limit would work? Not at all, and it may well be that the various repugnances I noted above will stand forever in the way of using an age limit. But in that case it will be necessary to come up with some plausible alternatives. Robert Veatch and Norman Daniels have suggested some interesting and alternative ways of using age, less stark than mine. They can be debated. Nancy S. Jecker and Robert A. Pearlman, after criticizing Harry R. Moody, Norman Daniels, and myself for our willingness to consider an age limit, conclude their article with a brief review of some possible alternatives—and find them full of problems as well! (See Jecker & Pearlman, 1989). No doubt anyway, as they say, we will have to explore those alternatives. I offer a simple test as we try to think about one alternative or another: If it seems to avoid the need for nasty choices altogether, or seems painless and congenial (like just cutting out unwanted treatment), we should have a hard time taking it seriously. In the best of all possible worlds, what the elderly want and need would fit perfectly with the available resources. Ours is not, nor is likely to be, such a world. Any solution that seems to imply such a world merits the same suspicion as offers of free trips to Europe or Florida just by placing a phone call.

Time and again I was accused of "blaming the elderly" for our present allocation problems. How nice it would be to find identifiable villains here, but I see no fault here *at all* with the elderly. Instead, we are only now beginning to see some of the costs and pitfalls of the great medical advances that have been made in recent decades, and some of the unforeseen and probably unforeseeable hazards of pursuing medical progress. It is the success of medicine, not its failures, that has created the problem of sustaining and paying for decent health care for the elderly. It is the success of the campaign against ageism, increasing the expectations of everyone for a medically and socially transformed old age, that have added to that problem. If there is any blame to be apportioned it should be directed at our dreams, some of which have come true. It is just that we did not know what that would mean. Now we are finding out.

REFERENCES

Anderson, P. (1991). On the "ragged edge" of medical progress: Daniel Callahan and problems of limits. Unpublished paper.

Barry, R. L., & Bradley, G. V. (Eds.). (1991). *Set no limits: A rebuttal to Daniel Callahan's proposal to limit health care for the elderly.* Urbana: University of Illinois Press.

Binstock, R. H., & Post, S. G. (Eds.). (1991). *Too old for health care: Controversies in medicine, law, economics, and ethics.* Baltimore: The Johns Hopkins University Press.

Breidenbaugh, M. Z., Sarsitis, I. M., & Milam, R. A. (1990). Medicare end stage renal disease population, *Health Care Financing Review, 12,* 101–104.

Callahan, D. (1987). *Setting limits: Medical goals in an aging society.* New York: Simon and Schuster.

Callahan, D. (1990). *What kind of life: The limits of medical progress.* New York: Simon and Schuster.

Callahan, D. (1993). *The troubled dream of life: Living with mortality.* New York: Simon and Schuster.

Chambers, C. V., Diamond, J. J., Perkel, R. L., & Lasch, L. A. (1994). Relationship of advance directives to hospital charges in a Medicare population. *Archives of Internal Medicine, 154,* 541–547.

Estes, C. L. (1988). Cost containment and the elderly: Conflict or challenge? *Journal of the American Medical Association, 36,* 68–72.

Hackler, C. (Ed.). (In press). *Health care for an aging population: Planning for the twenty-first century.* Albany: State University of New York Press.

Holahan, J., & Palmer, J. L. (1988). Medicare's fiscal problems: An imperative for reform. *Journal of Health, Politics, Policy and Law, 13,* 53–81.

Hollander, C. F., & Becker, H. A., (Eds.). (1987). *Growing old in the future.* Dordrecht: Martinius Nijhoff Publishers.

Homer, P., & Holstein, M., (Eds.). (1990). *A good old age: The paradox of setting limits.* New York: Simon and Schuster.

Hosking, M. P., Warner, M. A., Lobdell, C. M., Offord, K. P., & Melton, J. L. (1989). Outcome of surgery in patients 90 years of age and older. *Journal of the American Medical Association, 261,* 1909–1915.

Jecker, N. S., (Ed.). (1991). *Ethics and aging.* Clifton, NJ: Humana Press.

Jecker, N. S. (1991). Age-based rationing and women. *Journal of the American Medical Association, 266,* 3012–3015.

Jecker, N. S., & Pearlman, R. A. (1989). Ethical constraints on rationing medical care by age. *Journal of the American Geriatrics Society, 37,* 1067–1075.

Jouvenel, H. de. (1989). *Europe's ageing population: Trends and challenges to 2025.* Special co-publication of *Futures and Futuribles.* Guildford, UK: Butterworth.

Latta, V. B., & Keene, R. E. (1989). Leading surgical procedures for aged Medicare beneficiaries. *Health Care Financing Review, 11,* 99–100.

Lawlor, E. F. (1992). What kind of medicine? *The Gerontologist, 32,* 131–133.

Levinsky, N. G. (1990). Age as a criterion for rationing health care. *New England Journal of Medicine, 322,* 1813–1815.

Loriaux, (1990). Il Sera une fois... la revolution gruse jeux at enjeux autour d'une profunde mutation societale (Someday it will happen... the revolution of aging and the profound social change at stake). Université Catholique de Louvain. Louvain-la-Neuve, Claco: Institut de Démographie.

Manton, K. G., Corder, L., & Stallard, S. (1993). Changes in the use of personal assistance and special equipment from 1982 to 1989: Results from the 1982 and 1989 NLTCS. *The Gerontologist, 33,* 168–176.

Moody, H. R. (1991). Allocation, yes; Age-based rationing, no. In R. H. Binstock & S. G. Post, (Eds.), *Too Old for Health Care.* Baltimore: The Johns Hopkins University Press, pp. 180–203.

Preston, S. (1984). Children and the elderly: Divergent paths for America's dependents. *Demography, 21,* 455–491.

St. Louis University. (1989). Health care for the elderly. Symposium in the *St. Louis University Law Journal, 33,* 557–710.

Schneider, E. L., Guralnik, J. M. (1990). The aging of America: Impact on health care costs. *Journal of the American Medical Association, 263,* 2335–2340.

Schneiderman, L., Kronick, R., Kaplan, R. M., Anderson, J. P., & Langer, R. D. (1992). Effects of offering advance directives on medical treatment and costs. *Annals of Internal Medicine, 117,* 599–606.

Winslow, G. R., & Walters, J. W. (Eds.). (1993). *Facing limits: Ethics and health care for the elderly.* Boulder, CO: Westview Press.

Zweibel, N. R., Cassel, C. K., & Karvison, T. (1993). Public attitudes about the use of chronological age as a criterion for allocating health care resources. *The Gerontologist, 36,* 74–80.

NO

Ezekiel J. Emanuel and
Linda L. Emanuel

THE ECONOMICS OF DYING: THE ILLUSION OF COST SAVINGS AT THE END OF LIFE

For more than a decade, health policy analysts have noted—and some have decried—the high cost of dying.[1-7] With the acceleration of pressures on health care costs and calls for reform, considerably more attention has been focused on proposals to control costs at the end of life.[8] One proposal would require persons enrolling in a health care plan to complete an advance directive.[9,10] Others would require hospitals to establish guidelines to identify and reduce futile care.[11-13] Similar ideas have been expressed by members of President Bill Clinton's Health Care Task Force and by Joycelyn Elders, the surgeon general.[14]

Advance directives and hospice care were developed to ensure patients' autonomy and to provide high-quality care at the end of life. Compassion and dignity are sufficient justification for their use. Nevertheless, the persistent interest in saving money at the end of life through the use of advance directives and hospice care makes it imperative to assess how much money might realistically be saved.

COST AT THE END OF LIFE AND REASONS FOR COST CONTROL

Expenditures at the end of life seem disproportionately large. Although the precise numbers vary, studies consistently demonstrate that 27 to 30 percent of Medicare payments each year are for the 5 to 6 percent of Medicare beneficiaries who die in that year.[15-17] The latest available figures indicate that in 1988, the mean Medicare payment for the last year of life of a beneficiary who died was $13,316, as compared with $1,924 for all Medicare beneficiaries (a ratio of 6.9:1).[15] Payments for dying patients increase exponentially as death approaches, and payments during the last month of life constitute 40 percent of payments during the last year of life.[15] Identical trends and ratios have been found since the early 1960s.[6,15-17]

From Ezekiel J. Emanuel and Linda L. Emanuel, "The Economics of Dying: The Illusion of Cost Savings at the End of Life," *The New England Journal of Medicine*, vol. 330, no. 8 (February 24, 1994), pp. 540–544. Copyright © 1994 by The Massachusetts Medical Society. Reprinted by permission All rights reserved.

Many people believe that these expenditures are for the care of patients known in advance to be dying. The time of death is usually unpredictable, however, except perhaps when the patient has advanced cancer. There is no method to predict months or weeks in advance who will live and who will die. Consequently, it is difficult to know in advance what costs are for care at the end of life and what costs are for saving a life.[6,7] Only in retrospect, after a patient's death, can we identify the last year or month of life. Nevertheless, to many people, reducing expenditures at the end of life seems an easy and readily justifiable way of cutting wasteful spending and freeing resources to ensure universal access to health care.[9-11,18] General rules intended to curtail the use of unnecessary medical services have been shown to reduce both effective and wasteful services.[19] Consequently, there is some reluctance to limit interventions for relatively healthy people. Many believe, however, that interventions for patients whose death is imminent are inherently wasteful, since they neither cure nor ameliorate disease or disability.

Advance directives and hospice care have been proposed as methods of reducing medical costs at the end of life; both can transform "good ethics [into] good health economics."[9] In survey after survey, Americans indicate that they do not want to be kept alive if their disease is irreversible. If doctors would stop using high-technology interventions at the end of life, the argument goes, then we could simultaneously respect patients' autonomy and save tens of billions of dollars.[8-11,14] When we link ethics and economics to prevent futile care, it is claimed, "everyone wins—the patient, the family, and society as a whole."[11]

Despite the allure of these arguments, we are skeptical. Before making major changes in policy regarding the care of dying patients and formulating budget projections on the basis of cost savings of billions of dollars, we should review the economics of care at the end of life. The cost savings that could be achieved through the wider use of advance directives, hospice care, and curtailment of futile care have not been well studied. The available data suggest, however, that such savings would be less than many have imagined.

ADVANCE DIRECTIVES FOR HEALTH CARE AND COST SAVINGS

One study evaluating the effect of advance directives on costs randomly assigned outpatients to either a physician-initiated discussion of advance directives and encouragement to use them or no intervention.[20] There was no difference in medical costs or other variables between the groups: as the authors stated, "executing the California Durable Power of Attorney for Health Care and having a summary copy placed in the patient's medical record had no significant positive or negative effect on a patient's well-being, health status, medical treatments, or medical treatment charges."[20] Although this study involved small numbers of patients at only two hospitals and measured hospital charges rather than actual costs, similar preliminary results were reported in another study involving 854 patients who died at five medical centers.[21] Executing an advance directive did not significantly affect the cost of patients' terminal hospitalizations. The average hospital bill for those without an advance directive was $56,300, as compared with $61,589 for those with a living will and $58,346 for those with a durable power of attorney.[21] Additional studies are certainly needed, but these reports suggest that the wider use of advance directives is unlikely to produce dramatic cost savings.

HOSPICE CARE AND COST SAVINGS

Hospice patients refuse life-sustaining interventions, favor palliative care, and are often treated at home; they serve as another source of information on the magnitude of the potential savings from the reduced use of high-technology interventions at the end of life. A series of studies comparing hospice care and traditional care of terminally ill patients estimated that in the last month of life, home hospice care saves between 31 and 64 percent of medical care costs.[22-27] The difference is accounted for mostly by the reduced use of hospital services. Consequently, the savings for hospital-based hospice care are lower. However, the longer patients receive hospice care, the smaller the savings. As the National Hospice Study reported, for hospice patients "the longer the stay in hospice, the more likely [it was that] costs incurred exceeded those of conventional care patients in the last year of life; the economies associated with hospice occur primarily in the last weeks of life."[28] During the last six months of life, the mean medical costs for patients receiving hospice care at home are 27 percent less than for conventional care, and the savings with hospital-based hospice care are less than 15 percent.[22,24,26]

These studies may systematically overstate the savings associated with hospice care. Most have not been randomized and may have incorporated a selection bias,

since hospice patients by definition want less aggressive care. The one randomized study of hospice care found no cost savings for long-term hospice patients.[23] Patients receiving care in a hospice also tend to be from higher socioeconomic groups and to have informal support structures that enable them to obtain additional services, such as personal attendants not covered by Medicare, that are invisible in most cost estimates.[29] As rates of hospitalization decline, so, too, may the savings from hospice care.[22] Finally, an overwhelming majority of hospice patients have cancer, a fact that limits the generalizability of these data.[28]

FUTILE CARE AND COST SAVINGS

A related proposal to save money at the end of life is to reduce "futile care."[10,11] What constitutes futile care is controversial,[30-33] but the paradigmatic case is cardiopulmonary resuscitation for patients dying of cancer.[30-34] Unfortunately, there have been no studies of the financial consequences of eliminating resuscitation for patients with cancer. In a study of the cost of care for all patients with do-not-resuscitate (DNR) orders at a tertiary care hospital, almost 25 percent of whom had cancer, it was found that among patients who died, medical care for those with DNR orders cost about the same as for those without DNR orders: a mean of $62,594 for 616 patients with DNR orders as compared with $57,334 for 219 patients without DNR orders.[35]

Advocates of cost cutting have suggested extending the concept of futility to curtail marginally beneficial care.[10,11] Chemotherapy for unresectable [not removable] non-small-cell lung cancer is an example of marginal if not entirely futile therapy; it does not systematically enhance longevity, improve the quality of life, or palliate pain.[36,37] A randomized trial in Canada, comparing chemotherapy with high-quality supportive care for patients with non-small-cell lung cancer, found that the average cost of the supportive care was $8,595 (in 1984 Canadian dollars), whereas one chemotherapy regimen cost less ($7,645) and another regimen cost more ($12,232).[38] Some aspects of this study are controversial, and some costs were approximated because they were "not routinely identified in the Canadian health care system."[38,39] Nevertheless, the authors concluded that even if chemotherapy is expensive, "a policy of supportive care for patients with advanced non-small-cell lung cancer was associated with substantial costs."[38]

CAN WE SAVE ANY MONEY ON CARE AT THE END OF LIFE?

Can we realize any savings by the more frequent use of advance directives, hospice care, and less aggressive care at the end of life? We can estimate the proportion of health costs that might be saved in a best-case scenario—that is, if every American who died had executed an advance directive, refused aggressive care at the end of life, and elected to receive hospice care at home. The only reliable cost data for the last year of life are Medicare costs for patients 65 years of age or older; there are no reliable data on the total costs of health care for patients either over or under 65 who die. Consequently, many approximations are necessary in calculating the savings that can be realized.

In 1988, the mean annual cost per Medicare beneficiary who died during that year was $13,316.[15] Medicare primarily pays for acute care, however, and ac-

counts for only 45 percent of total health care costs for those 65 years old or older; the bulk of the excluded costs are for nursing home care.[49] The simplest way to estimate the additional health care costs for Medicare beneficiaries who die is to assume they use the same fraction of these other services that they do of services covered by Medicare. This means that patients 65 or older who die in a given year account for 27 percent of total health care expenditures—Medicare costs, nursing home costs, and the costs of other services for all patients 65 or older. Thus, we estimate that patients 65 years old or older who died in 1988 spent $29,295 for all their health care services, of which $13,316 was covered by Medicare.

How should we estimate costs during the last year of life for patients less than 65 years of age? Although costs for younger patients who die of cancer and the acquired immunodeficiency syndrome (AIDS) are probably substantially higher than costs for dying Medicare patients,[41] the costs for those who die of accidents, suicide, and homicide are probably less. Scitovsky showed that among a group of California patients who died, the mean total medical costs for the last year of life were about the same for those under 65 years of age as for those 65 to 79 years of age.[42] In 1988, the mean Medicare cost for 65-to-79-year-old patients who died was $15,346 (Lubitz J: personal communication). Assuming that this is 45 percent of total health care expenditures, we can estimate that the mean annual medical cost for patients under 65 who died in 1988 was $34,102.

We know that 2.17 million Americans died in 1988, of whom 1.49 million were Medicare beneficiaries. Using the hospice data, and assuming that the maximum we might save in health care costs during the last year of life by reducing interventions is 27 percent,[22,24,26] we can calculate how much could be saved if each of the 2.17 million Americans who died executed an advance directive, chose hospice care, and refused aggressive, in-hospital interventions at the end of life.... The total savings in health care expenditures would have been $18.1 billion in 1988, or 3.3 percent of all health care spending. In 1988, the savings in Medicare costs would have been $5.4 billion, or 6.1 percent of expenditures.[43] Since the percentage of health dollars spent on patients who died has been constant over 30 years, the savings as a percentage of total national health care costs and Medicare spending is unlikely to change over time.[6,15,44]

This calculation relies on best-case assumptions that err on the side of overestimating savings. We have extrapolated the savings for patients who receive hospice care to the use of advance directives and to the reduced use of futile interventions. Yet not everyone would refuse life-sustaining interventions in their advance directives, and futile interventions are hard to define, let alone stop. Moreover, achieving savings of any considerable magnitude depends on decreasing the numbers of days spent in the hospital, yet over the past decade there has already been a significant decline in both the number of hospital days for all patients and the proportion of costs for patients who die that are allocated to hospital care.[15] Furthermore, curtailing care at the end of life is likely to affect acute care and thus Medicare costs, but unlikely to decrease nursing home and other outpatient costs; indeed, it may even increase such costs. (Excluding nursing home costs would reduce the total savings from $18.1 billion to $15.9 billion, or 2.9 percent of total health care spending.)

Reducing health care expenditures by 3.3 percent cannot be dismissed lightly. Yet even with the most generous assumptions possible, the savings will be less than the scores of billions of dollars predicted by many commentators and the savings estimated from cutting administrative waste.[8–11,14,45]

WHY IS THERE NOT MUCH MONEY TO BE SAVED AT THE END OF LIFE?

Why, despite the high cost of dying documented for Medicare beneficiaries, is there not likely to be much in the way of cost savings from the use of advance directives, hospice care, and fewer high-technology interventions? One explanation is that the Medicare data produce a distorted image of the cost of dying. Commentators extrapolate the data for Medicare patients who die to the entire population.[8,10,11,14] Using 1990 expenditures, for example, Singer and Lowy calculate that "the care of patients who died" cost $184 billion (27 percent of the $661 billion spent on health care in 1990).[8] They suggest that $55 billion to $109 billion might be saved "from a policy of asking all patients about their wishes regarding life-sustaining treatment and incorporating those wishes into advance directives."

Although Medicare data on mortality and expenditures may be the only reliable figures available, they cannot be extrapolated without adjustment to the whole health care system. Less than 1 percent of the total American population dies each year, yet 5 to 6 percent of Medicare beneficiaries die. Five percent of Medicare patients may account for 27 percent of Medicare payments, but it is improbable that the less than 1 percent of the American population who die account for 27 percent of the total national spending on health care. We estimate that the 2.17 million Americans who die annually account for about 10 to 12 percent of health care expenditures.

It may be difficult to reduce substantially the percentage of health care expenditures spent on patients who die because humane care at the end of life is labor-intensive and therefore expensive. Even when patients refuse life-sustaining interventions, they do not necessarily require less medical care, just a different kind of care. High-quality palliative care —providing pain medications, helping in the activities of daily living, using radiation therapy for pain relief, and so on —requires skilled, and costly, personnel. Thus, even low-technology health care that is administered outside hospitals to terminally ill patients is not cheap.

Another explanation is related to the unpredictability of death. Since there are no reliable ways to identify the patients who will die,[6,44,46] it is not possible to say accurately months, weeks, or even days before death which patients will benefit from intensive interventions and which ones will receive "wasted" care. Retrospective cost studies will inflate costs at the end of life as compared with costs for patients known in advance to be dying because they include many patients receiving expensive care who are not expected to die yet do die. This clinical uncertainty also means that resources are initially expended until a patient's prognosis becomes clearer and physicians, patients, and the family are sure about either forging ahead with aggressive treatment or withdrawing it. This process is both ethically correct and what most Americans seem to desire.[47] Advance directives are unlikely to reduce this type of care, since physicians, patients, and family members are hesitant to discontinue therapy when there is a real chance of survival.

In addition, medical practice has changed over the past decade. For the vast majority of patients who die, DNR orders are already in place and other interventions are terminated. For instance, at Memorial Sloan-Kettering Cancer Center, 85 percent of patients with cancer who have cardiac arrest have DNR orders[48]; other institutions have reported rates of DNR orders among patients with cancer that are as high as 97 percent.[35] Currently, in tertiary care hospitals, between 60 and 80 percent of dying patients have DNR orders.[49-51] Admittedly, the decision to give a DNR order or withdraw life-sustaining treatment is usually made late in the course of a patient's illness. Nevertheless, given the steep rise in costs as death approaches, reducing care in these final days of life should yield the most savings.[15,35] As the data on hospice care demonstrate, there may be additional— but smaller—cost savings if the decision to stop treatment is pushed back several weeks.[22,24,26,28]

Finally, the increased use of living wills and health care proxy forms may not necessarily curtail the use of life-sustaining treatment. We have no empirical evidence that patients are getting substantially more treatment than they or their families want. Although there have been a few well-publicized cases in which physicians have treated patients against their wishes, these are probably unrepresentative.[52] Studies consistently show that physicians are more willing than patients and family members to withhold or withdraw life-sustaining treatments.[53,54] A large minority of people consistently want treatment even after they become incompetent or have a low chance of survival. For instance, about 20 percent of patients want life-sustaining therapy even if they are in a persistent vegetative state.[47] Similarly, about half of patients with AIDS want aggressive life-sustaining treatment, including admission to an intensive care unit and cardiopulmonary resuscitation, in circumstances in which they have a relatively poor chance of survival.[55,56] Thus, patients who complete advance directives may request more life-sustaining treatment than they currently receive, precluding any cost savings. In addition, studies demonstrate that family members are consistently more hesitant to withhold or withdraw life-sustaining treatment than the patients themselves.[53,54,57,58] Thus, if patients are encouraged to select proxy decision makers by executing durable powers of attorney, the cost savings may be minimal.

CONCLUSIONS

None of the individual studies of cost savings at the end of life associated with advance directives, hospice care, or the elimination of futile care are definitive. Yet they all point in the same direction: cost savings due to changes in practice at the end of life are not likely to be substantial. The amount that might be saved by reducing the use of aggressive life-sustaining interventions for dying patients is at most 3.3 percent of total national health care expenditures. In 1993, with $900 billion going to health care, this savings would amount to $29.7 billion. It is important to note that achieving such savings would not restrain the rate of growth in health

care spending over time.[59] Instead, this amount represents a fraction of the increase due to inflation in health care costs and less than the $50 billion to $90 billion needed to cover the uninsured population.

The unlikeliness of substantial savings in health care costs does not mean, however, that there are no good reasons to use advance directives, fund hospice care, and employ less aggressive life-sustaining treatments for dying patients. Respecting patients' wishes, reducing pain and suffering, and providing compassionate and dignified care at the end of life have overwhelming merit. But the hope of cutting the amount of money spent on life-sustaining interventions for the dying in order to reduce overall health care costs is probably vain. Our alternatives for achieving substantial savings seem limited to major changes in the financing and delivery of health care, difficult choices in the allocation of services, or both. Whatever we choose, we must stop deluding ourselves that advance directives and less aggressive care at the end of life will solve the financial problems of our health care system.

We are indebted to James Lubitz, M.P.H., Dan Brock, Ph.D., Joseph P. Newhouse, Ph.D., Rashi Fein, Ph.D., David Kidder, Ph.D., and Jane Weeks, M.D., for their comments on earlier drafts of the manuscript, and to the members of President Clinton's Health Care Task Force who discussed these issues with us.

REFERENCES

1. Leaf A. Medicine and the aged. N Engl J Med 1977;297:887–9O.

2. Turnbull AD, Carlon G, Baron R, Sichel W, Young C, Howland W. The inverse relationship

between cost and survival in the critically ill cancer patient. Crit Care Med 1979;7:20–3.

3. Ginzberg E. The high costs of dying. Inquiry 1980;17:293–5.

4. Shroeder SA, Showstack JA, Schwartz J. Survival of adult high-cost patients: report of a follow-up study from nine acute-care hospitals. JAMA 1981;245:1446–9.

5. Bayer R, Callahan D, Fletcher J, et al. The care of the terminally ill: mortality and economics. N Engl J Med 1983;309:1490–4.

6. Scitovsky AA. "The high cost of dying": what do the data show? Milbank Mem Fund Q Health Soc 1984;62:591–608.

7. Scitovsky AA, Capron AM. Medical care at the end of life: the interaction of economics and ethics. Annu Rev Public Health 1986;7:59–75.

8. Singer PA, Lowy FH. Rationing, patient preferences and cost of care at the end of life. Arch Intern Med 1992;152:478–80.

9. d'Oronzio JC. Good ethics, good health economics. New York Times. June 8, 1993:A25.

10. Fries JF, Koop CE, Beadle CE, et al. Reducing health care costs by reducing the need and demand for medical services. N Engl J Med 1993;329:321–5.

11. Lundberg GD. American health care system management objectives: the aura of inevitability becomes incarnate. JAMA 1993;269:2354–5.

12. Schneiderman LJ, Jecker N. Futility in practice. Arch intern Med 1993;153:437–41.

13. Murphy DJ, Finucane TE. New do-not-resuscitate policies: a first step in cost control. Arch Intern Med 1993;153:1641–8.

14. Godec MS. Your final 30 days—free. Washington Post. May 2, 1993:C3.

15. Lubitz JD, Riley GF. Trends in Medicare payments in the last year of life. N Engl J Med 1993;328:1092–6.

16. Lubitz J, Prihoda R. The use and costs of Medicare services in the last 2 years of life. Health Care Financ Rev 1984;5(3):117–31.

17. McCall N. Utilization and costs of Medicare services by beneficiaries in their last year of life. Med Care 1984;22:329–42.

18. Siu AL, Brook RH. Allocating health care resources: how can we ensure access to essential care? In: Ginzberg E, ed. Medicine and society: clinical decisions and societal values. Boulder, Colo.: Westview Press, 1987;20–33.

19. Siu AL, Sonnenberg FA, Manning WG, et al. Inappropriate use of hospitals in a randomized trial of health insurance plans. N Engl J Med 1986;315:1259–66.

20. Schneiderman LJ, Kronick R, Kaplan RM, Anderson JP, Langer RD. Effects of offering advance directives on medical treatments and costs. Ann Intern Med 1992;117:599–606.

21. Teno J, Lynn J, Phillips R, et al. Do advance directives save resources? Clin Res 1993;41:551A. abstract.

22. Kidder D. The effects of hospice coverage on Medicare expenditures. Health Serv Res 1992;27:195–217.

23. Kane RL, Wales J. Bernstein L, Leibowitz A, Kaplan S. A randomised controlled trial of hospice care. Lancet 1984;1:890–4.

24. Spector WD, Mor V. Utilization and charges for terminal cancer patients in Rhode Island. Inquiry 1984;21:328–37.

25. Hannan EL, O'Donnell JF. An evaluation of hospices in the New York State Hospice Demonstration Program. Inquiry 1984;21:338–48.

26. Mor V, Kidder D. Cost savings in hospice: final results of the National Hospice Study. Health Serv Res 1985;20:407–22.

27. Brooks CH, Smyth-Staruch K. Hospice home care cost savings to third-party insurers. Med Care 1984;22:691–703.

28. Greer DS, Mor V. An overview of National Hospice Study findings. J Chronic Dis 1986;39:5–7.

29. Moinpour CM, Polissar L. Factors affecting place of death of hospice and non-hospice cancer patients. Am J Public Health 1989;79:1549–51.

30. Schneiderman LJ, Jecker NS, Jonsen AR. Medical futility: its meaning and ethical implications. Ann Intern Med 1990;112:949–54.

31. Tomlinson T, Brody H. Futility and the ethics of resuscitation. JAMA 1990;264:1276–80.

32. Lantos JD, Singer PA, Walker RM, et al. The illusion of futility in clinical practice. Am J Med 1989;87:81–4.

33. Loewy EH, Carlson RA. Futility and its wider implications: a concept in need of further examination. Arch Intern Med 1993;153:429–31.

34. Blackhall LJ. Must we always use CPR? N Engl J Med 1987;317:1281–5.

35. Maksoud A, Jahnigen DW, Skibinski CI. Do not resuscitate orders and the cost of death. Arch Intern Med 1993;153:1249–53.

36. Ihde DC. Chemotherapy of lung cancer. N Engl J Med 1992;327:1434–41.

37. Ruckdeschel JC. Is chemotherapy for metastatic non-small cell lung cancer "worth it"? J Clin Oncol 1990;8:1293–6.

38. Jaakkimainen L, Goodwin PJ, Pater J, Warde P, Murray N, Rapp E. Counting the costs of chemotherapy in a National Cancer Institute of Canada randomized trial in nonsmall-cell lung cancer. J Clin Oncol 1990;8:1301–9.

39. Rapp E, Pater JL, Willan A, et al. chemotherapy can prolong survival in patients with advanced non-small-cell lung cancer—report of a Canadian multicenter randomized trial. J Clin Oncol 1988;6:633–41.

40. Waldo DR, Sonnefeld ST, McKusick DR, Arnett RH III. Health expenditures by age group, 1977 and 1987. Health Care Financ Rev 1989;10(4):111–20.

41. Riley G, Lubitz J, Prihoda R, Rabey E. The use and costs of Medicare services by cause of death. Inquiry 1987;24:233–44.

42. Scitovsky AA. Medical care in the last twelve months of life: the relation between age, functional status, and medical care expenditures. Milbank Q 1988;66:640–6O.

43. Levit KR, Lazenby HC, Cowan CA, Letsch SW. National health expenditures, 1990. Health Care Financ Rev 1991;13(1):29–54.

44. Newhouse JP. An iconoclastic view of health cost containment. Health Aff (Millwood) 1993;12: Suppl:152–71.

45. Woolhandler S, Himmelstein DU. The deteriorating administrative efficiency of the U.S. health care system. N Engl J Med 1991;324:1253–8.

46. Schapira DV, Studnicki J, Bradham DD, Wolff P, Jarrett A. Intensive care, survival, and expense of treating critically ill cancer patients. JAMA, 1993;269:783–6.

47. Emanuel LL, Barry MJ, Stoeckle JD, Ettelson LM, Emanuel EJ. Advance directives for medical care—a case for greater use. N Engl J Med 1991;324:889–95.

48. Vitelli CE, Cooper K, Rogatko A, Brennan MF. Cardiopulmonary resuscitation and the patient with cancer. J Clin Oncol 1991;9:111–5.

49. Gleeson K, Wise S. The do-not-resuscitate order: still too little too late. Arch Intern Med 1990;150:1057–60.

50. Smedira NG, Evans BH, Grais LS, et al. Withholding and withdrawal of life support from the critically ill. N Engl J Med 1990;322: 309–15.

51. Bedell SE, Pelle D, Maher PL, Cleary PD. Do-not-resuscitate orders for critically ill patients in the hospital: how are they used and what is their impact? JAMA 1986;256:233–7.

52. Emanuel EI. Who won't pull the plug? Washington Post. January 2, 1994:C3.

53. Seckler AB, Meier DE, Mulvihill M, Cammer Paris BE. Substituted judgment: how accurate are proxy predictions? Ann Intern Med 1991;115: 92–8.

54. Uhlmann RF, Pearlman RA, Cain KC. Physicians' and spouses' predictions of elderly patients resuscitation preferences. J Gerontol 1988;43(5):M115–M121.

55. Steinbrook R, Lo B, Moulton J, Saika G, Hollander H, Volberding PA. Preferences of homosexual men with AIDS for life-sustaining treatment. N Engl J Med 1986;314:457–60.

56. Haas JS, Weissman JS, Cleary PD, et al. Discussion of preferences for life-sustaining care by persons with AIDS: predictors of failure in patient-physician communication. Arch Intern Med 1993;153:1241–8.

57. Emanuel EJ, Emanuel LL. Proxy decision making for incompetent patients: an ethical and empirical analysis. JAMA 1992;267:2067–71.

58. Steiber SR. Right to die: public balks at deciding for others. Hospitals 1987;61:72.

59. Schwartz WB. The inevitable failure of current cost-containment strategies: why they can provide only temporary relief. JAMA 1987;257: 220–4.

POSTSCRIPT

Should Health Care for the Elderly Be Limited?

In October 1986 Dr. Thomas Starzl of Pittsburgh, Pennsylvania, transplanted a liver into a 76-year-old woman at a cost of over $200,000. Soon after that, Congress ordered organ transplantation to be covered under Medicare, which ensured that more older persons would receive this benefit. At the same time these events were taking place, a government campaign to contain medical costs was under way, with health care for the elderly targeted.

Not everyone agrees with this means of cost cutting. In "Public Attitudes About the Use of Chronological Age as a Criterion for Allocating Health Care Resources," *The Gerontologist* (February 1993), the authors report that the majority of older people surveyed accept the withholding of life-prolonging medical care from the hopelessly ill but that few would deny treatment on the basis of age alone. Two publications that express opposition to age-based health care rationing are Robert L. Barry and Gerard V. Bradley, eds., *Set No Limits: A Rebuttal to Daniel Callahan's Proposal to Limit Health Care for the Elderly* (University of Illinois Press, 1991) and Gerald R. Winslow and James W. Walters, eds., *Facing Limits: Ethics and Health Care for the Elderly* (Westview Press, 1992).

Currently, about 40 million Americans have no medical insurance and are at risk of being denied basic health care services. About 20 percent of all children have not had proper immunizations, and one-third of all pregnant women do not receive prenatal care during their first trimester. The federal government pays most of the health care costs of the elderly. While it may not meet the needs of all older people, the amount of medical aid that goes to the elderly is greater than any other demographic group, and the elderly have the highest disposable income. Daniel Callahan, in "Limiting Health Care for the Old?" *The Nation* (August 15/22, 1987), maintains that we must confront the realities of economics and limit health care. Callahan also writes on the allocation of health resources in "Allocating Health Resources," *Hastings Center Report* (April/May 1988) and "Debate: Response to Roger W. Hunt," *Journal of Medical Ethics* (vol. 19, 1993).

Most Americans have access to the best and most expensive medical care in the world. As these costs rise, some difficult decisions may have to be made regarding the allocation of these resources, whether by age, probability of beneficence, income, or other criteria. As the population ages and more health care dollars are spent on care during the last years of life, medical services for the elderly or the dying may become a natural target for reduction in order to balance the health care budget. Additional readings on this subject include

"Rationing, Patient Preferences and Cost of Care at the End of Life," *Archives of Internal Medicine* (vol. 152, 1992); "A Critique of Using Age to Ration Health Care," *Journal of Medical Ethics* (vol. 19, 1993); "Trends in Medicare Payments in the Last Year of Life," *The New England Journal of Medicine* (vol. 328, 1993); "Who Won't Pull the Plug?" *Washington Post* (January 2, 1994); and "What Do We Owe the Elderly: Allocating Social and Health Care Resources," *Hastings Center Report* (March/April 1994). Articles dealing with age bias include "Researchers Find Age Bias in Treatment of Severely Ill Patients," *AHA News* (September 23, 1996); "Controlling the Costs of Health Care for the Elderly: Fair Means and Foul," *The New England Journal of Medicine* (September 5, 1996); and "Recognizing Bedside Rationing: Clear Cases and Tough Calls," *Annals of Internal Medicine* (January 1, 1997).

ISSUE 4

Is Gun Control a Public Health Issue?

YES: Josh Sugarmann, from "Reverse Fire," *Mother Jones* (January/February 1994)

NO: Don B. Kates, Henry E. Schaffer, and William C. Waters IV, from "Public Health Pot Shots: How the CDC Succumbed to the Gun 'Epidemic,'" *Reason* (April 1997)

ISSUE SUMMARY

YES: Josh Sugarmann, executive director of the Violence Policy Center, an education foundation that researches firearm violence and advocates gun control, argues that guns increase the costs of hospitalization, rehabilitation, and lost wages, making them a serious public health issue.

NO: Attorney Don B. Kates, Professor Henry E. Schaffer and William C. Waters IV, a physician, counter that most gun-related violence is caused by aberrants, not ordinary gun owners.

More and more people in the United States are buying guns to protect themselves and their families in response to increasing crime rates. There are currently over 216 million firearms—close to 900,000 assault weapons—in private hands in the United States, more than double the number in 1970. Also, each year more than 24,000 Americans are killed with handguns in homicides, suicides, and accidents (an average of 65 people each day). Firearms are used in 70 percent of all murders committed in this country. These statistics raise important questions: Does gun ownership afford protection against crime or increase the risk of gun-related death? And are gun control and gun ownership public health concerns? Gun owners and opponents of gun control claim that weapons kept at home will prevent crime. Proponents of gun control claim that weapons kept at home are involved in too many fights causing injury or death, accidental shootings, and suicides.

To attempt to resolve these issues, Dr. Arthur Kellermann, an emergency room physician at the University of Tennessee, and his associates conducted a study, "Gun Ownership as a Risk Factor for Homicide in the Home," *The New England Journal of Medicine* (October 7, 1993). Dr. Kellermann's study concluded that people who keep guns in their homes are much more likely to kill or injure another family member than use the gun in self-defense against a criminal. Dr. Kellermann believes that a gun almost automatically makes any fight potentially more dangerous and the risks of having a gun outweigh the benefits. Many supporters of gun control claim that the study confirmed their warnings about the basic dangers of owning guns and keeping them in the home.

The contention that gun ownership is more dangerous than beneficial is not without its critics. The Kellermann study, for instance, only measured *risks* associated with gun ownership. He did not study cases in which guns actually deterred crime. Kellerman et al. also did not discuss the possibility that the guns may not have caused the violence; the violence may have caused the use of guns. For instance, in areas of high crime, citizens are more likely to arm themselves for self-protection.

Although it is unclear whether guns deter crime or cause it, gun control in one form or another has been around since the early part of this century. The first major gun control act strengthening restrictions on handguns followed the assassinations of John F. Kennedy, Dr. Martin Luther King Jr., and Robert Kennedy in the 1960s. Other laws banning the sale of handguns and the manufacture and sale of certain types of assault weapons followed. In 1993 President Clinton signed the Brady Bill, which imposed a five-day waiting period for handgun purchases. (The bill was named for James Brady, aide to former president Ronald Reagan. Both Brady and President Reagan were shot during an assassination attempt in the early 1980s). Unfortunately for gun control advocates, in June 1997 the Supreme Court ruled that the Brady gun control law violated "the very principle of separate state sovereignty" by requiring state officials to conduct background checks of prospective handgun buyers. In a 5-to-4 decision, the Court invalidated the background check of the 1993 law. This decision did not address, however, a separate portion of the Brady Bill that imposes a five-day waiting period before a gun sale can be completed.

Gun control is a controversial issue in the United States. Its opponents claim that it infringes on the constitutional rights of Americans to bear arms as granted by the Second Amendment. The gun lobby also pictures America under stricter gun controls as a country where honest citizens would be helpless against well-armed criminals. Many advocates of gun control, however, regard the deaths and injuries related to guns as a public health problem that can be treated only by getting rid of guns themselves.

In the following selections, Josh Sugarmann asserts that guns are definitely a public health issue and supports stricter gun control. He feels that guns offer no protective benefit even in homicide cases that followed forced entry. Don B. Kates, Henry E. Schaffer, and William C. Waters IV argue that violence is not a matter of honest citizens killing simply because a gun is nearby, but of criminals committing violent acts. The authors also claim that health organizations such as the Centers for Disease Control should focus on true public health issues and not veer off into social policy.

YES

Josh Sugarmann

REVERSE FIRE

For seven years gun-control advocates have lobbied for the Brady Bill, which mandates a national waiting period for buying handguns. But ironically, the bill's passage may actually benefit the gun industry. Oversold by its supporters, the Brady Bill has become synonymous in American minds with gun control itself. If violence continues once a national waiting period goes into effect (as it likely will), the gun lobby will offer the Brady Bill as proof that gun control doesn't work.

A LACK OF REGULATION

With its passage in 1993, gun-control advocates find themselves at a crossroads. We can continue to push legislation of dubious effectiveness. Or we can acknowledge that gun violence is a public-health crisis fueled by an inherently dangerous consumer product. To end the crisis, we have to regulate —or, in the case of handguns and assault weapons, completely ban—the product.

The romantic myths attached to gun ownership stop many people from thinking of them as a consumer product. As a result, the standard risk analysis applied to other potentially dangerous products—pesticides, prescription drugs, or toasters—has never been applied to firearms.

Yet guns are manufactured by corporations—with boards of directors, marketing plans, employees, and a bottom line—just like companies that manufacture toasters. What separates the gun industry from other manufacturers is lack of regulation.

For example, when a glut in the market caused handgun production to plummet from 2.6 million in 1982 to 1.4 million in 1986, the industry retooled its product line. To stimulate sales, manufacturers added firepower, technology, and capacity to their new models. The result: assault weapons, a switch from six-shot revolvers to high-capacity pistols, and increased use of plastics and high-tech additions like integral laser sights.

The industry was free to make these changes (most of which made the guns more dangerous) because guns that are 50 caliber or less and not fully automatic can be manufactured with virtually no restrictions. The Bureau of Alcohol, Tobacco, and Firearms (ATF) lacks even the common regulatory powers—including safety-standard setting and recall—granted government agencies such as the Consumer Product Safety Commission, the Food and Drug Administration, and the Environmental Protection Agency.

A DEADLY PRODUCT

Yet guns are the second most deadly consumer product (after cars) on the market. In Texas and Louisiana the firearms-related death rate already exceeds that for motor vehicles, and by the year 2000 firearms will likely supplant automobiles as the leading cause of product-related death throughout the United States.

But since Americans view firearm suicides, murders, and fatal accidents as separate problems, the enormity of America's gun crisis goes unrecognized. In 1990, American guns claimed an estimated 37,000 lives. Federal Bureau of Investigation data shows that gun murders that year reached an all-time high of 15,377; a record 12,489 involved handguns.

THE HUMAN TOLL

In 1990 (the most recent year for which statistics are available), 18,885 Americans took their own lives with firearms, and an estimated 13,030 of those deaths involved handguns. Unlike pills, gas, or razor blades—which are of limited effectiveness—guns are rarely forgiving. For example, self-inflicted cutting wounds account for 15 percent of all suicide attempts but only 1 percent of all successful suicides. Poisons and drugs account for 70 percent of suicide attempts but less than 12 percent of all suicides. Conversely, nonfatal, self-inflicted gunshot wounds are rare—yet three-fifths of all U.S. suicides involve firearms.

In addition to the human toll, the economic costs of not regulating guns are staggering. The Centers for Disease Control (CDC) estimated that the lifetime economic cost—hospitalization, rehabilitation, and lost wages—of firearms violence was $14.4 billion in 1985, making it the third most expensive injury category The average lifetime cost per person for each firearms fatality—$373,520 —was the highest of any injury.

Such human and economic costs are not tolerated for any other product. Many consumer products from lawn darts to the Dalkon Shield have been banned in the United States, even though they claimed only a fraction of the lives guns do in a day. The firearms industry is long overdue for the simple, regulatory oversight applied to other consumer products. For public safety, the ATF must be given authority to control the design, manufacture, distribution, and sale of firearms and ammunition.

Under such a plan, the ATF would subject each category of firearm and ammunition to an unreasonable-risk analysis to weed out products whose potential for harm outweighs any possible benefit. This would result in an immediate ban on the future production and sale of handguns and assault weapons because of their high risk and low utility.

Because they are easily concealed and accessed, handguns hold the dubious honor of being our number-one murder and suicide tool. Assault weapons—high-capacity, semiautomatic firearms designed primarily for the military and police—pose a public-safety risk as the result of their firepower. A 1989 study of ATF data conducted by Cox Newspapers found that assault firearms were twenty times more likely to turn up in crime traces than conventional firearms.

In addition, a regulatory approach to firearms would exert far greater control over the industry and its distribution network. It would not, however, affect the availability of standard sporting rifles and shotguns, which would continue to be sold because of their usefulness and relatively low risk.

A PUBLIC-HEALTH ISSUE

Such an approach is the industry's worst nightmare—conjuring images of an all-powerful "gun czar." And in a sense, gun manufacturers would be right: the ATF would become a gun czar in the same way that the EPA is a pesticide czar, the FDA is a prescription-drug-and-medical-device czar, and the Consumer Product Safety Commission is a toaster czar. Yet it is just such a regulatory approach that has dramatically reduced motor-vehicle deaths and injuries over the past twenty years.

Gun-control advocates cannot afford to spend another seven years battling over piecemeal measures that have little more to offer than good intentions. We are far past the point where registration, licensing, safety training, background checks, or waiting periods will have much effect on firearms violence. Tired of being shot and threatened, Americans are showing a deeper understanding of gun violence as a public-health issue, and are becoming aware of tide need to restrict specific categories of weapons.

As America's health-care debate continues, discussion of the role of guns—from the human price paid in mortality to the dollars-and-cents cost of uninsured gunshot victims—can only help clarify that gun violence is not a crime issue but a public-health issue. This shift in attitude is apparent in the firearms component of Bill Clinton's domestic violence prevention group, which is co-chaired not only by a representative from the Justice Department—as expected—but also by a CDC official.

Even if the only legacy of this current wave of revulsion is that gun violence will now be viewed as a public-health issue, America will still have taken a very large first step toward gun sanity.

NO

Don B. Kates, Henry E. Schaffer, and William C. Waters IV

PUBLIC HEALTH POT SHOTS: HOW THE CDC SUCCUMBED TO THE GUN "EPIDEMIC"

Last year Congress tried to take away $2.6 million from the U.S. Centers for Disease Control and Prevention. In budgetary terms, it was a pittance: 0.1 percent of the CDC's $2.2 billion allocation. Symbolically, however, it was important: $2.6 million was the amount the CDC's National Center for Injury Prevention and Control had spent in 1995 on studies of firearm injuries. Congressional critics, who charged that the center's research program was driven by an anti-gun prejudice, had previously sought to eliminate the NCIPC completely. "This research is designed to, and is used to, promote a campaign to reduce lawful firearms ownership in America," wrote 10 senators, including then–Majority Leader Bob Dole and current Majority Leader Trent Lott. "Funding redundant research initiatives, particularly those which are driven by a social-policy agenda, simply does not make sense."

After the NCIPC survived the 1995 budget process, opponents narrowed their focus, seeking to pull the plug on the gun research specifically, or at least to punish the CDC for continuing to fund it. At a May 1996 hearing, Rep. Jay Dickey (R-Ark.), co-sponsor of the amendment cutting the CDC's budget, chastised NCIPC Director Mark Rosenberg for treating guns as a "public health menace," suggesting that he was "working toward changing society's attitudes so that it becomes socially unacceptable to own handguns." In June the House Appropriations Committee adopted Dickey's amendment, which included a prohibition on the use of CDC funds "to advocate or promote gun control," and in July the full House rejected an attempt to restore the money.

Although the CDC ultimately got the $2.6 million back as part of a budget deal with the White House, the persistent assault on the agency's gun research created quite a stir. *New England Journal of Medicine* Editor Jerome Kassirer, who has published several of the CDC-funded gun studies, called it "an attack that strikes at the very heart of scientific research." Writing in *The Washington Post*, CDC Director David Satcher said criticism of the firearm research did not bode well for the country's future: "If we question the honesty of scientists who give every evidence of long deliberation on the issues before them, what are our expectations of anyone else? What hope is there for us as a society?" Frederick P. Rivara, a pediatrician who has received CDC money to do gun research, told *The Chronicle of Higher Education* that critics of the program were trying "to block scientific discovery because they don't like the results. This is a frightening trend for academic researchers. It's the equivalent of book burning."

That view was echoed by columnists and editorial writers throughout the country. In a *New York Times* column entitled "More N.R.A. Mischief," Bob Herbert defended the CDC's "rigorous, unbiased, scientific studies," suggesting that critics could not refute the results of the research and therefore had decided "to pull the plug on the funding and stop the effort altogether." Editorials offering the same interpretation appeared in *The Washington Post* ("NRA: Afraid of Facts"), *USA Today* ("Gun Lobby Keeps Rolling"), the *Los Angeles Times* ("NRA Aims at the Messenger"), *The Atlanta Journal* ("GOP Tries to Shoot the Messenger"), the *Sacramento Bee* ("Shooting the Messenger"), and the *Pittsburgh Post-Gazette* ("The Gun Epidemic").

Contrary to this picture of dispassionate scientists under assault by the Neanderthal NRA and its know-nothing allies in Congress, serious scholars have been criticizing the CDC's "public health" approach to gun research for years. In a presentation at the American Society of Criminology's 1994 meeting, for example, University of Illinois sociologist David Bordua and epidemiologist David Cowan called the public health literature on guns "advocacy based on po-

litical beliefs rather than scientific fact." Bordua and Cowan noted that *The New England Journal of Medicine* and the *Journal of the American Medical Association*, the main outlets for CDC-funded studies of firearms, are consistent supporters of strict gun control. They found that "reports with findings not supporting the position of the journal are rarely cited," "little is cited from the criminological or sociological field," and the articles that are cited "are almost always by medical or public health researchers."

Further, Bordua and Cowan said, "assumptions are presented as fact: that there is a causal association between gun ownership and the risk of violence, that this association is consistent across all demographic categories, and that additional legislation will reduce the prevalence of firearms and consequently reduce the incidence of violence." They concluded that "[i]ncestuous and selective literature citations may be acceptable for political tracts, but they introduce an artificial bias into scientific publications. Stating as fact associations which may be demonstrably false is not just unscientific, it is unprincipled." In a 1994 presentation to the Western Economics Association, State University of New York at Buffalo criminologist Lawrence Southwick compared public health firearm studies to popular articles produced by the gun lobby: "Generally the level of analysis done on each side is of a low quality.... The papers published in the medical literature (which are uniformly anti-gun) are particularly poor science."

* * *

As Bordua, Cowan, and Southwick observed, a prejudice against gun ownership pervades the public health field. Deborah Prothrow-Stith, dean of the Harvard School of Public Health, nicely summarizes the typical attitude of her colleagues in a recent book. "My own view on gun control is simple," she writes. "I hate guns and cannot imagine why anybody would want to own one. If I had my way, guns for sport would be registered, and all other guns would be banned." Opposition to gun ownership is also the official position of the U.S. Public Health Service, the CDC's parent agency. Since 1979, its goal has been "to reduce the number of handguns in private ownership," starting with a 25 percent reduction by the turn of the century.

Since 1985 the CDC has funded scores of firearm studies, all reaching conclusions that favor stricter gun control. But CDC officials insist they are not pursuing an anti-gun agenda. In a 1996 interview with the *Times-Picayune*, CDC spokeswoman Mary Fenley adamantly denied that the agency is "trying to eliminate guns." In a 1991 letter to CDC critic Dr. David Stolinsky, the NCIPC's Mark Rosenberg said "our scientific understanding of the role that firearms play in violent events is rudimentary." He added in a subsequent letter, "There is a strong need for further scientific investigations of the relationships among firearms ownership, firearms regulations and the risk of firearm-related injury. This is an area that has not been given adequate scrutiny. Hopefully, by addressing these important and appropriate scientific issues we will eventually arrive at conclusions which support effective, preventive actions."

Yet four years *earlier*, in a 1987 CDC report, Rosenberg thought the area adequately scrutinized, and his understanding sufficient, to urge confiscation of all firearms from "the general population," claiming "8,600 homicides and 5,370 sui-

cides could be avoided" each year. In 1993 *Rolling Stone* reported that Rosenberg "envisions a long term campaign, similar to [those concerning] tobacco use and auto safety, to convince Americans that guns are, first and foremost, a public health menace." In 1994 he told *The Washington Post*, "We need to revolutionize the way we look at guns, like what we did with cigarettes. Now it *[sic]* is dirty, deadly, and banned."

As Bordua and Cowan noted, one hallmark of the public health literature on guns is a tendency to ignore contrary scholarship. Among criminologists, Gary Kleck's encyclopedic *Point Blank: Guns and Violence in America* (1991) is universally recognized as the starting point for further research. Kleck, a professor of criminology at Florida State University, was initially a strong believer that gun ownership increased the incidence of homicide, but his research made him a skeptic. His book assembles strong evidence against the notion that reducing gun ownership is a good way to reduce violence. That may be why *Point Blank* is never cited in the CDC's own firearm publications or in articles reporting the results of CDC-funded gun studies.

Three Kleck studies, the first published in 1987, have found that guns are used in self-defense up to three times as often as they are used to commit crimes. These studies are so convincing that the doyen of American criminologists, Marvin Wolfgang, conceded in the Fall 1995 issue of *The Journal of Criminal Law and Criminology* that they pose a serious challenge to his own anti-gun views. "I am as strong a gun-control advocate as can be found among the criminologists in this country ... What troubles me is the article by Gary Kleck and Mark Gertz. The reason I am troubled is that they have provided an almost clear-cut case of methodologically sound research in support of something I have theoretically opposed for years, namely, the use of a gun against a criminal perpetrator."

Yet Rosenberg and his CDC colleague James Mercy, writing in *Health Affairs* in 1993, present the question "How frequently are guns used to successfully ward off potentially violent attacks?" as not just open but completely unresearched. They cite neither Kleck nor the various works on which he drew.

When CDC sources do cite adverse studies, they often get them wrong. In 1987 the National Institute of Justice hired two sociologists, James D. Wright and Peter H. Rossi, to assess the scholarly literature and produce an agenda for gun control. Wright and Rossi found the literature so biased and shoddy that it provided no basis for concluding anything positive about gun laws. Like Kleck, they were forced to give up their own prior faith in gun control as they researched the issue.

But that's not the story told by Dr. Arthur Kellermann, director of Emory University's Center for Injury Control and the CDC's favorite gun researcher. In a 1988 *New England Journal of Medicine* article, Kellermann and his co-authors cite Wright and Rossi's book *Under the Gun* to support the notion that "restricting access to handguns could substantially reduce our annual rate of homicide." What they actually said was: "There is no persuasive evidence that supports this view." In a 1992 *New England Journal of Medicine* article, Kellermann cites an *American Journal of Psychiatry* study to back up the claim "that limiting access to firearms could prevent many suicides." But the study actually found just the opposite—i.e., that

people who don't have guns find other ways to kill themselves.

At the same time that he misuses other people's work, Kellermann refuses to provide the full data for any of his studies so that scholars can evaluate his findings. His critics therefore can judge his results only from the partial data he chooses to publish. Consider a 1993 *New England Journal of Medicine* study that, according to press reports, "showed that keeping a gun in the home nearly triples the likelihood that someone in the household will be slain there." This claim cannot be verified because Kellerman will not release the data. Relying on independent sources to fill gaps in the published data, SUNY-Buffalo's Lawrence Southwick has speculated that Kellermann's full data set would actually vindicate defensive gun ownership. Such issues cannot be resolved without Kellermann's cooperation, but the CDC has refused to require its researchers to part with their data as a condition for taxpayer funding.

Even without access to secret data, it's clear that many of Kellermann's inferences are not justified. In a 1995 *JAMA* study that was funded by the CDC, he and his colleagues examined 198 incidents in which burglars entered occupied homes in Atlanta. They found that "only three individuals (1.5%) employed a firearm in self-defense"—from which they concluded that guns are rarely used for self-defense. On closer examination, however, Kellermann et al.'s data do not support that conclusion. In 42 percent of the incidents, there was no confrontation between victim and offender because "the offender(s) either left silently or fled when detected." When the burglar left silently, the victim was not even aware of the crime, so he did not have the opportunity to use a gun in self-defense (or to call the police, for that matter). The intruders who "fled when detected" show how defensive gun ownership can protect all victims, armed and unarmed alike, since the possibility of confronting an armed resident encourages burglars to flee.

These 83 no-confrontation incidents should be dropped from Kellermann et al.'s original list of 198 burglaries. Similarly, about 50 percent of U.S. homes do not contain guns, and in 70 percent of the homes that do, the guns are kept unloaded. After eliminating the burglaries where armed self-defense was simply not feasible, Kellermann's 198 incidents shrink to 17, and his 1.5 percent figure for defensive use rises to 17 percent. More important, this study covers only burglaries reported to the police. Since police catch only about 10 percent of home burglars, the only *good* reason to report a burglary is that police documentation is required to file an insurance claim. But if no property was lost because the burglar fled when the householder brandished a gun, why report the incident? And, aside from the inconvenience, there are strong reasons *not* to report: The gun may not be registered, or the householder may not be certain that guns can legally be used to repel unarmed burglars. Thus, for all Kellermann knows, successful gun use far exceeds the three incidents reported to police in his Atlanta study.

Similar sins of omission invalidate the conclusion of a 1986 *New England Journal of Medicine* study that Kellermann coauthored with University of Washington pathologist Donald T. Reay, another gun researcher who has enjoyed the CDC's support. (This particular study was funded by the Robert Wood Johnson Foundation.) Examining gunshot deaths in King County, Washington, from 1978 to 1983, Kellermann and Reay found that, of 398 people killed in a home where a gun was kept, only two were intruders shot while trying to get in. "We noted 43 suicides, criminal homicides, or accidental gunshot deaths involving a gun kept in the home for every case of homicide for self-protection," they wrote, concluding that "the advisability of keeping firearms in the home for protection must be questioned."

* * *

But since Kellermann and Reay considered only cases resulting in death, which Gary Kleck's research indicates are a tiny percentage of defensive gun uses, this conclusion does not follow. As the researchers themselves conceded, "Mortality studies such as ours do not include cases in which burglars or intruders are wounded or frightened away by the use or display of a firearm. Cases in which would-be intruders may have purposely avoided a house known to be armed are also not identified." By leaving out such cases, Kellermann and Reay excluded almost all of the lives saved, injuries avoided, and property protected by keeping a gun in the home. Yet advocates of gun control continue to use this study as the basis for claims such as, "A gun in the home is 43 times as likely to kill a family member as to be used in self-defense."

Another popular factoid—"having a gun in the home increases the risk of suicide by almost five times"—is also based on a Kellermann study, this one funded by the CDC and published by *The New England Journal of Medicine* in 1992. Kellermann and his colleagues matched each of 438 suicides to a "control" of the same race, sex, approximate age, and neighborhood. After controlling for arrests, drug abuse, living alone, and use of psychotropic medication (all of which were more common among the suicides), they found that a household with one or more guns was 4.8 times as likely to be the site of a suicide.

Although press reports about gun research commonly treat correlation and causation as one and the same, this association does not prove that having a gun in the house raises the risk of suicide. We can imagine alternative explanations: Perhaps gun ownership in this sample was associated with personality traits that were, in turn, related to suicide, or perhaps people who had contemplated suicide bought a gun for that reason. To put the association in perspective, it's worth noting that living alone and using illicit drugs were both better predictors of suicide than gun ownership was. That does not necessarily mean that living alone or using illegal drugs leads to suicide.

Furthermore, Kellermann and his colleagues selected their sample with an eye toward increasing the apparent role of gun ownership in suicide. They started by looking at all suicides that occurred during a 32-month period in King County, Washington, and Shelby County, Tennessee, but they excluded cases that occurred outside the home—nearly a third of the original sample. "Our study was restricted to suicides occurring in the victim's home," they explained with admirable frankness, "because a previous study has indicated that most suicides committed with guns occur there."

* * *

Kellermann also participated in CDC-funded research that simplistically compared homicide rates in Seattle and Vancouver, attributing the difference to Canada's stricter gun laws. This study, published in *The New England Journal of Medicine* in 1988, ignored important demographic differences between the two cities that help explain the much higher incidence of violence in Seattle. Furthermore, the researchers were aware of nationwide research that came to strikingly different conclusions about Canadian gun control, but they failed to inform their readers about that evidence.

Two years later in the same journal, the same research team compared suicide rates in Seattle and Vancouver. Unfazed by the fact that Seattle had a *lower* suicide rate, they emphasized that the rate was higher for one subgroup, adolescents and young men—a difference they attributed to lax American gun laws. Gary Mauser, a criminologist at Simon Fraser University, called the Seattle/Vancouver comparisons "a particularly egregious example" of "an abuse of scholarship, inventing, selecting, or misinterpreting data in order to validate *a priori* conclusions."

These and other studies funded by the CDC focus on the presence or absence of guns, rather than the characteristics of the people who use them. Indeed, the CDC's Rosenberg claims in the journal *Educational Horizons* that murderers are "ourselves—ordinary citizens, professionals, even health care workers": people who kill only because a gun happens to be available. Yet if there is one fact that has been incontestably established by homicide studies, it's that murderers are not ordinary gun owners but extreme aberrants whose life histories include drug abuse, serious accidents, felonies, and irrational violence. Unlike "ourselves," roughly 90 percent of adult murderers have significant criminal records, averaging an adult criminal career of six or more years with four major felonies.

Access to juvenile records would almost certainly show that the criminal careers of murderers stretch back into their adolescence. In *Murder in America* (1994), the criminologists Ronald W. Holmes and Stephen T. Holmes report that murderers generally "have histories of committing personal violence in childhood, against other children, siblings, and small animals." Murderers who don't have criminal records usually have histories of psychiatric treatment or domestic violence that did not lead to arrest.

Contrary to the impression fostered by Rosenberg and other opponents of gun ownership, the term "acquaintance homicide" does not mean killings that stem from ordinary family or neighborhood arguments. Typical acquaintance homicides include: an abusive man eventually killing a woman he has repeatedly assaulted; a drug user killing a dealer (or vice versa) in a robbery attempt; and gang members, drug dealers, and other criminals killing each other for reasons of economic rivalry or personal pique. According to a 1993 article in the *Journal of Trauma*, 80 percent of murders in Washington, D.C., are related to the drug trade, while "84% of [Philadelphia murder] victims in 1990 had antemortem drug use or criminal history." A 1994 article in *The New England Journal of Medicine* reported that 71 percent of Los Angeles children and adolescents injured in drive-by shootings "were documented members of violent street gangs." And University of North Carolina-Charlotte criminal justice scholars Richard Lumb and Paul C. Friday report that 71 percent of adult gunshot wound victims in Charlotte have criminal records.

As the English gun control analyst Colin Greenwood has noted, in any society there are always enough guns available, legally or illegally, to arm the violent. The true determinant of violence is the number of violent people, not the availability of a particular weapon. Guns contribute to murder in the trivial sense that they help violent people kill. But owning guns does not turn responsible, law-abiding people into killers. If the general availability of guns were as important a factor in violence as the CDC implies, the vast increase in firearm ownership during the past two decades should have led to a vast increase in homicide. The CDC suggested just that in a 1989 report to Congress, where it asserted that "[s]ince the early 1970s the year-to-year fluctuations in firearm availability has [sic] paralleled the numbers of homicides."

But this correlation was a fabrication: While the number of handguns rose 69 percent from 1974 to 1988, handgun murders actually dropped by 27 percent. Moreover, as U.S. handgun ownership more than doubled from the early 1970s through the 1990s, homicides held constant or declined for every major population group except young urban black men. The CDC can blame the homicide surge in this group on guns only by ignoring a crucial point: Gun ownership is far less common among urban blacks than among whites or rural blacks.

The CDC's reports and studies never give long-term trend data linking gun sales to murder rates, citing only carefully selected partial or short-term correlations. If murder went down in the first and second years, then back up in the third and fourth years, only the rise is mentioned. CDC publications focus on fluctuations and other unrepresentative phenomena to exaggerate the incidence of gun deaths and to conceal declines. Thus, in its *Advance Data from Vital and Health Statistics* (1994), the CDC melodramatically announces that gun deaths now "rival" driving fatalities, as if gun murders were increasing. But this trend simply reflects the fact that driving fatalities are declining more rapidly than murders.

While the CDC shows a selective interest in homicide trends, it tends to ignore trends in accidental gun deaths—with good reason. In the 25 years from 1968 to 1992, American gun ownership increased almost 135 percent (from 97 million to 222 million), with handgun ownership rising more than 300 percent. These huge increases coincided with a two-thirds *decline* in accidental gun fatalities. The CDC and the researchers it funds do not like to talk about this dramatic development, since it flies in the face of the assumption that more guns mean more deaths. They are especially reluctant to acknowledge the drop in accidental gun deaths because of the two most plausible explanations for it: the replacement of rifles and shotguns with the much safer handgun as the main weapon kept loaded for self-defense, and the NRA's impressive efforts in gun safety training.

* * *

The question is, why hasn't it been studied? The answer illustrates how the CDC's political agenda undermines its professed concern for saving lives. In the absence of an anti-gun animus, a two-thirds decrease in accidental gun deaths would surely have been a magnet for studies, especially since it coincided with a big increase in handgun ownership. But the CDC wants to reduce gun deaths

only by banning guns, not by promoting solutions that are consistent with more guns. So the absence of studies is an excuse to dismiss gun safety training rather than an incentive for research.

Taken by itself, any one of these flaws —omission of relevant evidence, misrepresentation of studies, questionable methodology, overreaching conclusions —could be addressed by a determination to do better in the future. But the consistent tendency to twist research in favor of an anti-gun agenda suggests that there is something inherently wrong with the CDC's approach in this area. Implicit in the decision to treat gun deaths as a "public health" problem is the notion that violence is a communicable disease that can be controlled by attacking the relevant pathogen.

Dr. Katherine Christoffel, head of the Handgun Epidemic Lowering Plan, a group that has received CDC support, stated this assumption plainly in a 1994 interview with *American Medical News*: "Guns are a virus that must be eradicated.... They are causing an epidemic of death by gunshot, which should be treated like any epidemic—you get rid of the virus.... Get rid of the guns, get rid of the bullets, and you get rid of the deaths."

In the same article, the CDC's Rosenberg said approvingly, "Kathy Christoffel is saying about firearms injuries what has been said for years about AIDS: that we can no longer be silent. That silence equals death and she's not willing to be silent anymore. She's asking for help." Similarly, in a 1993 *Atlanta Medicine* article on the public health approach to violence, Arthur Kellermann subtitled part of his discussion "The Bullet as Pathogen."

It is hardly surprising that research based on this paradigm would tend to indict gun ownership as a cause of death. The inadequacy of the disease metaphor, which some public health specialists seem to take quite literally, is readily apparent when we consider Koch's postulates, the criteria by which suspected pathogens are supposed to be judged: 1) The microorganism must be observed in all cases of the disease; 2) the microorganism must be isolated and grown in a pure culture medium; 3) microorganisms from the pure culture must reproduce the disease when inoculated in a test animal; and 4) the same kind of microorganism must be recovered from the experimentally diseased animal. A strict application of these criteria is clearly impossible in this case. But applying the postulates as an analogy, we can ask about the consistency of the relationship between guns and violence. Gun ownership usually does not result in violence, and violence frequently occurs in the absence of guns. Given these basic facts, depicting violence as a disease caused by the gun virus can only cloud our thinking.

It may also discredit the legitimate functions of public health. "The CDC has got to be careful that we don't get into social issues," Dr. C.J. Peters, head of the CDC's Special Pathogens Branch, told the *Pittsburgh Post-Gazette* last year, in the midst of the controversy over taxpayer-funded gun research. "If we're going to do that, we ought to start a center for social change. We should stay with medical issues."

If treating gun violence as a public health issue invites confusion and controversy, why is this approach so popular? The main function of the disease metaphor is to lend a patina of scientific credibility to the belief that guns cause violence—a belief that is hard to justify on empirical grounds. "We're trying to depoliticize the subject," Rosenberg told *USA Today* in 1995. "We're trying to transform it from politics to science." What they are actually trying to do is disguise politics as science.

POSTSCRIPT

Is Gun Control a Public Health Issue?

Between 1960 and 1970, both the murder rate in the United States and the rate of handgun ownership doubled. Was it coincidence that violence and gun ownership grew at nearly the same pace? Can it be assumed from this fact that more guns cause more violence? The conventional wisdom is that guns and violence are related in the same sense that owning a gun increases the risk that the *gun owner*, rather than the criminal, will be hurt.

In several major studies, Dr. Arthur Kellermann attempted to prove just that. In 1986 he published "Protection or Peril? An Analysis of Firearm-Related Deaths in the Home," *The New England Journal of Medicine* (vol. 314). His other publications on guns as a public health issue include "Validating Survey Responses to Questions About Gun Ownership Among Owners of Registered Handguns," *American Journal of Epidemiology* (vol. 131, 1990); "Men, Women, and Murder: Gender-Specific Differences in Rates of Fatal Violence and Victimization," *Journal of Trauma* (vol. 33, 1992); "Suicide in the Home in Relation to Gun Ownership," *The New England Journal of Medicine* (vol. 327, 1992); and "Gun Ownership as a Risk Factor for Homicide in the Home," *The New England Journal of Medicine* (vol. 329, 1993). Dr. Arthur Kellerman, quoted in "Should You Own a Gun?" *U.S. News and World Report* (August 15, 1994), says, "Most gun homicides occur in altercations among family members, friends or acquaintances. In a heated dispute, few carefully weigh the legal consequences of their actions. They are too busy reaching for a weapon. If it's a gun, death is more likely to result." Dr. Kellerman and his colleagues are not the only physicians who consider homicide and gun ownership public health issues. In *Mother Jones* (May/June 1993), Dr. Mark Rosenberg, an epidemiologist at the Centers for Disease Control, maintains that violence is a public health issue and that violence prevention should be pushed to the top of the public health agenda.

Is violence really a *health* issue? Each year, more than 500,000 Americans, including children, are brought to hospital emergency rooms for treatment of a violent injury. These injuries, including shootings and assaults, add over $5 billion dollars in direct medical costs to current health care expenditures. Lifetime costs of violent injuries, which include medical care and loss of productivity, is over $45 billion dollars. And since many gunshot victims are uninsured, the public at large pays the bill. Gunshot wounds can also strain the health care system by diverting resources away from other illnesses and injuries.

Articles on the relationship between guns and public health include "Homicide, Handguns, and the Crime Gun Hypothesis: Firearms Used in Fatal

Shootings of Law Enforcement Officers, 1980 to 1989," *American Journal of Public Health* (April 1994); "Firearm Violence and Public Health: Limiting the Availability of Guns," *Journal of the American Medical Association* (April 27, 1994); "Loaded Guns in the Home," *Journal of the American Medical Association* (June 10, 1992); "Handgun Control, M.D.," *Weekly Standard* (April 15, 1996); Gun Legislation Could Curb Youth Suicide," *Australian Nursing Journal* (November, 1996); and "Gun Violence Remains a Public Health Risk That's Still Hard to Track," *Nation's Health* (November, 1996).

Doctors who treat gunshot victims may feel that controlling gun ownership will reduce the number of shootings, but there is opposition to controlling the sale or possession of guns in this country. Despite this opposition, a majority of gun owners and the general public favor stricter gun controls, including safety classes for gun owners. Only 39 percent of the American public backs a total ban on handguns, according to an article in *USA Today* (December 17, 1993). And although gun control may save some lives, the availability of guns can never be truly stemmed. In "The False Promise of Gun Control," *The Atlantic Monthly* (March, 1994), law professor Daniel Polsby claims that gun control also diverts attention away from the roots of the crime problem in this country: lack of job opportunities, inadequate education, and the breakdown of families. Polsby compares gun control with Prohibition. Other articles that argue against gun control include "Security," *Forbes* (November 25, 1991); "The NRA: It's Not Pro-Gun, It's 'Anti-Crime,'" *Newsweek* (December 6, 1993); and "Gun Owners, YOU Are the Target," *American Hunter* (May 1994).

Overviews of the gun control issue include "Gun Control: Will It Help Reduce Violent Crime in the US?" *CQ Researcher* (June 10, 1994); *The Mounting Threat of Home Intruders: Weighing the Moral Option of Armed Self-Defense,"* (Charles C. Thomas Publishers, 1993); "Guns and Poses," *New Republic* (October 11, 1993); and "Struggling Against Common Sense: The Pluses and Minuses of Gun Control," *The World & I* (February 1997).

On the Internet . . .

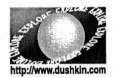

The Department of Health Fitness and the National Center for Health Fitness
International Institute for Health Promotion is a site for the National Center for Health Fitness at the American University. It includes a newsgroup and a health promotion clearinghouse. *http://www.healthy.american.edu/*

Wellness Web: The Patient's Network
Wellness Web supplies information on smoking, women's health, and related topics. It also offers references, screenings, resources, and what's new. *http://wellweb.com*

Center for Science in the Public Interest
This organization was founded by Dr. Michael Jacobson. The home page focuses on improving the nutritional quality of our food supply and on reducing the health problems caused by alcohol. The site has a health letter, a nutrition quiz, booze news, and links to other health sites. *http://www/cspinet.org/*

Stress and Stress Management
Defines stress, the psychological "fight or flight" response of the body to increased muscle tension, and recommendations for reducing negative effects of stress. *http://h-devil-www.mc.duke.edu/h-devil/emotion/stress.htm*

The Yoga Page
The Yoga Page is a Minnesota resource for information on yoga, health, and wellness. It also provides links to stress-reducing tips. *http://www.bowman-cline.com/yoga/index.htm*

PART 2

Mind/Body Relationship

Humans have long sought to extend life, eliminate disease, and prevent sickness. In modern times, people depend on technology to develop creative and innovative ways to improve health. However, as cures for diseases such as AIDS, cancer, and heart disease continue to elude scientists and doctors, many people question whether or not modern medicine has reached a plateau in improving health. As a result, over the last decade emphasis has been placed on prevention as a way to improve health. Although millions have made changes in their lifestyles in hopes of preventing the onset of disease, some scientists argue that people will always be plagued by illness and that overzealous emphasis on prevention and control is misplaced. The role of mind and body relationships is the key question regarding the issues debated in this section.

■ Should Healthy Behavior Be Mandated?

■ Can Spirituality Overcome Disease?

ISSUE 5

Should Healthy Behavior Be Mandated?

YES: Michael F. Jacobson, from "Prevention's the Issue: Your Money or Your Life Style," *The Nation* (July 13, 1992)

NO: Jacob Sullum, from "What the Doctor Orders," *Reason* (January 1996)

ISSUE SUMMARY

YES: Michael F. Jacobson, a microbiologist and the director of the Center for Science in the Public Interest, claims that federal policies emphasizing healthy behavior would not only improve public health but reduce health care spending.

NO: Journalist and author Jacob Sullum argues that, by treating risky behavior like a communicable disease, the public health establishment invites the government to meddle in our private lives.

During the past decade, there has been a movement towards self-care and prevention as a means to improve health. This movement has been based on several factors: many diseases such as cancer or heart disease have no "magic bullet" cure; health care costs have been spiraling; and it is cheaper, more humane, and more sensible, to try and prevent a disease rather than to attempt to cure it. If individuals could be encouraged to quit smoking, exercise, and eat low fat diets, a significantly lower number of cancers, heart disease, and other illnesses would develop.

While it makes sense to try to prevent a disease rather than to place emphasis on treatment, prevention may not always be possible. To prevent disease, health behavior changes are necessary, but these changes may be beyond the ability of some individuals, however motivated they may be. Not everyone, for instance, is physically capable of exercising or able to afford healthy food. Other factors can contribute to disease, many not modifiable. Individuals cannot change their age, gender, or heredity, which are all potential disease risk factors. There is also a limit as to how much an individual can affect environmental health risks including air pollution, exposure to pesticides, and toxic waste. Another issue is biological individuality. For instance, experts warn against eating too much salt because it it linked to high blood pressure in some individuals. Many people, however, are not affected by salt.

In the following selections, Michael Jacobson believes that the United States spends far too little on prevention of disease. He states that every year, hundreds of thousands of deaths would be avoided and billions of dollars would be saved if Americans practiced healthier behaviors and if government policies were oriented toward health and prevention.

Jacob Sullum argues that even when people are aware of the hazards of smoking, poor diet, and so on, many will continue to engage in these behaviors. Public health officials should accept that individuals' choices, no matter how unhealthy, should be respected.

YES

Michael F. Jacobson

PREVENTION'S THE ISSUE: YOUR MONEY OR YOUR LIFE STYLE

To listen to the presidential hopefuls, including those who fell by the wayside earlier this year, you'd think that America's health care crisis is solely one of access and payment. Lost in the duels over "play or pay," "single payer" and "small-group-market insurance reform" is the fact that a good chunk of our health costs are preventable. Every year, hundreds of thousands of deaths could be avoided and billions of dollars saved if Americans lived a little differently and if federal tax and other policies were reoriented toward health. But we hear nothing about this from Bush, Clinton or Perot.

Consider booze. Alcoholic beverages cause more devastation in our society than any other product. For starters, booze accounts for 100,000 deaths each year due to cancer, auto crashes, liver cirrhosis, stroke, etc. According to the National Institute on Alcohol Abuse and Alcoholism, drinking is a factor in half of all homicides and in three out of ten suicides. Alcoholism is a major cause of family violence, birth defects, workplace injuries and other tragedies. Cigarettes may kill more people, but alcohol ruins more lives, beginning even in grade-school years, and destroys millions of families. For candidates who claim to be "pro-family," attention to alcoholism is mandatory.

The direct and indirect costs to society of alcohol problems total more than $100 billion each year. By contrast, state and federal excise taxes on alcohol amount to only about $15 billion. Should taxpayers be subsidizing the booze barons?

Former Surgeon General C. Everett Koop's 1988 Workshop on Drunk Driving reported that raising excise taxes "could have the largest long-term effect on alcohol-impaired driving of all policy and program options available." The workshop recommended raising beer and wine taxes to equal the higher liquor rate and to make up for the inflation that since 1970 has severely eroded the value of tax revenues.

The Koop workshop's recommendation would generate more than $16 billion in new revenues annually. Part of that sum could be applied to treating and preventing alcoholism, with the remainder funding critical health and social programs. But even if not one dime were applied to alcohol programs, the higher prices caused by the tax hike would slash alcohol consumption by almost 10 percent—and by even more among grade school and high school students. That's a lot fewer car crashes and teen pregnancies, less mental retardation and lower health care costs.

While tax hikes are generally considered political poison, polls show that the vast majority of Americans support higher alcohol and tobacco taxes. Any regressiveness could be cured by lowering income-tax rates for low-income families.

On another front, a broad coalition, which includes groups ranging from the Christian Life Commission of the Southern Baptist Convention to Public Citizen, from the National P.T.A. to the American Medical Association, is calling for reforms of alcohol advertising. With support from such unlikely bedfellows as Senator Strom Thurmond [R-South Carolina] and Representative Joseph Kennedy [D-Massachusetts], the coalition is seeking legislation that would require health information in all alcohol ads. Currently, TV commercials imply that beer is the elixir of health and key to social and sexual success, while magazine ads and billboards suggest that the road to economic success is paved with empty liquor bottles.

Beyond supporting higher excise taxes and restrictions on advertising, the presidential candidates should be calling for educational programs in schools and the mass media, universally available treatment for alcoholism and other drug addictions, and the prohibition of alcohol purchases and alcohol advertising as tax-deductible business expenses (the last measure alone would raise $2 billion annually).

* * *

As with alcoholic beverages, higher taxes and comprehensive educational campaigns could save billions in medical treatment for victims of tobacco smoke. In a 1988 referendum, Californians voted to boost the state tax on cigarettes from 10 cents per pack to 35 cents. One-fourth of the revenues—$115 million in 1991—was earmarked for tobacco research and aggressive antismoking campaigns. The result: Cigarette smoking declined by 17 percent between 1987 and 1990, a far sharper decline than in any other state. One-third of California's quitters said the state's antismoking ads were the main reason they stopped.

The Canadians, too, have gotten serious about smoking. They raised taxes so that an average pack now costs U.S. $4.72, compared with $1.73 in the United States. As a direct result, 16 percent fewer Canadians smoked in 1991 than in 1990; a decline in lung-cancer, emphysema and heart-disease death rates will surely follow.

Although Congress has voted modest increases in tobacco taxes, they barely keep up with recent inflation. Boosting the tax from the current 20 cents a pack to, say, $1.20 a pack would generate about $21 billion in needed revenues and cut smoking rates by more than 15 percent. Boosting the tax by $2 would still leave the price of a pack less than it is in Canada and bring in more than $30 billion in new revenues.

As for cigarette advertising, Congress has considered tighter restrictions, but without presidential leadership that notion has died a quiet death on Capitol Hill.

* * *

Diet is a third area where federal action could save untold lives and dollars. Fatty, salty diets promote obesity, diabetes, stroke, heart disease and certain cancers. Those diet-related diseases cause hundreds of thousands of premature deaths each year. Surgeons perform about 400,000 coronary bypass operations annually at a cost of more than $13 billion.

If we really wanted to cut health care costs we'd be better off training dietitians than surgeons. If more people followed a diet based on grains, beans and vegetables rather than on meat, eggs and dairy products, we could save thousands of lives and billions of dollars. But the federal government is doing precious little to convey that critical information to Americans. President Bush's only comment on health and nutrition has been to ridicule broccoli and carrots. The Agriculture Department now facilitates programs that enable the meat, dairy and egg industries to spend tens of millions of dollars each year on advertising and public-relations campaigns intended to boost sales. (The department also gave $200 million last year to McDonald's, Gallo, Seagram and dozens of other companies to promote sales abroad of their sometimes less than salubrious products.)

The government could be, but isn't, serving healthy meals to employees and others in government cafeterias, federal prisons, military bases, senior citizen centers and school food programs. While the Food and Drug Administration has sought to implement a law that would require better nutrition labeling on thousands of foods and that would cut down on diet-related illnesses, the food industry, with the help of Vice President Quayle's Competitiveness Council, is seeking a one-year delay.

* * *

The need to prevent serious health problems extends into many spheres of our lives and our economy. Workers need to be far better protected from dangerous machinery and chemicals. Farmers need to be encouraged to reduce their use of dangerous pesticides, veterinary drugs and chemical fertilizers in order to safeguard their health and that of consumers. Manufacturing facilities and hazardous-waste dumps threaten the health of nearby communities. The lifesaving Special Supplemental Food Program for Women, Infants and Children must be extended to every needy mother and child. Childhood immunization campaigns, a fundamental aspect of public health, must be fully funded to reverse, for example, the sixfold increase in measles cases that occurred between 1985 and 1989.

Even more broadly, poverty itself correlates with poor health and must be eliminated. A concern for health must be factored into every aspect of a government's policies. All Cabinet secretaries, not just the Secretary of Health and Human Services, must realize that their actions can improve or worsen the public's health.

Yet the presidential candidates are totally neglecting the prevention side of the health issue. It is certainly true that a disease-based economy provides thousands of jobs for physicians, nurses, advertising executives, ranchers, candy manufacturers, tobacco growers, cigarette makers, brewers, vintners, broadcasters, athletes, medical-equipment manufacturers and other potential political supporters.

The long list of industries nourished by, and that nurture, Americans' pathogenic life style makes it difficult for many political candidates to advocate cutting health care costs by improving the public's health. PAC [political action committee] contributions speak louder than words. For instance, in the 1989–90 election cycle, alcoholic-beverage companies, trade associations and executives doled out more than $2.8 million in the form of PAC contributions, honorariums and private donations to members of Congress.

In 1991 Americans spent almost $738 billion on health. Thirty-six million of us lacked health insurance. We certainly do need to obtain universal insurance coverage and control skyrocketing costs of drugs, exorbitant doctors' bills, superfluous operations and unnecessary insurance agents and bill collectors. But disease prevention is even more important, whether you're a cold-blooded economist concerned about the budget or a parent concerned about a child's health. Some individuals, without any encouragement from Uncle Sam, will discard their cigarettes, double cheeseburgers and liquor. But many millions more would do so—leading to a healthier populace and a healthier economy—if our political candidates and elected officials advocated policies that advanced the most sensible way to control the costs of illness: promoting health.

NO

Jacob Sullum

WHAT THE DOCTOR ORDERS

In the introduction to the first major American book on public health, U.S. Army surgeon John S. Billings explained the field's concerns: "Whatever can cause, or help to cause, discomfort, pain, sickness, death, vice, or crime—and whatever has a tendency to avert, destroy, or diminish such causes—are matters of interest to the sanitarian; and the powers of science and the arts, great as they are, are taxed to the uttermost to afford even an approximate solution to the problems with which he is concerned."

Despite this ambitious mandate—and the book's impressive length (nearly 1,500 pages in two volumes)—*A Treatise on Hygiene and Public Health* had little to say about the issues that occupy today's public health professionals. There were no sections on smoking, alcoholism, drug abuse, obesity, vehicular accidents, mental illness, suicide, homicide, domestic violence, or unwanted pregnancy. Published in 1879, the book was instead concerned with such things as compiling vital statistics, preventing the spread of disease, abating public nuisances, and assuring wholesome food, clean drinking water, and sanitary living conditions.

A century later, public health textbooks discuss the control of communicable diseases mainly as history. The field's present and future lie elsewhere. "The entire spectrum of 'social ailments,' such as drug abuse, venereal disease, mental illness, suicide, and accidents, includes problems appropriate to public health activity," explains Jack Smolensky in *Principles of Community Health* (1977). "The greatest potential for improving the health of the American people is to be found in what they do and don't do to and for themselves." Similarly, *Introduction to Public Health* (1978), by Daniel M. Wilner, Rosabelle Price Walkley, and Edward J. O'Neill, notes that the field, which once "had much narrower interests," now "includes the *social and behavioral aspects of life* —endangered by contemporary stresses, addictive diseases, and emotional instability."

The extent of the shift can be sensed by perusing a few issues of the American Public Health Association's journal. In 1911, when the journal was first published, typical articles included "Modern Methods of Controlling the Spread of Asiatic Cholera," "Sanitation of Bakeries and Restaurant Kitchens," and "The Need of Exact Accounting for Still-Births." Issues published in 1995 offered "Menthol vs. Nonmenthol Cigarettes: Effects on Smoking Behavior," "Correlates of College Student Binge Drinking," and "Violence by Male Partners Against Women During the Childbearing Year: A Contextual Analysis." The journal also covers strictly medical issues, of course, and even runs articles on traditional public health topics such as vaccination, nutrition, and infant mortality. But the amount of space taken up by studies of social problems and behavioral issues is striking.

In a sense, the change in focus is understandable. After all, Americans are not dying the way they once did. The chapter on infant mortality in *A Treatise on Hygiene and Public Health* reports that during the late 1860s and early 1870s, two-fifths to one-half of children in major American cities died before reaching the age of 5. The major killers included measles, scarlet fever, smallpox, diptheria, whooping cough, bronchitis, pneumonia, tuberculosis, and "diarrheal diseases." Largely because of such afflictions, life expectancy at birth was only 49 in 1900, compared to roughly 75 today, while the annual death rate was 17 per 1,000, compared to about half that today. Beginning in the 1870s, the discovery that infectious diseases were caused by specific microorganisms made it possible to control them through vaccination, antibiotics, better sanitation, water purification, and elimination of carriers such as rats and mosquitoes. At the same time, improvements in nutrition and living conditions increased resistance to infection. Although it is difficult to separate the effects of public health programs from the effects of rising affluence and changing patterns of work,

there's no question that disease-control efforts have had an important impact on the length and quality of life.

Americans no longer live in terror of smallpox or cholera. Despite occasional outbreaks of infectious diseases such as rabies and tuberculosis, the fear of epidemics that was once an accepted part of life is virtually unknown. The one major exception is AIDS, which is not readily transmitted and remains largely confined to a few high-risk groups. For the most part, Americans die of things you can't catch: cancer, heart disease, trauma. Accordingly, the public health establishment is focusing on those causes and the factors underlying them. Having vanquished most true epidemics, it has turned its attention to metaphorical "epidemics" such as smoking, obesity, and suicide. Along the way, the public health establishment has become the most influential lobby for ever-increasing government control over Americans' personal choices.

* * *

By the late 1930s, with the importance of infectious diseases declining, public health specialists started taking an interest in chronic conditions. "The public health establishment requires an issue that has salience in the public press, outside of the scientific community, in order to maintain support," says Barbara Rosenkrantz, professor emeritus of the history of science at Harvard. "Public health only becomes interesting when there are real problems."

The interest in chronic diseases led to lifestyle-oriented medical research that began in earnest after World War II. The Framingham heart study, a large-scale, long-term project that has helped identify risk factors for heart disease, began in 1948 and produced its first report in the early 1950s. The first influential studies linking cigarette smoking to lung cancer appeared about the same time. Philip Cole, a professor of epidemiology at the University of Alabama, Birmingham, argues that concern about smoking and other causes of non-infectious disease is "very much within the classical tradition of public health, even though it does not speak to the issue of contagion." He distinguishes this interest, manifested in the work of researchers and the recommendations of physicians, from "a continued effort on the part of government to usurp control of individuals' lives," a trend that worries him.

But the concerns of public health practitioners have a way of influencing public policy. Surgeons general of the U.S. Public Health Service have become official nags, urging us to shape up so we can reach the health goals they have set for the nation. The wide domain of public health allows them to champion whatever causes interest them. C. Everett Koop said we should achieve "a smoke-free society" by the year 2000. Antonia Novello condemned liquor and beer advertising that she found distasteful. Joycelyn Elders pontificated about gun control and masturbation. The circumstances of Elders's departure and the battle over her successor show that both liberals and conservatives take the top public health job quite seriously.

The key event that elevated the surgeon general's prestige and visibility occurred in 1964, when Luther M. Terry released the report of his Advisory Committee on Smoking and Health. The document, which declared that "cigarette smoking is a health hazard of sufficient importance in the United States to warrant appropriate remedial action," heralded the decline of the U.S. tobacco industry and the beginning of the contemporary anti-smoking movement. It helped put risky behavior at the top of the public health agenda.

The involvement of physicians in the auto-safety movement of the late 1960s and early '70s also helped legitimize the expansion of public health. "The automobile is the etiological agent in an epidemic accounting for some 50,000 deaths and 4 million injuries each year," wrote Seymour Charles of Physicians for Automotive Safety and John States of the American Association of Automotive Medicine in the July 4, 1966, issue of the *Journal of the American Medical Association*. They cited drunk-driving laws, seat-belt requirements, and other mandated design changes as examples of "preventive medicine." Today, advocates of a public health approach to violence cite the medicalization of traffic accidents as a precedent.

The establishment of Medicare and Medicaid in 1965 reinforced the argument that government should take an interest in the personal habits of its citizens because risky behavior might affect the public treasury. In a 1976 essay commissioned by *Time*, Dr. John H. Knowles, president of the Rockefeller Foundation, reviewed the rise of taxpayer-funded health insurance and declared that "the cost of sloth, gluttony, alcoholic overuse, reckless driving, sexual intemperance, and smoking is now a national, not an individual responsibility." Writing in *Daedalus* the following year, he said, "I believe that the idea of a 'right' to health should be replaced by the idea of an individual moral obligation to preserve one's own health—a public duty if you will."

In 1979, the surgeon general released *Healthy People*, a report that broke new ground by setting specific goals for reductions in mortality. "We are killing ourselves by our own careless habits," wrote Joseph Califano, then secretary of health, education, and welfare, calling for "a second public health revolution" (the first being the triumph over infectious diseases). *Healthy People*, which estimated that "perhaps as much as half of U.S. mortality in 1976 was due to unhealthy behavior or lifestyle," advised Americans to quit smoking, drink less, exercise more, fasten their seat belts, stop driving so fast, and cut down on fat, salt, and sugar. It also recommended motorcycle-helmet laws and gun control to improve public health.

Healthy People drew on a "national prevention strategy" developed by the U.S. Center for Disease Control (now the Centers for Disease Control and Prevention [CDC]), an agency whose evolution reflects the expanding interests of public health. Established during World War II as a unit of the U.S. Public Health Service charged with malaria control in war areas, it became the Communicable Disease Center in 1946. By the end of the 1950s the CDC had acquired exclusive federal authority over communicable diseases. In the 1960s it took on a wide range of projects, including family planning and overseas smallpox control. In the early to mid-1970s it absorbed the Public Health Service's nutrition program, the National Institute of Occupational Safety and Health, and the National Clearinghouse on Smoking and Health. It also took over federal programs dealing with lead poisoning, urban rat control, and water fluoridation. In the late 1970s the CDC drew up a list of its main priorities, the most serious health problems facing the country. The list included smoking, alcohol abuse, un-

wanted pregnancies, car accidents, workplace injuries, environmental hazards, social disorders, suicide, homicide, mental illness, and stress. Today only one of the CDC's seven "centers" deals with the agency's original task, control of infectious diseases..

A cynic would view the CDC's growth as a classic example of bureaucratic survival: If the problem you were charged with solving starts to get better, find new problems that will continue to justify your budget. More generally, it is easy to dismiss public health's ever-expanding agenda as a bid for funding, power, and status. Yet the field's practitioners argue, with evident sincerity, that they are simply adapting to changing patterns of morbidity and mortality. Without speculating about motivation, we can ask whether it makes sense to apply the methods of disease control to problems that are not caused by germs. If it doesn't, much of what is done in the name of public health today is seriously misguided.

* * *

The question is especially important because public health generally implies government action. That used to mean keeping statistics, imposing quarantines, requiring vaccination of children, providing purified water, building sewer systems, inspecting restaurants, regulating emissions from factories, and reviewing drugs for safety. Nowadays it means, among other things, raising alcohol taxes, restricting cigarette ads, banning guns, arresting marijuana growers, and forcing people to buckle their seat belts. These measures are attempts to control illness and injury by controlling behavior thought to be associated with them. The idea is straightforward: Less drinking means less cirrhosis of the liver, less smoking means less lung cancer, less gun ownership means less suicide.

Whether or not these expectations are justified, treating behavior as if it were a communicable disease is problematic. First of all, behavior cannot be transmitted to other people against their will. Second, people do not choose to be sick, but they do choose to engage in risky behavior. The choice implies that the behavior, unlike a viral or bacterial infection, has value. It also implies that attempts to control the behavior will be resisted.

Resistance to public health measures is not new. Such interventions were often criticized, sometimes justifiably, as inappropriate exercises of government power. But in the past, public health officials could argue that they were protecting people from external threats: carriers of contagious diseases, fumes from the local glue factory, contaminated water, food poisoning, dangerous quack remedies. By contrast, the new enemies of public health come from within; the aim is to protect people from themselves rather than each other. The implications of this distinction can be better understood by considering a few of the "epidemics" that have taken the place of smallpox and cholera.

Smoking. In the public health literature, smoking is not an activity or even a habit. It is "the greatest community health hazard," "the single most important preventable cause of death," "the plague of our time," "the global tobacco epidemic." The disease metaphor has been used so much that it is now taken literally. The foreword to the 1988 surgeon general's report on nicotine addiction informs us, "Tobacco use is a dis-order which can be remedied through medical attention." This definition was not always so casually accepted. In the 1977 monograph, *Tobacco Use as a Mental Disorder*, published by the National Institute on Drug Abuse, Jerome H. Jaffe noted that "a behavior that merely predisposes to other medical illnesses is not necessarily, in and of itself, a disease or disorder. ... We certainly would not want to consider skiing as a mental disorder, although it clearly raises the likelihood of developing several well-defined orthopedic disorders. Risk taking, *per se*, is not a mental disorder."

Yet today public health professionals consider smoking itself a disease, something inherently undesirable that happens to unwilling victims. "Free will is not within the power of most smokers," writes former CDC Director William Foege in "The Growing Brown Plague," a 1990 editorial in the *Journal of the American Medical Association*. If it were, they certainly would choose not to smoke. As Scott Ballin, chairman of the Coalition on Smoking or Health, explains, "The product has no potential benefits.... It's addictive, so people don't have the choice to smoke or not to smoke."

These statements are part of a catechism intended to explain why so many people continue to smoke, when clearly they shouldn't. That catechism does not admit the possibility that smoking might offer some people benefits that in their minds outweigh its hazards. This blindness is inherent in the public health perspective, which seeks collective prescriptions that do not take account of individual tastes and preferences. It recognizes one supreme value—health—that cannot be trumped by other considerations.

Having promoted smoking from risk factor to disease, the public health establishment now targets alleged risk factors for smoking, most notably cigarette advertising. "If exposure to cigarette advertising is a risk factor for disease," writes Rep. Henry Waxman (D-Calif.) in a 1991 *JAMA* editorial, "it is incumbent on the public and elected officials to deal with it as we would the vector of any other pathogen." In other words, banning cigarette ads is like draining the swamps where the mosquitoes that carry malaria breed. That seems to be the assumption underlying the Clinton administration's proposed restrictions on tobacco advertising.

The alarm about the danger posed by cigarette advertising is based largely on well-publicized studies in medical journals that prove less than the researchers' conclusions and accompanying editorials imply. A typical example is the 1991 *JAMA* study cited by the Clinton administration. The researchers reported that 6-year-olds were as likely to match Joe Camel with a pack of cigarettes as they were to match the Disney Channel logo with Mickey Mouse. "Given the serious consequences of smoking," they wrote, "the exposure of children to environmental tobacco advertising may represent an important health risk. ..." But recognizing Joe Camel is not tantamount to smoking, any more than recognizing the logos for Ford and Chevrolet (which most of the kids in the study did) is tantamount to driving.

The same issue of *JAMA* carried an article reporting that Camel's market share among smokers under the age of 18 increased from 0.5 percent in 1988 to nearly 33 percent in 1991. The authors attributed the change to the Joe Camel campaign and concluded that "a total ban of tobacco advertising and promotions... can be based on sound scientific reasoning." Yet during the period covered by the study, smoking among minors actually *fell*. So while Joe Camel may have had something to do with the shift in brand preferences (a shift that also occurred in other age groups, though less dramatically), he cannot be blamed for convincing more kids to smoke.

Jean J. Boddewyn, a marketing professor at Baruch College who is skeptical of the alleged link between tobacco advertising and consumption levels, has argued that medical journals are not an appropriate venue for such research. Writing in the December 1993 issue of the *Journal of Advertising*, he suggests that medical editors and reviewers lack expertise in the area and are too quick to publish articles that reflect badly on the tobacco industry. "How would the [*Journal of Advertising*'s] reputation fare," he wonders, "if it published an article on the *health consequences of smoking*, after asking only advertising specialists to review it?" Boddewyn also complains that articles on tobacco advertising in medical journals rarely refer to relevant sources outside the public health literature.

Alcohol Abuse. Like smoking, alcohol abuse is considered a disease within the public health field. *Community Health* (1978), by C. L. Anderson, Richard F. Morton, and Lawrence W. Green, calls alcoholism "an inborn defect of metabolism," while *Introduction to Public Health* defines it as "the progressive chronic illness characterized by habitual heavy drinking that interferes with numerous... aspects of an individual's life." This view of alcoholism remains controversial, but it has a long pedigree, dating back to Benjamin Rush in the 18th century. As *Introduction to Public Health* concedes, however, "alcohol in moderation appears to do the body no permanent harm."

Nevertheless, heavy taxation of alcoholic beverages is a standard public health prescription for alcohol abuse. Restrictions on sales and advertising are also popular. Advocates of such measures hope to reduce overall consumption of alcohol and thereby reduce alcohol abuse. "The cost of alcohol should be greatly increased by taxation," *Community Health* recommends. "There is an excellent correlation between a low relative price, high consumption, and high cirrhotic mortality in international comparisons." In fact, it is not clear that reducing overall consumption would have much of an impact on alcohol abuse. It is precisely the people who have the biggest problems with alcohol who would be most resistant to changes in price or availability. Furthermore, societies or ethnic groups with relatively low drinking rates may have relatively high rates of abuse, and vice versa.

Assuming a tax hike did reduce alcohol problems, it would not necessarily be justified even on utilitarian grounds. Since moderate drinkers far outnumber alcoholics, their foregone pleasure might well outweigh the benefits of less alcohol abuse. As in the case of smoking, the public health paradigm simply ignores this issue.

Drug Abuse. In the early 1970s a debate raged in academic journals about the merits of studying illegal drug use as if it were an epidemic. Critics of this approach noted that illegal drug use is not caught like a virus; it is volitional behavior. Proponents of the disease model said this didn't matter.

Community Health explains: "If drug abuse is seen as a practice that is transmitted from one person to another, it may be considered for operational purposes as a contagious illness. This approach makes it possible to apply to its study the methods and terminology used in the epidemiology of infectious diseases. In the epidemiological model the infectious agent is heroin, the host and reservoir are both man, and the vector is the drug-using peer.... The disease presents all the well-known characteristics of epidemics, including rapid spread, clear geographic bounds, and certain age groups and strata of the population being more affected than others."

But these criteria apply to many phenomena that we do not treat as epidemics, including clothing fashions, recreational trends, rumors, jokes, and political ideas. Clearly, not everything that spreads from person to person is an epidemic.

Presumably, an epidemic has to be something bad. Oddly, however, *bad* is defined not by the individuals involved but by the epidemiologist. A happy, productive, well-adjusted user of illegal drugs is still sick, still part of an epidemic, even though he doesn't realize it. Alternatively, as former drug czar William Bennett has argued, the moderate drug user is an asymptomatic carrier—a Typhoid Mary—spreading misery to others by setting a bad example, even though he feels fine. (Indeed, by doing well while doing drugs, he is a more serious threat in this regard than the addict in the gutter.) Either way, the user has to be isolated and cured, whether he likes it or not.

To be fair, it should be noted that many public health specialists do not toe the official government line, which defines any use of illegal drugs as abuse. They often acknowledge that prohibition has side effects and that the distinctions made by the law do not necessarily correspond with the objective hazards of various drugs. Defining drug use as a public health problem, rather than a crime, they tend to support "harm reduction" measures such as legal availability of syringes and needles, the use of medical marijuana, and "treatment" as an alternative to prison.

Still, the medical model has coercive implications, especially if "denial" is understood as one component of the "disease." Smolensky says law enforcement agencies should "ignore the user, since his is a medical problem which requires prevention, therapy, or rehabilitation, and is not a criminal act." This begs the question of what happens when the user resists "prevention, therapy, or rehabilitation."

Obesity. If smoking, alcohol abuse, and illegal drug use can be diseases, surely obesity can. It carries substantial health risks, and people who are fat generally don't want to be. They find it difficult to lose weight, and when they do succeed they often relapse. When deprived of food, they suffer strong cravings and other withdrawal symptoms.

Recently, the "epidemic of obesity" has been trumpeted repeatedly on the front page of *The New York Times*. The first story, which appeared in July 1994, was prompted by a study from the National Center for Health Statistics that found the share of American adults who are overweight increased from a quarter to a third between 1980 and 1991. "The government is not doing enough," complained Assistant Secretary of Health Philip R. Lee. "We don't have a coherent, across-the-board policy." The second story, published last September, reported on a *New England Journal of Medicine* study that found gaining as little as 11 to 18 pounds was associated with a higher risk of heart disease—or, as the headline on the jump page put it, "Even Moderate Weight Gains Can Be Deadly." The study attributed 300,000 deaths a year to obesity, including a third of cancer deaths and most deaths from cardiovascular disease. The lead researcher, JoAnn E. Manson, said, "It won't be long before obesity surpasses cigarette smoking as a cause of death in this country."

If, as Assistant Secretary Lee recommends, the government decides to do more about obesity—the second most important preventable cause of death in this country (soon to be the first)— what would "a coherent, across-the-board policy" look like? As early as June 1975, in its *Forward Plan for Health*, the U.S. Public Health Service was suggesting "strong regulations to control the advertisement of food products, especially those of high sugar content or little nutritional value." But surely we can do better than that. A tax on high-fat foods would help cover the cost of obesity-related illness and disability, while deterring overconsumption of ice cream and steak. Of course, such a tax would be paid by the lean as well as the overweight. It might be more fair and efficient to tax people for every pound over their ideal weight. Such a market-based system would make the obese realize the costs they impose on society and give them an incentive to slim down. Last year I suggested this plan in *National Review,* and the magazine received a couple of letters from readers who took it seriously. Fortunately, they were outraged; but I can't shake the thought that somewhere in Washington a public health bureaucrat read the item and said, "Hmmm...."

Violence. In *Sentinel for Health: A History of the Centers for Disease Control*, Elizabeth W. Etheridge notes that CDC Director William Foege encountered resistance when he pushed the boundaries of public health in the late 1970s. "Of all the areas," she writes, "violence was the most controversial and the one the public health community found hardest to accept." The opposition to this idea is not surprising. Even people who are willing to redefine risky habits as diseases may be troubled by the denial of individual responsibility implicit in treating assault and murder like an outbreak of influenza.

Focusing on guns is one way of obscuring the moral issues raised by the public health approach to violence. As Chicago pediatrician Katherine Cristoffel, founder of the HELP (Handgun Epidemic Lowering Plan) Network, explained in a 1994 *American Medical News* article: "Gun violence should be treated like polio and tuberculosis and every other epidemic. Guns are a virus that must be eradicated." She drew a parallel with the campaign against smoking: "It is possible to ban guns. There's a precedent in cigarette smoking. Before the surgeon general's report, it was a moral issue, a personal rights issue. But once it was declared a public health issue, there was a dramatic change.... Get rid of cigarettes, get rid of secondhand smoke, and you get rid of lung disease. It's the same with guns. Get rid of the guns, get rid of the bullets, and you get rid of the deaths."

This is not merely the opinion of a few wild-eyed activists. The public health establishment has consistently endorsed stricter gun control, treating firearms as a "risk factor," a "pathogen," a "social ill" to be minimized or eliminated. According to *Healthy People*, the 1979 surgeon general's report, "Measures that could reduce risk of firearm deaths and injuries range from encouraging safer storage and use to a ban on private ownership. Evidence from England suggests that prohibiting possession of handguns would reduce the number of deaths and injuries, particularly those unrelated to criminal assaults." In 1979 the CDC endorsed the goal of reducing the number of privately owned handguns, with an initial target of a 25 percent decrease by 2000. In 1992 C. Everett Koop declared violence "a public health emergency" and, in response, endorsed a national licensing system for gun owners.

Public health research on firearms, much of it funded by the CDC, has attracted a great deal of publicity, generating many of the factoids that supporters of gun control are fond of citing. Consider the claim that "a gun in the home is 43 times as likely to kill a family member as to be used in self-defense." This is based on a 1986 study by Arthur L. Kellermann and Donald T. Reay published in the *New England Journal of Medicine*. Examining gunshot deaths in King County, Washington, from 1978 to 1983, Kellermann and Reay found that, of 398 people killed in the home where the gun was kept, only two were intruders shot while trying to get in. "We noted 43 suicides, criminal homicides, or accidental gunshot deaths involving a gun kept in the home for every case of homicide for self-protection," they wrote. It's not a good idea, they suggested, to keep a gun at home.

But since Kellermann and Reay considered only cases resulting in death, which surveys indicate are a tiny percentage of defensive gun uses, this conclusion does not follow at all. "Mortality studies such as ours do not include cases in which burglars or intruders are wounded or frightened away by the use or display of a firearm," they conceded. "Cases in which would-be intruders may have purposely avoided a house known to be armed are also not identified." By leaving out such cases, Kellermann and Reay excluded almost all of the lives saved, injuries avoided, and property protected by keeping a gun in the home.

In contrast with the criminological literature, where scholars on both sides of the issue carry on a lively debate, studies published in the *New England Journal of Medicine, JAMA,* and other medical or public health journals almost invariably condemn gun ownership and advocate stricter gun control. As with the studies of tobacco advertising, the public health researchers rarely cite scholars from other disciplines, preferring to stay within a field where almost everyone agrees that guns are bad.

* * *

The public health research on gun ownership, like the research on other kinds of "unhealthy" behavior, is driven by the expectation that people will change their ways once they realize the risks they are taking. *Healthy People* notes that "formidable obstacles" stand in the way of improved public health, "Prominent among them are individual attitudes toward the changes necessary for better health," it says. "Though opinion polls note greater interest in healthier lifestyles, many people remain apathetic and unmotivated.... Some consider activities to promote health moralistic rather than scientific; still others are wary of measures which they feel may infringe on personal liberties.

However, *the scientific basis for suggested measures has grown so compelling, it is likely that such biases will begin to shift."* (Emphasis added.) In other words, only those ignorant of the scientific evidence could possibly oppose the public health agenda.

This assumption is central to the public health mentality. Back in 1879, John S. Billings stated it quite candidly: "By some writers, as Wilhelm von Humboldt and John Stuart Mill, it is denied that the State should directly attempt to improve the physical welfare of its citizens, on the ground that such interference will probably do more harm than good. But all admit that the State should extend special protection to those who are incapable of judging their own best interests, or of taking care of themselves, such as the insane, persons of feeble intellect, or children; and we have seen that in sanitary matters the public at large are thus incompetent."

Billings was defending traditional public health measures aimed at preventing the spread of infectious diseases and controlling health hazards such as rotting animal carcasses. It is reasonable to expect that such measures will be welcomed by the intended beneficiaries, once they understand the aim. The same cannot be said of public health's new targets. Even when they know about the relevant hazards (and assuming the information is accurate), many people will continue to smoke, drink, take illegal drugs, eat fatty foods, buy guns, speed, eschew seat belts and motorcycle helmets, and otherwise behave in ways frowned upon by the public health establishment. This is not because they misunderstand; it's because, for the sake of pleasure, utility, or convenience, they are prepared to accept the risks. When public health experts assume that these decisions are wrong, they do indeed treat adults like incompetent children.

One such expert, writing in the *New England Journal of Medicine* 20 years ago, declared, "It is a crime to commit suicide quickly. However, to kill oneself slowly by means of an unhealthy life style is readily condoned and even encouraged." The article prompted a response from Robert F. Meenan, a professor at the University of California School of Medicine in San Francisco, who observed: "Health professionals are trained to supply the individual with medical facts and opinions. However, they have no personal attributes, knowledge, or training that qualifies them to dictate the preferences of others. Nevertheless, doctors generally assume that the high priority that they place on health should be shared by others. They find it hard to accept that some people may opt for a brief, intense existence full of unhealthy practices. Such individuals are pejoratively labeled 'noncompliant' and pressures are applied on them to reorder their priorities."

* * *

More than 75 years ago, H. L. Mencken complained about this tendency to impose a moral value—the paramount importance of health—in the guise of medical science. "Hygiene is the corruption of medicine by morality," he wrote in 1919. "It is impossible to find a hygienist who does not debase his theory of the healthful with a theory of the virtuous." The public health establishment seeks government power to impose its vision of virtue on the rest of America.

And public health doctrine admits no limits. *Principles of Community Health* tells us that "the most widely accepted definition of individual health is that of the World Health Organization: 'Health is a state of complete physical, mental, and social well-being and not merely the absence of disease or infirmity.' " A government empowered to maximize "health" is a totalitarian government.

In response to such concerns, the public health establishment argues that government intervention is justified because individual decisions about risk affect other people. "Motorcyclists often contend that helmet laws infringe on personal liberties," notes *Healthy People*, "and opponents of mandatory laws argue that since other people usually are not endangered, the individual motorcyclist should be allowed personal responsibility for risk. But the high cost of disabling and fatal injuries, the burden on families, and the demands on medical care resources are borne by society as a whole." This familiar line of reasoning implies that all resources—including not just taxpayer-funded welfare and health care but private savings, insurance coverage, and charity—are part of a common pool owned by "society as a whole" and guarded by the government. Similarly, "social cost" calculations for tobacco and alcohol count medical expenses, regardless of who pays them or under what circumstances, and "lost productivity," as if every individual owes a full lifetime of income (at the highest possible wage?) to "society as a whole."

As Faith T. Fitzgerald, a professor at the University of California, Davis, Medical Center, writes in the *New England Journal of Medicine*: "Both health care providers and the commonwealth now have a vested interest in certain forms of behavior, previously considered a person's private business, if the behavior impairs a person's 'health.' Certain failures of self-care have become, in a sense, crimes against society, because society has to pay for their consequences. ... In effect, we have said that people owe it to society to stop misbehaving, and we use illness as evidence of misbehavior."

Most public health practitioners would presumably recoil at the full implications of the argument that government should override individual decisions affecting health because such decisions have an impact on "society as a whole." They are no doubt surprised and offended to be called "health fascists," when their goal is to extend and improve people's lives. But some defenders of the public health movement recognize that its aims are fundamentally collectivist and cannot be reconciled with the American tradition of limited government. In 1975 Dan E. Beauchamp, then an assistant professor of public health at the University of North Carolina and currently a professor in the School of Public Health at the State University of New York at Albany, presented a paper at the annual meeting of the American Public Health Association in which he argued that "the radical individualism inherent in the market model" is the biggest obstacle to improving public health.

"The historic dream of public health that preventable death and disability ought to be minimized is a dream of social justice," Beauchamp said. "We are far from recognizing the principle that death and disability are collective problems and that all persons are entitled to health protection." He rejected "the ultimately arbitrary distinction between voluntary and involuntary hazards" and complained that "the primary duty to avert disease and injury still rests with the individual." He called upon public health practitioners to challenge "the powerful sway market-justice holds over our imagination, granting fundamental freedom to all individuals to be left alone." Of all the risk factors for disease and injury, freedom may be the most important.

POSTSCRIPT

Should Healthy Behavior Be Mandated?

Although no one claims that smoking and high fat diets are safe and unrelated to disease, an overemphasis on disease prevention through individual health behaviors may be misused and exaggerated. Professors Lenn and Madeleine Goodman indicate agreement in their article "Prevention—How Misuse of a Concept Undercuts Its Worth," *Hastings Center Report* (April 1986). The Goodmans feel that shifting the responsibility of health and well-being onto the individual relieves the government and health care industry of their responsibility to provide education, a clean environment, research into disease causes, and adequate health care for everyone. They also believe that a healthy lifestyle does not guarantee good health and longevity. In "Pleasure & Its Perils," *National Review* (May 1, 1995), physician Perr Skrabanek agrees. In "A Matter of Taste," *National Review* (May 1, 1995), editor Jacob Sullum maintains that zealots such as Michael Jacobson attempt to interfere in personal food and health habits.

Although a good diet and exercise are important to help prevent disease, they clearly do not guarantee health. Many other unmodifiable risk factors can also produce disease. Cardiologist Henry Solomon, in *The Exercise Myth* (Harcourt Brace Jovanovich, 1984), argues that even exercise will not necessarily prevent diseases or improve longevity. Solomon believes that heredity is as much responsible for a long life as are healthy behaviors. Thomas Moore makes the same point with regard to cholesterol reduction in *Heart Failure* (Random House, 1989). He claims that diet does not reduce serum cholesterol for many people and that heredity is as important as lifestyle in maintaining and controlling cholesterol. These writers argue that disease prevention via a healthy lifestyle may not be a valid way to maintain wellness.

Although it is clear that we cannot always keep ourselves well via healthy behaviors, many writers claim that individuals, not doctors or government, can maintain health. Donald Ardell, in *High Level Wellness* (Ten Speed Press, 1986), maintains that individuals can join the ranks of those who look to themselves rather than to their physicians for the maintenance of their health. He claims that what an individual can do for his or her own benefit is enormous; what medicine can do is quite limited. Other articles related to individual health behaviors and wellness include "The Progressive: Michael Jacobson," *The Progressive* (September 1994); "Managing Stress and Living Longer," *USA Today Magazine* (May 1990); "Pressure Treatment: How Exercise Can Help You Control Your Blood Pressure," *Walking* (June 1992); and "Are We Meeting Our Goals for Health?" *New Choice* (March 1994).

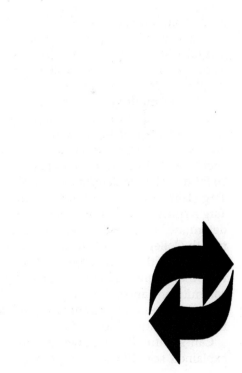

ISSUE 6

Can Spirituality Overcome Disease?

YES: Herbert Benson and Marg Stark, from *Timeless Healing: The Power and Biology of Belief* (Scribner, 1996)

NO: William B. Lindley, from "Prayer and Healing," *Truth Seeker* (vol. 122, no. 2, 1995)

ISSUE SUMMARY

YES: Herbert Benson, associate professor of medicine at Harvard Medical School, and journalist Marg Stark contend that faith and spirituality will enhance and prolong life.

NO: William B. Lindley, associate editor of *Truth Seeker*, counters that there is no scientific way to determine that spirituality can heal.

Practitioners of holistic medicine believe that people must be responsible for their own health by practicing healthy behaviors and maintaining positive attitudes instead of relying on health providers. They also believe that physical disease has both behavioral, psychological, and spiritual components. These spiritual components can be explained by the relationship between beliefs, mental attitude, and the immune system. Until recently, few studies existed to prove a relationship between spirituality—a feeling of connectedness to the greater Self—and health.

Much of modern medicine has spent the past century ridding itself of mysticism and relying on science. Twenty years ago, no legitimate physician would have dared to study the effects of spirituality on disease. Recently, however, at the California Pacific Medical Center in San Francisco, Dr. Elisabeth Targ, clinical director of psychosocial oncology research, has recruited 20 faith healers to determine if prayer can affect the outcome of disease. Dr. Targ claims that her preliminary results are encouraging. In addition to Dr. Targ's study, other research has shown that religion and spirituality can help determine health and well-being. According to a 1995 investigation at Dartmouth College, one of the strongest predictors of success after open-heart surgery was the level of comfort patients derived from religion and spirituality. Other recent studies have linked health with church attendance, religious commitment, and spirituality. There are, however, other studies that have not been as successful; a recent one involving the effects of prayer on alcoholics found no relationship.

Can spirituality or prayer in relation to health and healing actually be explained scientifically? Prayer or a sense of spirituality may function in a similar manner as stress management or relaxation. Spirituality or prayer may cause the release of hormones that help lower blood pressure or produce other benefits. Though science may never be able to exactly determine the benefits of spirituality, the fact is it does appear to help some people.

In the following selections, Herbert Benson and Marg Stark believe that spirituality can have a significant influence over the body. William B. Lindley argues that people do not become ill because their mental states, psyches, or attitudes negatively affect their biological systems.

YES

Herbert Benson and Marg Stark

TIMELESS HEALING: THE POWER AND BIOLOGY OF BELIEF

At one time or another, I'm sure nearly everyone experiences extraordinary and magical events, the converging of time and circumstance so logic-defiant that one cannot help but feel these events were divinely directed. It could be a chance reunion with a long-lost friend, a life change that comes at precisely the time you need it, or an image you see in a cloud formation. It could be a clergyperson's sermon that seems eerily relevant to the problems you've been facing, something as dramatic as hearing a voice speak to you inspirationally or as quiet as a bliss that envelops you suddenly. Whatever the form, the more the incident means to us, the more we attach sacred status to it in our lives. We shake our heads, asking, "What are the chances?" all the while feeling a profound reverberation within that perhaps life is not random, that perhaps these are tangible signs that a mystical force contours our life.

But it's possible that the reverberation you feel within when an experience you deem magical or spiritual occurs may not be just emotional but physical as well. Not only did my research—and that of my colleagues—reveal that 25% of people feel more spiritual as the result of the elicitation of the relaxation response, but it showed that those same people have fewer medical symptoms than do those who reported no increase in spirituality from the elicitation.

I decided to call the combined force of these internal influences the *faith factor*—remembered wellness and the elicitation of the relaxation response. But it became clear that a person's religious convictions or life philosophy enhanced the average effects of the relaxation response in three ways: (1) People who chose an appropriate focus, that which drew upon their deepest philosophic or religious convictions, were more apt to adhere to the elicitation routine, looking forward to it and enjoying it; (2) affirmative beliefs of any kind brought forth remembered wellness, reviving top-down, nerve-cell firing patterns in the brain that were associated with wellness; (3) when present, faith in an eternal or life-transcending force seemed to make the fullest use of remembered wellness because it is a supremely soothing belief, disconnecting unhealthy logic and worries.

I already knew that eliciting the relaxation response could "disconnect" everyday thoughts and worries, calming people's bodies and minds more quickly and to a degree otherwise unachievable. It appeared that beliefs added to the response transported the mind/body even more dramatically, quieting worries and fears significantly better than the relaxation response alone. And I speculated that religious faith was more influential than other affirmative beliefs.

I want to emphasize that the benefits of the faith factor are not the exclusive domain of the devout. People don't have to have a professed belief in God to reap the psychological and physical rewards of the faith factor. With lead investigator Dr. Jared D. Kass, a professor at Lesley College Graduate School of Arts and Sciences in Cambridge, MA, my colleagues and I developed a questionnaire to quantify and describe the spiritual feelings that accompanied the relaxation response, to document their frequency and potential health effects.

Based on the survey responses, we calculated "spirituality scores." But because virtually all of our survey respondents reported a "belief in God," this statement could not be used to differentiate people. It was the more amorphous feeling of spirituality that could be linked to better psychological and physical well-being. However, there is one group that does seem more likely to have spiritual encounters. Indeed, women had higher spirituality scores than men, for reasons we don't yet understand.

As subjective as remembered wellness is, there are some definitive things I can say about incorporating healing beliefs and faith into your life. These are some of the principles and practical lessons I've drawn from my long medical quest for lasting truths. I hope they prove helpful to you:

Let Faith, the Ultimate Belief, Heal You. According to medical research, faith in God is good for us, and this benefit is not exclusive to one denomination or theology. You can believe in God in a quiet, introspective way or declare your convictions out loud to the world—either way, you'll still reap the physiologic rewards.

For many reasons, religious activity and churchgoing are also healthy. Religious groups encourage all kinds of health-affirming activities—fellowship and socializing perhaps first among them, but also prayer, volunteerism, familiar rituals and music. Prayer, in particular, appears to be therapeutic, the specifics of which science will continue to explore.

Trust Your Instincts More Often. People describe the process of finding out what is important to them, of tapping into their beliefs, in very different ways, sometimes calling it "soul-searching," "mulling it over," "listening to one's heart," "going inside of one's self," "praying," or "sleeping on it." Some people act on instincts or common sense; others find a truth or intuition emerges slowly. But most people know when something "feels right." Most people have a kind of internal radar that occasionally calls out to them.

The next time you're faced with a major decision, medical or otherwise, ask yourself, "What would I do if the choice were entirely up to me?" I'm not suggesting that you make decisions based on this factor alone, but at least let belief be a player. Honor your convictions and perceptions enough to make them a part of a hearty intellectual argument.

Let your instincts guide you. Follow them up with research. Put your health in good, trustworthy hands. Let your health have time to correct itself. Invest remembered wellness and a reasonable application of self-care, medications and surgery for maximum health returns.

Practice and Apply Self-Care Regularly. Work with your doctor, and with unconventional practitioners if you so choose, to learn self-care habits. I consider self-care anything an individual can do, independent of doctors or healers, to enhance his or her health. This includes mind/body reactions such as remembered wellness, the relaxation response and the faith factor. It also embraces good nutrition, exercise and other means of stress management.

I use the term "self-care" because it puts the onus on you, it shifts the emphasis from your role as passive patient to active participant—a shift that medicine has not always encouraged. However, I caution against becoming self-absorbed in self-care. Don't become fixated on your health or on the avoidance of aging, illness or death. Make your daily elicitation of the relaxation response, your jog or your salad at lunch a no-brainer, which you do not analyze or overthink. Simply delight in the event itself.

It's almost always valuable to seek the assistance of your physician to determine the difference between a condition that will benefit from self-care exclusively and one that requires drugs or procedures to treat. Learning about your body is an evolutionary process. You'll work toward a more independent attitude. Become acquainted with the warning signs of heart attacks, strokes, cancer and other life-threatening diseases. Over time, you'll develop a sense of what symptoms are important—those that are extreme or don't go away.

How influential can a coordinated contingent of self-care habits be? We honestly don't know, but *Prevention* advisor Dean Ornish, MD, president of the Preventive Medicine Research Institute in Sausalito, CA, found that heart disease could not only be relieved but reversed when patients made significant changes in diet, exercise and stress management. Our two programs will soon be compared in a groundbreaking research project sponsored by the Commonwealth of Massachusetts Group Insurance Commission and the John Hancock Insurance Company. In this comparison, patients with heart disease will be divided between our two clinics in hopes that we can gauge the adherence to and results of various self-care components and other treatments.

Beware of People with All the Answers. Be careful of any physician, nontraditional healer, spiritual guide, mind/body guru, or any adviser who claims to have all the answers or wants others to think so. Besides love and sex, writers and lecturers today take up few topics with as much evangelistic zeal as health and spirituality. It is no small task shielding these very personal matters from unhealthy speculation and overanalysis, but start with tuning out overly confident or all-knowing mentors and guides. Value your emotions and intuitions the same way your brain does; don't let someone manipulate your wiring for his or her gain.

Mind/body medicine should remind us of the precious nature of our minds, and of the importance of critiquing the messages we allow to become actualized in our brains/bodies.

Whether or not you believe in God, I believe that we are all wired to crave meaning in life, to assign profound power and sacredness to human experiences, and sometimes even to lend "god" status or "godliness" to humans and human endeavors. Be wary of this tendency, because it may rob spiritual life of its grandeur and of the wonderful transcendent qualities that cannot be accessed entirely by human intellect, and because it makes us very susceptible to human manipulation. Not only is your body a temple, but your mind is an architect, busy transforming the ideas you feed it. Protect it from those who exploit the power of remembered wellness for personal gain.

Remember that the 'Nocebo' is Equally Powerful. Unfortunately, remembered wellness has a flip side. It can have negative side effects, called the *nocebo* (as opposed to placebo). Our agitated minds may inappropriately trigger the fight-or-flight response in the body. Similarly, automatic negative thoughts, bad moods and compulsive worrying eventually take up physical residence in our bodies. Extreme examples of the nocebo effect include voodoo death, belief-engendered death, mass psychogenic illness, false memories and "memories" of alien abductions. People who dwell on worst-case scenarios, who exaggerate risks, or who project doubt and undue worry keep the nocebo effect busy in their physiologies. They signal their brains to send help when no physical sickness is present, persuading the body to get sick when there is no biologic reason sickness should occur.

Remember that Immortality is Impossible. While it's healthy to listen to your heart, it's also harmful to deny or duck the truth. No one lives forever. No matter how well-versed you become in mind/body medicine, no matter how far medical progress may be able to set back the clock, death is, like illness and pain, an unfortunate but natural fact of life.

I must sound as if I'm talking in circles, first telling you not to let a diagnosis define you, then warning you not to fall prey to denial. Nonetheless, some lecturers and New Age entrepreneurs imply that all disease is curable and that we can avoid death and aging if we only believe. These salespeople do great harm to people by fostering guilt, and they damage the field of mind/body medicine, which is legitimately trying to establish its findings and change the way Western medicine is practiced. No evidence exists that death can be denied its eventual toll.

Indeed, fear of death can bring out the worst in people, but the realization that death is an inevitable, natural occurrence can also propel healthy, impassioned living.

Living well, exercising and eating appropriately, seeing doctors when you need to but not overrelying on the medical system—these are all proven buffers against disease and illness.

Believe in Something Good. Even though we do not necessarily need all the pills and procedures that conventional medicine and unconventional medicine give us, these medicinal symbols retain an aura of effectiveness and often appease our desire for action. While we must learn to use medicine more appropriately for the conditions it can help, and to wean ourselves from excessive spending on unnecessary therapies, we'll often need some catalysts for belief, even if belief is really the healer.

So remember the vigor from the time you felt healthiest in your life. Remember the blessing your mother said to you before you left for school, the smell of incense at church, or the tranquility you felt picking up stones from the beach on Cape Cod. Remember the time the penicillin vanquished your ear infection, or the time the surgeon removed the splinter from deep in your foot and your pain immediately ceased. Remember how full-throated you sang in the choir or how long you stayed on the dance floor of a nightclub. Remember the doctor who really cared about you or the chaplain who prayed with you in the hospital. Remember the way you felt when you made love to your husband or wife, and the way you felt when your daughter or son was born.

Then let go, and believe. You've read all about your physiology, you've surrounded yourself with good caregivers who help you take a moderate, balanced approach to your health and health care. Now it's time to enjoy your endowment, this wiring for faith that makes the power of remembered wellness so enduring.

Believe in something good if you can. Or even better, believe in something better than anything you can fathom. Because for us mortals, this is very profound medicine.

NO

William B. Lindley

PRAYER AND HEALING

I was raised in Christian Science. That gives me somewhat of an inside perspective on prayer and healing. However, the Christian Science experience is far from typical. The "Scientific Statement of Being" begins: "There is no life, truth, intelligence nor substance in matter." Most Christians who offer prayers of petition for the healing of an illness believe that their bodies are real and the illness is real, but they want supernatural intervention, the sort of thing Jesus is reported to have done in the gospels. Christian Science, interpreting Jesus' work quite differently insists that reality lies elsewhere. The analogue to prayer is "knowing the truth." Christian Science insists that miracles are not "supernatural, but divinely natural."

As I grew up and matter made more sense to me, I drifted away from Christian Science. Then I began hearing about natural, nonmiraculous analogues to what I had been taught: psychosomatic diseases and cures, the placebo effect, and, more recently, the neurochemical connections between mood and the immune system. These, along with "spontaneous remission" of cancers, were attempts to explain "miracles" without invoking the supernatural or the paranormal. (Note that "spontaneous" (natural), and "God did it" (supernatural), are "explanations" that explain nothing. There's no "how.") Believers in miracles—evangelicals, Christian Scientists, miscellaneous New Agers, and so forth—continue as before.

PRAYER AND HEALING

Healing Words by Larry Dossey, M.D., is a book devoted to prayer and healing, and its author believes firmly that prayer (communication with "the Absolute") brings about beneficial effects that are real and substantial and supernatural or paranormal in character. However, when he raises the question, "What is prayer?", the answer is so far-ranging that all sorts of things that would not ordinarily be considered prayer are included. He rejects the Christian concept of prayer! Of course he doesn't use such strong language as "reject," preferring slippery words like "redefine," tentative" and "reevaluate." He has a chart contrasting the "traditional Western model" with the "modern" model of prayer. Probably over 95% of the prayers for healing that are made in the United States would be of the "old" model, which Dossey considers obsolete. Interestingly enough, Christian Science prayer would fall under the 5% that he would approve of.

Even though Dossey seems to think little of traditional prayer, his citations of many experiments that allegedly demonstrate the efficacy of prayer do not indicate whether the style of prayer was traditional or otherwise. (He clearly expresses his opinion that all kinds work, some better than others.) The experiments are broken down into various categories of what was prayed over—barley seeds(!), mice, people, etc.—but not into categories of what kind of prayer was made.

Sometimes Dossey seems to be unaware of the implications of what he says. For example, he quotes psychologist Lawrence LeShan to the effect that healing through prayer is effective in perhaps 15 to 20% of cases and that nobody can tell in advance which cases will have happy outcomes. Somewhat disheartened by this, Dossey goes on to claim that prayer works anyway. Then he mentions the "bizarre," "perverted" use of prayer by high school football teams in Texas, where, of course, they offer up highly unsportsmanlike prayers for victory. Such prayers obviously "work" 50% of the time. (We might cut this to 48% or so for tie games.) Thus one can conclude that prayer for victory in football is three times as efficacious as prayer for healing!

THE PROBLEMS OF PRAYER

Dossey wisely reminds us that if all prayers for healing led to success, population growth would be even more catastrophic than it is; 100% success rates for other kinds of prayer could have other horrible long-term effects. (Billy Graham put it a little differently: "God answers all prayers; sometimes the answer is 'no.'") However, once this is admitted—and note that it flatly contradicts Jesus' promise in Matthew 7:7,8: "Ask, and it will be given you; search, and you will find; knock, and the door will be opened for you. For everyone who asks receives, and everyone who searches finds, and for everyone who knocks, the door will be opened"—the result is indistinguishable from that of no prayer at all.

Another problem is the intent of the person praying. Others who have faced the incoherent attempts to define prayer have said that the essence of prayer, whether there be a Supreme Being or not, is that the person praying must intend, or want, or be praying for, a particular happy ending to the current crisis. However, Dossey rejects the concept of intent. He states: "For reasons I shall discuss later, never once did I pray for specific outcomes—for cancers to go away, for heart attacks to be healed, for diabetes to vanish." He reports on an interesting group, Spindrift, that provides many "proofs" that prayer works. This group had a number of Christian Scientists in it. (One was a Christian Science practitioner whose "license" was revoked after The First Church of Christ, Scientist found out what he was up to.) Spindrift took up the question of directed vs. undirected prayer, and found that the undirected prayer worked somewhat better. Most of the other experiments by other groups, for example, with barley seeds, were directed—the intent to have the seeds flourish was in the minds of the people who prayed over them.

PRAYER EXPERIMENTS

Let's take a closer look at those experiments. There is a long list of them. The compiler is Daniel J. Benor, M.D. He published his survey in the journal *Complementary Medical Research* in 1990. The activity is called "spiritual healing," and this is defined as "the intentional influence of one or more people upon another living system without utilizing known physical means of intervention." (Note how this differs from the Spindrift effort cited above and from Dossey's preference for nondirected prayer.) Of 131 trials, five involved water, with three showing "significant results," but what was being prayed for in the water cases is not mentioned. There were ten trials of "enzymes," including trypsin, dopamine, and noradrenaline. (Are these enzymes? I think not.) There were seven trials on fungi and yeasts, with some prayers being for, some against, the prosperous growth of the culture. Similarly for the ten trials on bacteria, mainly E. coli and salmonella. Cells in vitro (tube or glass dish) were prayed over, including four trials on snail pacemaker cells. There were 19 trials on plants and seeds, including five on the above-mentioned barley seeds. Three of these involved different kinds of person praying: one with neurotic depression, one with psychotic depression, and one with a green thumb. As you might guess, the last showed the strongest beneficial effect. Other plants and seeds prayed over include: rye grass, wheat seeds, radish seeds, mung beans, potatoes and corn. The prayer trials on animals include 14 on anesthetized mice, with a variety of experimental conditions and effects sought. Humans were also prayed over for a total of 38 of the 131 trials. Some of the conditions prayed over are obviously psychosomatic, some less so. Clearly there is an enthusiastic "spiritual healing research" community doing many things we wouldn't ordinarily think of.

Something I was unable to find in all this is any breakdown by religion of the person praying. Christians would consider it vital to ask whether the words "In Jesus' name we pray, amen" were spoken. If they weren't, the Christians would be extremely skeptical of the efficacy of the prayers. If they were confronted by overwhelming evidence that a non-Christian prayer was highly effective, they would suspect Satanism and look for evidence of it. Similarly perhaps for Muslims. Catholics might accept evidence of efficacy of prayers invoking the Trinity while being skeptical of those with Protestant prayer tags. Regrettably, the 131 trials provide us with no information along these lines

Another missing factor that I regret is a detailed skeptical review of the experimental methodology of some of the more impressive trials. The Committee for the Scientific Investigation of Claims of the Paranormal seems to be silent in this area. While they have offered some criticism of Therapeutic Touch, they seem to be silent on the question of religious prayer healing, except in "revivals," where some noteworthy frauds have been exposed. This is part of a pattern. Most of the subjects discussed in the *Skeptical Inquirer* are New Age phenomena, such as crop circles, UFOs, pyramid power, astrology, and so on. CSICOP seems to be leaving Christianity alone, at least for the time being. Dossey's book cries for skeptical attention. As in the other cases, such attention would have to be very painstaking, time-consuming, and expensive.

Meanwhile, prayers for healing continue, some effectively utilizing known psychosomatic processes, others producing remarkable placebo effects (the same thing, except that we don't know what's happening), and many more where supernatural claims are made, as well as those disappointing cases where God seems to have said "no."

POSTSCRIPT

Can Spirituality Overcome Disease?

Can we influence the course of illness? Can emotions, stress management, and prayer prevent or cure disease? In a telephone poll of 1,004 Americans conducted by TIME/CNN in June 1996, 82 percent believed in the healing power of personal prayer. Three-fourths felt that praying for someone else could help cure their illness. Interestingly, fewer than two-thirds of doctors say they believe in God. Dr. Herbert Benson, who developed the "relaxation response," thinks there is a strong link between religious commitment and good health. He believes that people do not have to have a professed belief in God to reap the psychological and physical rewards of the "faith factor." Benson defined the faith factor as the combined force of the relaxation response and the placebo effect.

Dr. Bernard Siegel, writing in his bestseller *Love, Medicine and Miracles* (Harper & Row, 1986), claims that there are no "incurable diseases, only incurable people" and that illness is a personality flaw. In "Welcome to the Mind/Body Revolution," *Psychology Today* (July/August 1993) author Marc Barash further discusses how the mind and immune system influence each other. Journalist Susan Chollar claims that in treating cancer, "evidence grows that emotions can alter the course of the disease." See "Mind Over Cancer," *American Health* (November 1994).

In *You Don't Have to Die: Unraveling the AIDS Myth* (Burton Goldberg Group, 1994), a chapter entitled "Mind-Body Medicine" discusses the body's innate healing capabilities and the role of self-responsibility in the healing process. A long-term AIDS survivor who traveled the country interviewing other long-term survivors found that the one thing they all shared was the belief that AIDS was survivable. They all also accepted the reality of their diagnosis, but refused to see their condition as a death sentence.

Readings that address these issues include "The Greatest Story Never Told," *Utne Reader* (March/April 1997); "Commentary: Into the Heart of Healing," *Making the Rounds in Health, Faith and Ethics* (May 20, 1996); "Faith and Healing," *Time* (June 24, 1996); "Healing Power of Prayer," *Family Circle* (January 9, 1996); "The New Millennium," *Fate* (May 1995); and "Mysterious Remission," *Vogue* (March 1995), which discusses cancer remission.

On the Internet . . .

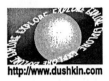

Nicotine and Tobacco Network

Kids and Smoking presents a directory of resources related to children and smoking issues from the University of Arizona. It offers information on pregnancy and tobacco use, tobacco use prevention, and tobacco use by teens. The site is arranged according to age group. It includes information on tobacco advertising and teens and specific no-smoking campaigns and links to other related sites. *http://www.ahsc.arizona.edu/nicnet/topkid.htm*

National Institute on Alcohol Abuse and Alcoholism

Offers an overview of the history of the organization as well as online publications and databases. *http://www.niaaa.nih.gov*

Action on Smoking and Health (ASH)

Describes ASH, an organization that is devoted to the problems of smoking and nonsmokers' rights and provides scientific, medical, legal, legislative, historical, and other information about smoking. Includes recent press releases, copies of the ASH newsletter, selections from the EPA's report on involuntary smoking and hyperlinks to smoking-related sites. *http://www.setinc.com/ash/ashhome.html*

Drug Education

Drug education page includes a set of materials with opinions on how to deal with the drug problems in our society. The site includes references from professional journals and links to other relevant sites. *http://www.magic.mb.ca/~lampi/new_drugs.html*

Internet Resources on Substance Abuse and Addiction

Posts a driectory of Web pages devoted to substance abuse and addiction, compiled by the Canadian Centre on Substance Abuse (CCSA) in Ottawa, Ontario. Provides Telnet access to several library catalogs and notes related listservers. Offers links to sites about AIDS, crime, fetal alcohol syndrome, gambling, impaired driving, mental health, self-help, tobacco, and treatment, *http://www.ccsa.ca/classed.htm*

PART 3

Substance Use and Abuse

While millions of Americans use and abuse drugs ranging from marijuana to alcohol and tobacco, experts continue to seek solutions for the related problems and to find causes of addiction. According to some reports, marijuana helps AIDS and cancer patients' symptoms and some people feel that this use of the drug should be legalized. Although excessive drinking is clearly associated with health problems, there are researchers who claim that moderate alcohol consumption may actually benefit health. Smoking has become an issue of personal rights as well as health. Nonsmokers claim that secondhand smoke is a hazard to their well-being. The issues in this section deal with the complex concerns about drugs in our society.

■ Is Secondhand Smoke a Proven Health Risk for Nonsmokers?

■ Should Moderate Use of Alcohol Be Recommended?

■ Is Marijuana Dangerous and Addictive?

ISSUE 7

Is Secondhand Smoke a Proven Health Risk for Nonsmokers?

YES: Editors of *Consumer Reports,* **from "Secondhand Smoke: Is It a Hazard?"** *Consumer Reports* (January 1995)

NO: Jacob Sullum, from "Just How Bad Is Secondhand Smoke?" *National Review* (May 16, 1994)

ISSUE SUMMARY

YES: The editors of *Consumer Reports* argue that there is sound scientific data proving that the health of nonsmokers suffers when they are forced to breathe tobacco smoke. They point out that many studies make a consistent case that secondhand smoke causes lung cancer and other illnesses.

NO: Editor and journalist Jacob Sullum argues that there is no evidence that secondhand smoking carries the dangers associated with actually smoking. He accuses the Environmental Protection Agency (EPA) of making inappropriate assumptions and manipulating data to arrive at a predetermined conclusion that is not accurate.

Smoking has become an established part of our culture. When cigarette manufacturing became a major industry at the turn of the century, the typical smoker was a middle-class working man. Beginning in the 1920s, however, cigarettes began to seem sophisticated and even fashionable, and women, too, started to smoke in increasing numbers. As advertising successfully penetrated the youth market and encouraged more and more young people to take up smoking, the number of smokers increased, and by 1964, 40 percent of the adult population smoked.

In 1964 the first major blow to smoking occurred: Then–surgeon general of the United States, Luther L. Terry, made his now-famous report positively linking smoking to lung cancer, heart disease, and other ailments. Other reports and stronger warnings on cigarette packs have contributed to the steady decline of smoking in the United States. In June 1997 the tobacco industry was dealt a new blow. Under a $368 billion agreement between the tobacco companies and state authorities, advertising figures like Joe Camel and the Marlboro Man will be gone; so will cigarette vending machines, tobacco billboard ads, and the sponsorship of sporting events by tobacco companies. Cigarette packs may soon feature even stronger warnings such as "Cigarettes cause cancer." The tobacco deal will also settle the pending

40 state lawsuits and 17 class-action suits to recoup the health care costs of smokers. Currently, despite all the health warnings, approximately 45 million Americans continue to smoke.

Although the health effects of cigarette smoking are well known, until 1981 the risks associated with breathing others' smoke, or *secondhand smoke*, were not as clear. A Japanese study completed during that year showed that nonsmoking women who were married to smokers had a higher risk of lung cancer than those who were married to nonsmokers. This study indicated that breathing in cigarette smoke on a daily basis is a significant risk factor for lung cancer. Since the publication of the Japanese study, secondhand smoke —also called *environmental tobacco smoke* or *passive smoke*—has been linked to numerous other diseases such as lung cancer, heart disease, asthma, and other upper respiratory diseases. The children of smokers are particularly vulnerable.

Based on the Japanese study and 30 other investigations, the EPA issued a report entitled *Respiratory Health Effects of Passive Smoking: Lung Cancer and Other Disorders* in the early 1990s, which "concluded that the widespread exposure to environmental tobacco smoke in the United States presents a serious and substantial public health impact."

As a result of these health risks, nonsmokers' complaints about smokers, and the EPA report, most states now restrict smoking in public places. In addition, smoking is banned on most domestic airplane flights and in many workplaces.

Although the nonsmoking majority may welcome these restrictions, there has been doubt cast as to the scientific validity of the research on secondhand smoke. John C. Luik, a senior associate of the Niagara Institute, claims that the substance of the EPA's report is flawed and that the agency only looked at studies involving smoking spouses and not workplace situations. Luik maintains that most of the studies involving secondhand smoke in the workplace have failed to find a statistically significant relationship between exposure to cigarette smoke and lung cancer among nonsmokers. Luik, in "Pandora's Box: The Dangers of Politically Corrupted Science for Democratic Public Policy," *Bostonia* (Winter 1993–1994), also argues that none of the studies used by the EPA, on the health risks of nonsmoking spouses living with a smoker, showed a strong relative risk for the nonsmokers.

In the following selections, the editors of *Consumer Reports* claim that the tobacco companies are doing exactly what they did with actual smoking: they are utilizing a small amount of scientific uncertainty along with a large amount of public relations to suggest that there is still a question as to whether or not passive smoking is harmful. The authors cite numerous well-designed studies that prove that exposure to others' smoke can cause lung cancer, heart disease, asthma, and bronchitis. Jacob Sullum agrees with Luik that public policy restricting smoking in public places is based on inaccurate data. He claims that the risks of inhaling secondhand smoke are overrated and inaccurate.

YES   Editors of *Consumer Reports*

SECONDHAND SMOKE: IS IT A HAZARD?

In the 1950's and 60's, as scientists piled up a mountain of evidence on the life-threatening health consequences of smoking, the tobacco industry mounted a fierce and sophisticated campaign to keep doubt alive in the public mind.

The effort ultimately flopped; even scientists funded by tobacco-industry money today concede that smoking is bad for you. But it did succeed in putting off that day of reckoning when everyone acknowledged the hazard. That delay bought many years of robust sales.

The industry is at it again, only this time the target is secondhand smoke. A review of the record shows that tobacco companies are doing exactly what they did with "firsthand" smoke: They're using a little bit of scientific uncertainty and a lot of public relations to suggest there is still a serious debate about the health hazards of breathing smoke from other people's cigarettes.

At one time, such a controversy was real. When we reported on the subject 10 years ago, we described the evidence as "sparse and often conflicting." That's no longer true. A number of studies make a consistent case that secondhand smoke, like firsthand smoke, causes lung cancer. Many reputable groups that have inspected the evidence have reached this conclusion, including the U.S. Surgeon General's office, the National Research Council, the National Institute of Occupational Safety and Health, the International Agency for Research on Cancer, and the U.S. Occupational Safety and Health Administration (OSHA).

Other studies have found strong links between passive smoking and a host of other ills, such as asthma and bronchitis in children. Furthermore, evidence is accumulating that secondhand smoke contributes to the development of heart disease.

Early in 1993, the U.S. Environmental Protection Agency [EPA], after a painstaking and wide-ranging scientific review, declared secondhand smoke a known—not just "probable," or "possible"—human carcinogen. The EPA estimated that such smoke is responsible for several thousand cases of lung cancer in U.S. nonsmokers each year. Passive smoke joins a select company of only about a dozen other environmental pollutants in this risk category.

For the $48-billion U.S. tobacco industry, the EPA decision has been the worst setback since 1964, when the Surgeon General first declared that smoking causes cancer.

The EPA decision added momentum to widespread efforts to limit or ban smoking in public or at work. It gave employers a reason to fear workers' compensation claims based on exposure to workplace smoke. Businesses and organizations ranging from Taco Bell to the U.S. military have already banned or restricted smoking in their facilities. Seventy percent of the nation's shopping malls are now smoke-free.

Several states, including California, Maryland, Utah, Vermont, and Washington, have proposed or enacted strict controls on workplace smoking. As this report went to press, OSHA was considering nationwide rules that would, in effect, ban smoking on the job except in specially ventilated areas. Pending in the courts are at least two lawsuits brought against tobacco companies by relatives of nonsmokers who died of lung cancer after long exposure to secondhand smoke at work.

All those developments have helped to turn smoking from a public activity to a practice increasingly indulged in private. What's more they have helped persuade many smokers to cut back or quit. The smoking rate has dropped significantly, from one in three adults in 1980 to one in four today, cutting deeply into the tobacco industry's domestic market.

The industry is fighting back. It has sued in Federal court in an effort to overturn the EPA's decision. It has spent millions to block or roll back state and local public-smoking restrictions. Its public-relations firms are creating bogus "grassroots" organizations as fronts for lobbying against smoking restrictions. (See "Public-Interest Pretenders," *Consumer Reports*, May 1994.)

In its most visible effort, a months-long national advertising campaign, the industry has attempted to spread doubt about the science behind the EPA decision and to recast the issue of secondhand smoke as one of individual rights versus an overzealous government agency.

THE EVIDENCE?

For years, researchers have accumulated information about the effects of the compounds in secondhand smoke. Cigarette smoke and tars condensed from it induce cancer in laboratory animals. The smoke causes genetic mutations in bacteria, another common test for carcinogenic potential. And several of its components are known or probable human carcinogens.

If scientists had only this animal and laboratory evidence to go on, secondhand smoke would still qualify as a "probable" or "possible" human carcinogen. But in addition, tobacco smoke is among a handful of substances—asbestos, vinyl chloride, and radon are others—for which abundant human evidence exists. That evidence comes from epidemiology, the study of disease patterns in human populations. It's the scientific field responsible for identifying all the know human carcinogens.

There are 33 published epidemiological studies of secondhand smoke, 13 of which were conducted in the U.S. Most used standard epidemiological technique: They looked at nonsmoking women who developed lung cancer, to see whether they were more likely to be married to smokers than were women who didn't get the disease. (Other researchers studied cancer rates in people exposed to smoke at work or from other family members; a few also studied husbands of women smokers.)

In all such studies, it is difficult to accurately measure every variable. Most of the smoking occurred decades ago, and the details can't be learned. Some women whose husbands didn't smoke might still have breathed smoke at work or with friends. And some wives of smokers might have been able to avoid their spouses' smoke. But both of those factors would tend to hide any true relationship between exposure and disease. So, if anything, the studies should underestimate the risk of secondhand smoke.

Nevertheless, 26 of the 33 studies indicated a link between secondhand smoke and lung cancer. Those studies estimated that people breathing secondhand smoke were 8 to 150 percent more likely to get lung cancer sometime later. Of the remaining seven studies, one found no connection with lung-cancer rates. Six suggested that people exposed to secondhand smoke had *lower* rates of lung cancer, although no one suggests passive smoking really reduces the risk.

Seven of the 26 positive studies included enough subjects, and found a sufficient effect, to attain "statistical significance"—meaning there was no more than a 5 percent probability that the results in those studies occurred by chance. In contrast, just one of the negative studies reached statistical significance.

STRENGTH IN NUMBERS

The nonsignificant studies can still be valuable when combined with all the rest for analysis. This technique, called meta-analysis, is commonly used with carefully designed clinical trials of drugs. But its use in epidemiology is controversial, since no two studies have identical designs and the analysts must make certain assumptions as they combine data. So, the result of a meta-analysis is supporting evidence but is not definitive by itself.

Six different meta-analyses have been carried out on the secondhand-smoke studies. Every one of them yielded a statistically significant increase in lung-cancer risk of approximately 20 to 40 percent. The EPA's study is the most recent of these meta-analyses. It found an increased risk of 19 percent among U.S. nonsmokers married to smokers.

More evidence for a link between cancer and secondhand smoke comes from 19 of the studies, which grouped subjects into exposure categories. In every one of those, women exposed to the most smoke for the most years had higher cancer risks that women exposed to less smoke. That dose-response relationship —an increase in risk with an increase in exposure—is an important indication of a true cause-effect relationship.

Evidence for a dose-response relationship got important support from the most recent secondhand-smoke study, published last summer by epidemiologist Elizabeth Fontham of Louisiana State University Medical Center. The largest such study ever done, it's also considered by experts in the field to be the best in design and execution. Fontham found increased risks of lung cancer with increasing exposure to secondhand smoke, whether it took place at home, at work, or in a social setting. A spouse's smoking alone produced an overall 30 percent increase in lung-cancer risk. Women with the greatest lifetime exposure— from smoking by parents, husbands, friends, and coworkers—had a 225 percent increase in risk. (That's much less than the hazard posed by active smoking, which confers a 1,100 to 2,400 percent increase in lung-cancer risk.)

For any given nonsmoker, the lifetime risk of getting lung cancer remains small —4 to 5 in 1,000 ordinarily, 6 to 7 in 1,000 if he or she has a smoking spouse. But exposure to secondhand smoke is so commonplace that, according to the EPA's calculations, it produces an extra 3000 lung-cancer deaths among adults in the U.S. each year.

That makes secondhand smoke the third-ranking known cause of lung cancer, after active smoking and indoor radon.

LUNG PROBLEMS

Despite all the attention given to lung cancer, it may not be the most significant health effect of secondhand smoke. Two others stand out as well—respiratory disorders in children and heart disease in adults.

The ill effects of smoke on children begin even before birth, since many of the components of smoke reach the developing fetus through the mother. Infants born to smoking mothers weigh less and have weaker lungs than unexposed newborns. Regardless of birth weight, babies born to smoking mothers are more likely to die in infancy than unexposed infants.

Whether from these prenatal effects or from secondhand exposure to smoke after birth, children reared around smoking parents have about twice as many respiratory infections—bronchitis and croup, for example—as the children of non-smokers. After reviewing a number of studies, the EPA's risk analysis concluded that secondhand smoke causes an extra 150,000 to 300,000 respiratory infections a

year among the nation's 5.5 million children under the age of 18 months.

Asthma, the other major childhood respiratory ailment, also turns out to be about twice as common in children exposed to high levels of secondhand smoke. Wheezing from asthma and cough from bronchial irritation occur more frequently among children of smokers. And among children with asthma, living with smoking parents markedly worsens the disease. The EPA blames secondhand smoke for causing between 8,000 and 26,000 new cases of childhood asthma a year, and for aggravating the condition in about 200,000 children. "Children just should not be around people smoking," says Ross Brownson, professor of epidemiology at the St. Louis University School of Public Health.

HEART DISEASE

The epidemiological evidence on secondhand smoke and heart disease is not as abundant as that on lung cancer, and the experts are still debating the implications. But about a dozen studies exist, and they consistently show an elevated risk. Among nonsmokers who are exposed to their spouses' smoke, the chance of death from heart disease increases by about 30 percent. (The effects of active smoking on the heart were established some years ago. Smoking about doubles a person's chance of dying from a cardiovascular condition.)

Although the heart-disease evidence isn't as strong as that for lung cancer, a number of authorities have already declared secondhand smoke a risk factor for heart disease. They include the states of California and Maryland, OSHA, the American Heart Association, and the American College of Cardiology. They point not only to the epidemiological evidence, but to animal studies, which have shown that exposure to specific elements of secondhand smoke causes blood to clot more easily and damages arterial linings—two critical steps in the development of heart disease. In addition, human studies show that the carbon monoxide in secondhand smoke decreases the supply of oxygen reaching the heart muscle, which could cause serious problems for someone with coronary heart disease.

If exposure to secondhand smoke does increase the risk of heart disease by 30 percent, then it is causing an estimated 35,000 to 40,000 heart-disease deaths a year in the U.S.—about 10 times the number of lung-cancer deaths attributed to secondhand smoke. That would make the annual toll from secondhand smoke comparable to that from motor-vehicle accidents.

THE INDUSTRY'S CAMPAIGN

The tobacco industry foresaw the health debate over secondhand smoke—and the problems it would cause for cigarette makers. In 1978, a Roper poll commissioned by the Tobacco Institute, the industry's trade group, called growing public concern about secondhand smoke "the most dangerous development yet to the viability of the tobacco industry" and recommended "developing and widely publicizing clear-cut, credible medical evidence that passive smoking is not harmful."

In 1986, Imperial Tobacco Ltd., Canada's largest cigarette company, commissioned a secret study on how to combat the growing success of antismoking activists. The study documents, made public in the course of a lawsuit, lay out in prescient detail the industry's current strategy on secondhand smoke:

"Passive smoking [should be] used as the focal point.... Of all the health issues surrounding smoking... the one which the tobacco industry has the most chance of winning [is] that the evidence proclaimed by the antigroup is flawed.... It is highly desirable to control the focus of the debate." The document goes on to urge "an attack on the credibility of evidence presented to date." The ideal advocate would be a medical professional, the report said, but "the challenge will be to find a sympathetic doctor who can be demonstrated to take a largely independent stance."

The recommended message on secondhand smoke: "Now that you have seen that all which has been said is not true, let's be adult and get down to the real business, a respect for each other's choices and space."

Whether or not U.S. tobacco companies ever saw the Canadian report, their current public-relations campaign is following its advice.

INFLUENCING SCIENCE

In its efforts to construct the sort of "credible medical evidence" its pollsters recommended, the tobacco industry has commissioned research from sympathetic scientists, sponsored scientific meetings carefully tailored to bring out their point of view, and published the results in the medical literature.

The research support comes through various channels: direct grants from companies or industry-funded research institutes—such as the Council for Tobacco Research and the Center for Indoor Air Research—and consulting contracts from tobacco companies, public-relations firms, and law firms. To get favorable research on the record, the industry has borrowed a technique from the pharmaceutical industry: sponsoring scientific symposia and seeing to it that their findings end up on medical library shelves.

Lisa Bero, a health policy analyst at the University of California, San Francisco, has documented the results of such symposia. She identified four symposia on passive smoking held between 1974 and 1990 that were paid for by the tobacco industry. She then compared the articles generated by the symposia with a random sample of articles on secondhand smoke that appeared in other scientific journals over the same period.

Only 4 percent of the articles from the industry-funded symposia said that passive smoking was unhealthful, compared with 65 percent of the other journal articles. Fully 72 percent of symposia reports argued that secondhand smoke wasn't harmful, compared with 20 percent of independent journal articles. (The balance of the articles were neutral.) The symposium reports did not undergo the standard scientific process of peer review, meaning they were not scrutinized by other experts in the field. Instead, they were published as non-peer-reviewed supplements to journals, or as freestanding books or monographs. Nevertheless, they can be found in the computerized databases of the medical literature. That makes them available for citation by others.

This careful construction of a citable scientific record came in handy when the tobacco industry set out to attack early drafts of the EPA's report on secondhand smoke. Bero found that two-thirds of comments critical of the report came from industry scientists, who drew heavily on industry-generated literature. The Tobacco Institute's own submission, for instance, cited 32 papers from symposia, but only seven peer-reviewed articles.

As the industry has learned, however, research support doesn't guarantee that a scientist will go along with the company line. At least five members of an independent scientific advisory board that reviewed the EPA report had ties to industry research groups, either as advisers or grant recipients, including a scientist awarded a $1.2-million grant from Philip Morris [the largest cigarette manufacturer in the United States] during the review period. Yet the board unanimously agreed that passive smoking was a cancer risk.

PUBLIC PERSUASION

In a public-relations campaign, scientific articles don't mean much if only scientists read them. The industry is bringing its perspective to a much wider audience, with the help of a few journalists. This became clear when we studied industry-generated material on secondhand smoke and looked over newspaper and magazine articles sympathetic to the industry's position.

To read this material is to enter a house of mirrors that endlessly reflects the same set of opinions, voiced by the same few people, again and again. A person who saw nothing else could conclude that there were only four or five scientists in all of North America qualified to speak about secondhand smoke—all of them skeptical of its danger.

You can see how this works by tracing the public utterances of one of those scientists, Gary Huber, a lung specialist at the University of Texas. Shook, Hardy & Bacon, the tobacco industry's longtime law firm, pays Huber's university to support his group's compilation of research on lung disease. Despite this, he told us, his views are his own.

In 1991, Huber wrote an article for *Consumers' Research*—a small-circulation magazine not connected to *Consumer Reports*—in which he argued that the scientific evidence on the hazards of passive smoking is "shoddy and poorly conceived." He felt the epidemiological studies were too weak and the composition of secondhand smoke too poorly understood to reach a conclusion on any risk.

In early 1993, Huber was prominently quoted in an article in *Investor's Business Daily*. Writer Michael Fumento stated that "many in the scientific and medical community" dispute the EPA's opinion. All five scientists quoted to back up this viewpoint have received some type of industry support.

Both Huber's and Fumento's articles became, in turn, sources for a series of opinion pieces written by another journalist, Jacob Sullum. In *The Wall Street Journal* and *Forbes Media Critic*, Sullum built on Fumento's arguments and quoted three of the same scientists, including Huber. When we asked the Tobacco Institute for material on secondhand smoke, it sent us a packet that included Fumento's article.

R. J. Reynolds reprinted Sullum's *Wall Street Journal* article nationwide in a full-page ad. The ad's headline: "If We Said It, You Might Not Believe It." Philip Morris went even further, buying full-page ads in major national publications for six straight days to reprint Sullum's longer *Forbes Media Critic* article.

The effect: Huber's argument has undoubtedly now been seen by millions more people than ever read the original EPA report, never mind any of the hundreds of scientific articles on the subject in medical journals.

The industry's strategy has been effective. John Pierce, a researcher at the University of California, San Diego, who specializes in tobacco issues, checked the calls made to a statewide smokers' hotline immediately after the Reynolds and Philip Morris ads started appearing in print. Although the hotline was intended to give support to smokers who wanted to quit, the calls coming in during that period were overwhelmingly accusatory. "We had a whole heap of people calling us, asking why we were misleading them," Pierce recalls. "There are all too many people willing to believe the industry when it says this thing's not really bad for you."

ATTACKING THE SCIENCE

The heart of the cigarette makers' campaign appears to be their attack on the scientific methods used to measure the risk of secondhand smoke. In its advertising, its public statements, and its lawsuit against the EPA, the industry argues that the agency "cherry-picked" data to reach a foregone conclusion and violated the rules of statistical analysis. That's a clever strategy; it takes advantage of the public's unfamiliarity with research methods and the common perception that one week's scientific report will be debunked the following week.

To evaluate the industry arguments, we consulted CU's own professional statisticians and also turned to Charles Hennekens and Julie Buring, epidemiologists at Harvard Medical School and coauthors of a leading edidemiology textbook. They have no ties to the tobacco industry, and their own research includes studying various causes of heart disease and cancer. Here's what they said about the criticisms.

Pooling Studies   The industry argues that the EPA had no business pooling smaller studies, many failing the "statistical significance" test, into one large collection of data. This is the meta-analysis technique we described above. "They've combined studies as different as night and day, which is not an accepted way to do a meta-analysis," says Walker Merryman, vice president of the Tobacco Institute.

In truth, the EPA made an effort to compare comparable studies. It sorted them by country or region, excluded the poorest-quality studies, and then pooled data only within each geographical group. The pooled results for Greece, Hong Kong, Japan, and the U.S. all showed statistically significant risk increases. The pooled results from Western Europe and China, though positive, didn't reach significance.

"Having a number of studies that show similar results but are not large enough individually to be statistically significant on their own is exactly the situation where meta-analysis is appropriate," Buring says.

The Significance Level   When they analyze their data, most researchers try to set their "statistical significance" hurdle at 5 percent. In everyday language, that means there is less than a 5 percent probability the results occurred by happenstance.

However, the tobacco industry argues that the EPA lowered its hurdle to 10 percent when it pooled the various studies. Jacob Sullum said it "in effect doubles the odds of being wrong." An industry scientific consultant called it a "confidence game."

But here too, the EPA played fair. It did set a 5 percent significance level. The agency used a standard statistical technique, called a one-tailed test, that allowed a 5 percent chance of wrongly concluding that secondhand smoke increases the risk of cancer. This technique, taught in every introductory statistics course, is appropriate when, as in this case, there is already independent evidence that a substance is harmful.

What's more, when Hennekens and Buring analyzed pooled data from the 11 U.S. studies on which the EPA relied most heavily, they found that the data do meet the even tougher standard the critics are demanding.

Confounding Factors   Since epidemiologists can't control everything that happens in the lives of their subjects, they have to be wary of confounding factors, possible alternative causes for the results. Relatively small risks, like that from secondhand smoke, are especially vulnerable to confounding.

The tobacco industry and its defenders have raised just such a possibility. "There are numerous, and in many cases unaccounted for, factors which makes the whole process exceedingly difficult," Merryman says. "Since we're dealing with an issue of such magnitude, I think it's proper to insist they be accounted for." The critics have usually focused on diet or socioeconomic status, both of which have been linked to the incidence of cancer. If people exposed to secondhand smoke were more likely to be poor or to have poor diets, data could be muddied.

In fact, the EPA considered possible confounding factors. Five of the studies it analyzed included information on diet. None of those five studies suggested that diet could account for the increased risk in people exposed to secondhand smoke.

The studies the EPA relied on didn't record socioeconomic status, but Fontham's newer study did—and found no link to risk. She also looked at diet and found that a diet high in fruits and vegetables did seem to protect people from lung cancer. But even after accounting for that, there was still a significant relationship between secondhand smoke and lung cancer.

Epidemiologists readily concede they can never account for all the factors that affect health. But since studies done in many countries with different cultures and habits all point to an elevated risk, confounding factors are not likely to be the explanation.

The 'Excluded' Studies The industry has repeatedly implied that the EPA ignored two 1992 studies because they didn't support the agency's conclusions. In fact, both studies were published during the seven-month period after the EPA report was written but before the agency released it. And neither study suggests the EPA is wrong.

In one, University of South Florida researcher Heather Stockwell found that nonsmoking women married to smokers had a 60 percent higher risk of lung cancer than women married to nonsmokers. The most highly exposed group—women exposed for 40 years or more—had a 130 percent increase in risk. In the other study, Ross Brownson, then of the Missouri Department of Health, found no risk increase for all exposed women as a group—but the most highly exposed had a 30 percent increase.

Both the EPA and the industry have calculated, but not published, re-analyses that include all the new studies. The EPA says it still finds a statistically significant risk; R. J. Reynolds says it doesn't.

THE BOTTOM LINE

There's no question that all epidemiological studies have a built-in imprecision, Buring told us. "But when you see different investigators, using different definitions and study designs, all showing similar results, then you have to believe there's something going on."

The case against secondhand smoke has reached that point. Short of conducting an impossible experiment—deliberately exposing thousands of people to secondhand smoke for decades, to see what happens—this is about as good as the human evidence on secondhand smoke is likely to get.

When those results are combined with the laboratory studies, the abundant evidence that firsthand smoke causes cancer, and the evidence for a dose-response relationship, the health implications are clear—and the EPA's conclusion inescapable.

"If we didn't have the tobacco companies spending millions of dollars to confuse the facts, this issue would be an open-and-shut case," says Stanton Glantz, a longtime tobacco researcher at the University of California, San Francisco. "The fact is that passive smoking causes lung cancer."

Your personal risk? Since the amount of smoke inhaled appears related to the risk of disease, there probably is a minimal hazard from brief exposure. But steady doses of secondhand smoke at home or on the job aren't so benign.

A nonsmoker's individual risk of dying from lung cancer, normally small, is increased slightly by living or working for years among people who smoke heavily. And although the individual risk is relatively small, the numbers add up to an issue of public health. Thousands of people in the U.S. may be dying or made sick every year from other people's smoking.

James Repace and Alfred Lowrey, two statistical researchers who study the effects of secondhand smoke, have concluded that a lifetime increase in lung-cancer risk of 1 in 1,000 could be caused by long-term occupational exposure to air containing more than 6.8 micrograms of nicotine per cubic meter of air. (The nicotine itself doesn't cause lung disease but is a marker for smoke concentration.) Concentrations that heavy occur regularly in many homes and workplaces.

For its study, the EPA found 19 reports of measurements of nicotine levels in enclosed spaces where people smoked. Nicotine levels in homes of smokers had averages that ranged from study to study, between 2 and about 11 micrograms; in offices, the range of averages was about 1 to 13. Restaurants were even smokier, with averages between about 6 and 18 micrograms.

WHAT SHOULD BE DONE

If secondhand tobacco smoke were not connected to the profits of a powerful industry, we doubt there would be much argument about drastically restricting people's exposure to it.

The lifetime added risk of developing lung cancer from prolonged exposure to secondhand smoke is roughly 1 in 1,000—1,000 times greater than the one-in-a-million lifetime cancer risk considered unacceptable for many other environmental contaminants. Even in small doses, it can be an uncomfortable irritant, at the very least.

In response to the data, the tobacco industry has accelerated its campaign against public smoking restrictions. For instance, five companies together laid out nearly $8-million last year in an unsuccessful effort to persuade California voters to approve a smoking-control law that would have invalidated stronger state and local restrictions.

The 1994 elections greatly improved the industry's legislative prospects. Out as chairman of the House Subcommittee on Health and Environment is Democrat Henry Waxman of California. His hearings last year produced the widely seen image of tobacco-company chiefs swearing they didn't think cigarettes were addictive. His likely replacement is Republican Thomas Bliley. The major employer in Bliley's Virginia district is Philip Morris, and Bliley has already said, "I don't think we need any more legislation concerning tobacco."

We disagree. We believe nonsmokers have a right to breathe smoke-free air, and we have long favored restrictions on where people may smoke. The medical evidence makes it imperative to impose such limits. In particular, we support measures to keep smoke out of the workplace—not just offices and factories but also restaurants, stores, and public transportation, because of the risk to the millions of Americans who work there, too.

We support OSHA's efforts to limit workplace smoking to certain ventilated rooms. OSHA calculates that over the next 45 years a workplace smoking ban would eliminate between 5,500 and 32,500 lung-cancer deaths and 98,000 to 578,000 deaths from heart disease. (The variation comes from uncertainty about current levels of exposure to secondhand smoke.)

That makes control of smoke one of the great public-health bargains. Getting rid of workplace smoke requires posting signs, putting a few chairs and an ashtray outdoors, or putting an appropriate ventilation fan into a special smoking room —an improvement that OSHA estimates would cost $4,000 per building. In contrast, the bill for removing asbestos from a commercial building averages $300,000.

NO   Jacob Sullum

JUST HOW BAD IS
SECONDHAND SMOKE?

"Secondhand Smoke Kills." So says a billboard on Pico Boulevard in Los Angeles that I pass every day on the way to work. I'm still not convinced. But most Americans seem to be: a CNN / *Time* poll conducted in March found that 78 per cent believe secondhand smoke is "very" or "somewhat" harmful.

That idea was endorsed by the U.S. Environmental Protection Agency [EPA] last year, when it declared secondhand smoke "a known human lung carcinogen." Since then the EPA's report has helped justify smoking bans throughout the country: in cities such as Los Angeles and San Francisco (likely to be joined soon by New York); in Maryland, Vermont, and Washington state; and in government offices, including the Defense Department. On March 25, the Occupational Safety and Health Administration proposed a ban on smoking in workplaces, including bars and restaurants. A bill introduced by Representative Henry Waxman (D., Calif.) would go even further, banning smoking in almost every building except residences.

Most supporters of such measures probably believe that the EPA's report presents definitive scientific evidence that "secondhand smoke kills." But a closer look shows that the EPA manipulated data and finessed important points to arrive at a predetermined conclusion. The agency compromised science to support the political crusade against smoking.

The first line of defense for people who want to avoid scrutiny of the case against secondhand smoke (a/k/a environmental tobacco smoke, or ETS) is to argue by analogy. "We know that tobacco smoke causes disease and can kill you," says Scott Ballin, chairman of the Coalition on Smoking or Health. "It makes sense that a person who doesn't smoke cigarettes, who's sitting next to a smoker and inhaling the smoke, is also at some risk." The EPA offers a similar argument, devoting a chapter of its report on ETS to the evidence that smoking causes cancer.

Although superficially plausible, this analogy is misleading. A smoker breathes in hot, concentrated tobacco smoke and holds it in his lungs before exhaling. A nonsmoker in the vicinity, by contrast, breathes air that includes minute quantities of residual chemicals from tobacco smoke. "ETS is so highly diluted that it is not even appropriate to call it smoke," says Gary Huber, a professor of medicine at the University of Texas Health Science Center, writing with two colleagues in the July 1991 *Consumers' Research.* Furthermore, since many of the compounds in tobacco smoke are unstable, it is not safe to assume even that a nonsmoker is exposed to the same chemicals as a smoker. Of 50 biologically active substances thought to be present in ETS, Huber and his colleagues report, only 14 have actually been detected.

Even if exposure to ETS were analogous to smoking, the doses involved are so small that it's not clear they would have any effect. Many chemicals that are hazardous or even fatal above a certain level are harmless (or beneficial) in smaller doses. James Enstrom, a professor of epidemiology at UCLA, estimates that someone exposed to ETS would be taking in the equivalent of a few cigarettes a year, perhaps one-hundredth of a cigarette a day. Yet studies of smoking have never looked at people who smoke that little; the lowest-exposure groups have been subjects who smoke up to five cigarettes a day.

THE EPA'S SMOKING GUN

So it's not reasonable to conclude that ETS must be dangerous because smoking is dangerous. You have to look at the research that deals specifically with ETS. The EPA's finding is based on 30 epidemiological studies that compared lung-cancer rates among nonsmokers (mainly women) who lived with smokers to lung-cancer rates among nonsmokers who lived with nonsmokers. None of the studies measured actual exposure to ETS; they simply assumed that people who lived with smokers were more exposed than people who didn't. In most of these studies, lung cancer was somewhat more common among the subject living with smokers, but in only 6 cases were the results statistically significant.

This is a crucial point. In any study that compares a group exposed to a suspected risk factor with a control group, the luck of the draw may result in a difference between the two groups that does not reflect a difference between the populations the groups are supposed to represent. Researchers do statistical tests to account for the possibility of such a fluke. By convention, epidemiologists call a result significant when the probability that it occurred purely by chance is 5 per cent or less. By this standard, 80 per cent of the studies discussed by the EPA did not find a statistically significant link between ETS and lung cancer.

But the EPA, which had always used the conventional definition of statistical significance in its risk assessments, adopted a different standard for the report on ETS. It considered a result significant if the probability that it occurred purely by chance was 10 per cent or less. This change essentially doubles the odds of being wrong. "The justification for this usage," according to the report itself, "is based on the *a priori* hypothesis... that a positive association exists between exposure to ETS and lung cancer." Of course, the EPA was supposed to *test* that hypothesis, not simply assume that it is true.

Instead of presenting results from the epidemiological studies as they originally appeared, the EPA recalculated them using the less rigorous standard. As a report from the Congressional Research

Service drily notes, "it is unusual to return to a study after the fact, lower the required significance level, and declare its results to be supportive rather than unsupportive of the effect one's theory suggests should be present."

Even after the EPA massaged the data, the vast majority of the studies still did not show a significant association between ETS and lung cancer. Of the 11 U.S. studies, only 1 yielded a result that was significant according to the looser definition. (According to the usual definition, none of them did.) To bolster the evidence, the EPA did a "meta-analysis" of these studies. Dr. Enstrom notes that this technique was originally intended for clinical trials that assess the impact of a drug or procedure by randomly assigning subjects to treatment and control groups. By contrast, the data analyzed by the EPA came from retrospective case-control studies that "matched" people with lung cancer to people without lung cancer. Enstrom says using meta-analysis for such studies "is not a particularly meaningful exercise," because the studies are apt to differ in the way they define exposure, the confounding variables they take into account, the types of cancer they include, and so on.

In any event, the EPA's conclusion —that living with a smoker raises a woman's risk of getting lung cancer by 19 per cent—is justified only according to the definition of statistical significance adopted especially for these data. By the usual standard, even the meta-analysis does not support the claim that ETS causes lung cancer. Furthermore, the EPA excluded from its analysis a major U.S. study, published in the November 1992 *American Journal of Public Health*, that failed to find a significant link between ETS and lung cancer. Given the large size of the study, it could well have changed the outcome of the meta-analysis, so that the result would not have been significant even by the EPA's revised standard.

SMALL CLAIMS

Despite this "fancy statistical footwork," as a July 1992 article in *Science* described it, the EPA was able to claim only a weak association between ETS and lung cancer. With a risk increase as low as 19 per cent, it is difficult to rule out the possibility that other factors were at work. "At least 20 confounding variables have been identified as important to the development of lung cancer," write Huber et al. "No reported study comes anywhere close to controlling, or even mentioning, half of these."

Smokers tend to differ from nonsmokers in many ways—including diet, socioeconomic status, risk-taking behavior, and exercise—and it is likely that the spouses of smokers share these characteristics to some extent. "If wives of smokers share in poor health habits or other factors that could contribute to illness," the Congressional Research Service notes, "statistical associations found between disease and passive smoking could be incidental or misleading."

Misclassification could also account for some or all of the observed differences between wives of smokers and wives of nonsmokers. It's possible that some of the subjects thought to be nonsmokers were actually smokers or former smokers. Since spouses of smokers are more likely to be smokers themselves, such errors would have biased the results. The EPA adjusted the data to account for this effect, but it's impossible to say whether it fully compensated for misclassification.

These issues are especially important when the relationship between a suspected risk factor and a disease is weak. Based on the 11 U.S. studies, the EPA concluded that a woman who lives with a smoker is 1.19 times as likely to get lung cancer as a woman who lives with a nonsmoker. This ratio did not rise above 2.1 to 1 in any of the U.S. studies. In previous risk assessments, the EPA has seen such weak associations as cause for skepticism. When the agency examined the alleged connection between electromagnetic fields and cancer, for example, it said, "the association is not strong enough to constitute a proven causal relationship, largely because the relative risks in the published reports have seldom exceeded 3.0."

This concern did not prevent the EPA from reaching a firm conclusion about ETS, even though the agency recognized the limitations of the data. The head of the Scientific Advisory Board that reviewed the report conceded: "This is a classic case where the evidence is not all that strong."

The evidence is especially unimpressive when compared to the evidence that smoking causes lung cancer. In the latter case, there are thousands of studies, and virtually all of them have found a positive association, statistically significant in the vast majority of cases. And the associations are sizable: a typical female smoker is about 10 times as likely to get lung cancer as a female nonsmoker; for men the ratio is more like 20 to 1; and among heavy smokers, the figures are even higher. "The data on active smoking are so much stronger," Enstrom says. "That should be the focus of attention, not something which is so small and has the potential to be confounded by so many different things. I personally am baffled as to why people give it so much credibility."

PROTECTED FROM THEMSELVES

The explanation may be that the EPA's conclusion about ETS is useful in a way that the evidence about smoking is not. Although the share of adults who smoke has dropped from about 40 per cent to about 25 per cent since 1965, some 50 million Americans continue to smoke. And as Duke University economist W. Kip Viscusi shows in his recent book *Smoking: Making the Risky Decision*, this is not because they are ignorant about the health effects. Rather, they are willing to accept the risks in exchange for the benefits of smoking. From a "public-health" perspective, this is intolerable; no one should be allowed to make such a foolish decision. But the idea of protecting people from themselves still arouses considerable opposition in this country. Hence antismoking activists and public-health officials need a different excuse for restricting smoking: it endangers innocent bystanders.

When EPA Administrator Carol Browner testified in favor of Waxman's Smoke-Free Environment Act in February, she relied heavily on the ETS report. But the main benefit that she claimed for the bill was its expected impact on smokers. "The reduction in smoker mortality due to smokers who quit, cut back, or do not start is estimated to range from about 33,000 to 99,000 lives per year," she said. And six surgeons general, reported the *New York Times*, "echoed the theme that this simple measure could do more for the public health than any other bill in years."

If your main goal is improving "the public health," you may be inclined to shade the truth a bit if it helps to make smoking less acceptable and more inconvenient. Marc Lalonde, Canada's former minister of national health and welfare, offered a rationale for such a strategy in a highly influential 1974 report: "Science is full of 'ifs,' 'buts,' and 'maybes,' while messages designed to influence the public must be loud, clear, and unequivocal.... The scientific 'yes, but' is essential to research, but for modifying human behavior of the population it sometimes produces the 'uncertain sound.' This is all the excuse needed by many to cultivate and tolerate an environment and lifestyle that is hazardous to health."

Writing about the ETS controversy in *Toxicologic Pathology*, Yale University epidemiologist Alvan Feinstein quotes a colleague who appears to have been influenced by the Lalonde Doctrine: "Yes, it's rotten science, but it's in a worthy cause. It will help us get rid of cigarettes and become a smoke-free society."

This seems to be the attitude that the EPA brought to its risk assessment.

In June 1990 the agency released the first draft of *Environmental Tobacco Smoke: A Guide to Workplace Smoking Policies*, intended to advise employers to institute smoking restrictions. Yet this was three and a half years before the EPA officially determined that ETS was a health hazard. In a letter to Representative Thomas J. Bliley Jr., (R., Va.), then EPA Administrator William Reilly admitted that "beginning the development of an Agency risk assessment after the commencement of work on the draft policy guide gave the appearance of the very situation—i.e., policy leading science—that I am committed to avoid."

Reilly was so committed to avoiding this appearance that he decided not to release the final version of the policy guide, even though it was ready by December 1992. As he explained to the *Wall Street Journal*, putting out the guide along with the risk assessment would "look like we're trying to torque the science." But don't worry. Miss Browner, Mr. Reilly's successor, released the handy pamphlet last July.

POSTSCRIPT

Is Secondhand Smoke a Proven Health Risk for Nonsmokers?

The tobacco industry not only supports smokers' rights to smoke in public but also claims that passive smoking is not harmful. To justify the claim that passive smoking is harmless to health, industry representatives argue that the research is inconclusive and lacking in validity. The industry used similar tactics to try and persuade smokers that smoking had not been proven harmful to health after the surgeon general's proclamation that it had in 1964. The industry has more recently attacked research linking secondhand smoke with cancer, heart disease, and other health problems.

In addition to maintaining that secondhand smoke is not harmful, the tobacco industry holds that laws restricting smoking in public places violate smokers' civil rights; after all, smokers are taxpayers too. Also, smoking is a personal choice, and the industry contends that the government has no right to restrict when and where smokers may light up. Articles supporting this view include "Smoke and Mirrors," by Jacob Sullum, *Reason* (February 1991); "Zealots Against Science," *The American Spectator* (July 1990); "Coping With Smoking," by Tibor Machan, *Freeman* (April 1989); and "The Health Police Are Blowing Smoke," *Fortune* (April 25, 1988). Other writers also claim that proposed bans on tobacco advertising would be an example of unwanted government paternalism. See John Luik, "Tobacco Advertising Bans and the Dark Face of Government Paternalism," *International Journal of Advertising* (vol. 12, 1993).

Because public smoking is an issue of both health and personal rights, it generates many arguments. Both nonsmokers and smokers claim that their rights are violated when one group's desires are allowed to prevail over the other's. In the battle over smoking, nonsmokers cite research showing that long-term exposure to passive smoke increases the risk of many illnesses, including heart disease and lung cancer. Researchers claim that passive tobacco smoke contains over 40 cancer-causing chemicals and is responsible for as many as 50,000 deaths each year. A recent study, "Environmental Tobacco Smoke and Lung Cancer in Nonsmoking Women: A Multicenter Study," *Journal of the American Medical Association* (June 8, 1994), confirms these findings: researchers found that nonsmoking women living with smoking spouses faced a 30 percent higher risk of developing lung cancer than nonsmoking women living with nonsmokers.

Numerous research studies have indicated that passive smoking is a health risk. The landmark investigation, which concluded that nonsmoking wives of smoking spouses have a higher risk of developing lung cancer, found that only a fraction of female lung cancer patients actually smoked cigarettes. It was concluded that the women who developed lung cancer were exposed to high levels of secondhand smoke from their husbands' cigarettes. See "Non-Smoking Wives of Heavy Smokers Have a Higher Risk of Lung Cancer: A Study from Japan," *British Medical Journal* (January 17, 1981). This classic study was followed by many others, all reaching the same conclusion: exposure to passive smoke is a risk for lung cancer and other smoking-related diseases. Further readings include "Mortal Sins," *National Review* (May 19, 1997), an article about the morality of sex and smoking. See also "Smoking Wars," *National Review* (July 29, 1996); "Where There's Smoke There's P. J. O'Rourke," *The American Spectator* (July 1996); "Urine Tests Confirm Fears About Passive Smoking," *New Scientist* (January 29, 1994); "Threat from Passive Smoking Is Upgraded," *Science News* (June 11, 1994); and "Passive Smoke and Lung Cancer," *American Health* (September 1994). In "Last Drag," *Across the Board* (March 1996), Jacob Sullum discusses the consequences of a total ban on cigarettes by the government.

Since the classic Japanese study of 1981, it has been confirmed that smoking is harmful not only to the smoker but also to the persons surrounding the smoker. Yet, numerous writers continue to support the right to smoke in public and continue to question the validity of the scientific research, accusing the EPA of manipulating data. However, as the nonsmoking majority continue to vocally support a ban on public smoking, more and more work sites, public buildings, and retail establishments are restricting indoor smoking.

ISSUE 8

Should Moderate Use of Alcohol Be Recommended?

YES: Dave Shiflett, from "Here's to Your Health," *The American Spectator* (October 1996)

NO: Meir J. Stampfer, Eric B. Rimm, and Diana Chapman Walsh, from "Alcohol, the Heart, and Public Policy," *American Journal of Public Health* (June 1993)

ISSUE SUMMARY

YES: Writer Dave Shiflett claims that for years the antidrinking establishment has insisted that even moderate drinking is bad for health despite the fact that science indicates otherwise.

NO: Physicians Meir J. Stampfer and Eric B. Rimm and professor Diana Chapman Walsh argue that encouraging the use of alcohol, even in moderation, could lead to an increase in its consumption, with potentially dangerous results.

Moderate drinking has been associated with many positive health effects, including a reduction of heart disease, overall longevity, better circulation, and less stress. More than 100 studies have found that alcohol reduces the risk of coronary heart disease and that moderate drinkers live longer, healthier lives than nondrinkers. Alcohol reduces the risk of heart problems due to its apparent ability to elevate levels of HDLs (the "good" cholesterol) and to prevent blood clots from forming. The studies all found these results among individuals who consumed a moderate amount of alcohol, or less than two drinks per day.

Moderate alcohol consumption appears to offer health benefits, but excessive usage—over two drinks per day—increases the risk of cancer, cirrhosis of the liver, and other health problems, and leads to alcoholism. Alcoholism is a factor in automobile fatalities, family dysfunction, and crime. Should moderate consumption actually be recommended to reduce heart disease if the use could lead to excessive drinking?

A core of this debate is the definition of moderate consumption. Moderation is two or less drinks per day to a researcher, but may be considerably more to actual drinkers. Some individuals abstain from drinking all week and have several drinks on Friday night. Are they drinking moderately? An additional issue is how much does a person need to drink to achieve the benefits of alcohol? Should alcohol be promoted at the expense of other activities that promote a healthy heart such as exercise and smoking cessation? And what about those individuals such as pregnant women who should not drink at all?

Beyond two drinks a day, alcohol has direct adverse effects on the heart. With as many as four drinks a day, men are less likely to die of heart disease than a nondrinker, but these men are at increased risk of death from other illnesses. Specifically, they have a greater probability of dying from cancer of the esophagus and stomach as well as from cirrhosis of the liver and from being involved in automobile accidents. In France, where the average citizen drinks eight to ten times as much wine as Americans, the rates of cirrhosis of the liver, accidents, and suicides are higher than in the United States. Women are also at risk—studies have shown that alcohol increases the risk of breast cancer. For many women, the hazards of drinking outweigh the benefits.

Promoting alcohol in moderation to reduce heart disease may help save lives. On the other hand, researchers agree that no one should start drinking for the express purpose of reducing this risk. The potential for alcohol abuse is too high, and there are much safer and healthier ways to protect the heart. For instance, although alcohol boosts HDLs, exercising and losing excess weight raise them even more. Exercise, in addition to elevating HDLs, also reduces the risk of diabetes, lowers blood pressure, and improves circulation. Exercise does not carry the health risks of alcohol.

In the following articles, writer Dave Shiflett claims that science has indicated that moderate drinking is beneficial, but the government busybodies keep insisting that it is harmful. Meir J. Stampfer, Eric B. Rimm, and Diana Chapman Walsh argue that the benefits of moderate drinking over abstinence are unclear. They also are against promoting the message that moderate consumption is beneficial because of the ambiguity of the concept of "moderate" and the potential for alcohol abuse.

YES

Dave Shiflett

HERE'S TO YOUR HEALTH

Said Aristotle unto Plato,
"Have another sweet potato?"
Said Plato unto Aristotle,
"Thank you, I prefer the bottle."

—Owen Wister

Were America's students still burdened with the duty of rote memorization, we can nevertheless be assured they wouldn't be asked to learn a ditty so dangerous as Mr. Wister's. Quite the contrary. Anyone who spouted such sentiments in a contemporary classroom might find that the rules against washing out young mouths with soap can be lifted on special occasions.

Consider the case of poor Shannon Eierman, a 16-year-old honor student and all-county softball player at Atholton (Md.) High School. On a school ski trip to Vermont in February of this year [1996], Eierman walked into the room of some friends and discovered they were drinking beer. Hoping to avoid trouble, she grabbed two beers and began pouring them out.

Too late. Chaperones suddenly appeared; soon a dozen or so of the young-sters had been relieved of their ski passes and forced to write detailed accounts of their transgressions. Seven of the guilty, including Eierman, were suspended from school, she for five days. Shannon was also forced to attend an alcohol treatment program and was banned from extracurricular activities for two quarters—a punishment that may have cost her a sports scholarship.

It could have been worse. Shannon had actually received the minimum punishment under Howard County's "zero tolerance" program. As the *Washington Post* reported, "Last year, Howard officials provoked an uproar when they suspended students who drank a glass of wine with dinner in France on a school trip."

For a generation steeped in mescaline, marijuana, and tequila shooters, the baby boomers take a fanatically harsh stance on beer drinking by their children—harsher, indeed, than the stiff old Puritans who proclaimed drink a "gift from God." Students who bring even a non-alcoholic beer to a Fairfax

County (Va.) school face suspension, even though those concoctions' alcohol content is only .5 percent (By way of comparison, one study indicates that after three days in the refrigerator, Dole pineapple juice becomes .34 percent alcohol.)

And nationwide, alcohol education campaigns have not shied from comparing booze use to cocaine snorting. Indeed, one poster, featuring a bottle of beer tipped by a hypodermic needle, carries this message: "Beer contains alcohol. Alcohol is a drug. Alcohol is the number one drug problem in the country. Not marijuana. Not cocaine. Alcohol. Talk to your kids about alcohol."

In fidelity to Uncle Sam's auntish predilections, the latest edition of the official United States nutritional guidelines warns that drinking can lead to high blood pressure, cancer, "accidents, violence, suicides, birth defects, and overall mortality." Yet the guidelines also declare, in a stunning turnaround, that "moderate drinking is associated with lower risk for Coronary Heart Disease in some individuals." This is a significant change from earlier statements that alcohol had "no benefit" and suggestions to avoid any level of drinking whatsoever. It also gives rise to an amusing paradox: While the federal government says moderate alcohol intake can prolong life, public schools and the government-funded "anti-abuse" apparatus treat alcohol like rat poison. All of which raises at least two interesting questions: What does the scientific evidence tell us, and what effect does this evidence have on public policy?

* * *

There is nothing new about health claims for alcohol. Among the most extravagant were made on behalf of distilled spirits by one Hieronymous Brunschwig, who practiced medicine in fifteenth-century Germany:

> It eases diseases coming of cold. It comforts the heart. It heals all old and new sores on the head. It causes a good color in a person. It heals baldness and causes the hair well to grow, and kills lice and fleas. It cures lethargy.... It eases the pain in the teeth, and causes sweet breath. It heals the canker in the mouth, in the teeth, in the lips, and in the tongue. It causes the heavy tongue to become light and well-speaking. It heals the short breath. It causes good digestion and appetite for to eat, and takes away all belching. It draws the wind out of the body.

Nowadays the claims are not quite so grandiose, yet the idea is the same: Moderate drinking is good for most people. A March 1996 article in the *British Medical Journal* offered this overview: "The inverse association between moderate alcohol consumption and coronary heart disease is well established. Evidence for a causal interpretation comes from over 60 ecological, case-control, and cohort studies."

Indeed, anyone requesting similar evidence will have it delivered by the truckload. The Harvard Medical School analyzed 200 studies and found that moderate drinking is associated with as much as a 45 percent reduced risk of heart disease. The Honolulu Heart Study put the decrease at 50 percent. When "60 Minutes" did a story on the subject, it broadcast this hearty endorsement by Dr. Curtis Ellison of the Boston School of Medicine: "I think the data are now so convincing that the total morality rates are lower among moderate drinkers. It seems quite clear that we should not do anything that would decrease moderate drinkers in the population."

So convinced is the British government of the benefits of moderate drinking that it actually suggests that older abstainers abandon their teetotaling. The UK guidelines, called "Sensible Drinking," make these recommendations for men:

- The health benefit from drinking relates to men aged over 40 and the major part of this can be obtained at levels as low as one unit a day with the maximum health advantage lying between one and two units a day.

- Regular consumption of between three and four units a day by men of all ages will not accrue significant health risks.

- Consistently drinking four or more units a day is not advised as a sensible drinking level because of the progressive health risk it carries.

Because women tend to be lighter than men, and because their bodies contain a lower proportion of water which results in higher tissue concentration of alcohol, their guidelines are somewhat more stringent:

- The health benefit from drinking for women relates to post-menopausal women and the major part of this can be obtained at levels as low as one unit a day, with the maximum health advantage lying between one and two units a day.

- Regular consumption of between two and three units a day by women of all ages will not accrue any significant health risk.

- Consistently drinking three or more units a day is not advised as a sensible drinking level because of the progressive health risk it carries.

The good news doesn't stop there. In what will probably be a shock to Americans of both sexes, the UK guidelines even dismiss the idea that pregnant women should abstain: "In the light of the evidence received, our conclusion is that, to minimize risk to the developing fetus, women who are trying to become pregnant or are at any stage of pregnancy, should not drink more than 1 or 2 units of alcohol once or twice a week, and should avoid episodes of intoxication."

From reduction in cholesterol gallstones to lower rates of Ischaemic stroke, "Sensible Drinking" finds many benefits to moderate tippling, including this stunner: "Drinking in the range of 7 units to 40 units a week lowers the risk of [Coronary Heart Disease] by between 30% and 50%." (A British drink is somewhat smaller than an American drink: about 9–10 grams of alcohol vs. 12–14grams.)

American advocates of healthy drinking have been singing the same song for many years, though not under government auspices. Lewis Perdue, author of *The French Paradox and Beyond* and publisher of *Healthy Drinking* magazine, notes a 1991 Harvard study which found that male doctors who drank on average one-half to one drink per day had 21 percent less coronary artery disease than abstainers, or a relative risk of .79 for the drinkers compared to 1.00 for abstainers. "The relative risk," Perdue crows, "continued to drop with increased consumption. Men who consumed one to one and a half drinks per day reduced their Coronary Artery Disease risk by 32 percent, three to four and a half per day reduced it by 43 percent, and those drinking more than four and a half drinks per day reduced their risk by 59 percent."

Perdue admits that there are tradeoffs, even for those who favor moderate drinking. "The World Health Association's statistics for 1989 showed that the U.S. death rate from cirrhosis was 17 per 100,000 while cardiovascular disease killed 464 per 100,000. By contrast, the same study shows France with almost double the cirrhosis rate—31 per 100,000 —but with cardiovascular rates at only 310 per 100,000. Using these figures, it is not hard to see that if the U.S. rates were normalized with those of France, 14 more people per 100,000 would die of cirrhosis, but 154 fewer people would die of cardiovascular disease, a net savings of 140 people per 100,000 population who would live longer in order to die of something else."

* * *

While there is solid scientific consensus on the benefits of moderate drinking, don't expect a quick change in American attitudes about alcohol, or national policies. The chief reason is that American society has had an uneven relationship with alcohol. Sometimes they love it. Other times they can't pour it down the gutters quickly enough. Contemporary policies tend to reflect the latter passion.

David Hanson, a professor of sociology at SUNY-Potsdam and author of *Preventing Alcohol Abuse*, writes that while beer drinking even by the very young was common early in our history, an increasing concern with public drunkenness led to social crackdowns of a somewhat Muslim nature starting in the early nineteenth century. By the 1830's, a temperance movement had taken hold that pushed for total abstinence; by 1855, thirteen of the then forty states and territories had instituted prohibition.

If those were tough days for bartenders, they were terrific for the writers of tracts. The Women's Christian Temper-

ance Union, Hanson reports, pumped out over 1 billion pages of anti-alcohol propaganda between 1865 and 1925. When the Anti-Saloon League began publishing operations in 1909, it quickly rose to a level of 250 million book pages per month. Among the warnings:

- "The majority of beer drinkers die from dropsy."
- "It turns the blood to water."
- "A cat or dog may be killed by causing it to drink a small quantity of alcohol. A boy once drank whisky from a flask he had found, and died in a few hours..."
- "When alcohol is constantly used, it may slowly change the muscles of the heart into fat.... It is sometimes so soft that a finger could easily be pushed through its walls."

Today's tract writers work for lobbying organizations, federal agencies, and other special interest groups, but their end goal —"no use" of alcohol—remains the same. Not surprisingly, extremism in the defense of abstinence is not considered a vice. In one of its official publications, the federal Center For Substance Abuse Prevention (CSAP), which supports anti-drinking programs throughout the country, was generous to the point of praise about the work of Artfux, a group that (illegally) defaces alcohol-advertising billboards: "While Artfux recognized that the billboards were private property, these artists viewed their actions as the lesser of two evils.... Furthermore, Artfux contended that they were providing health information that was hidden from the public by the alcohol and tobacco industries."

This sort of vandalism is not so lightly brushed aside when it is aimed at abortion providers and the like, but is indicative of the fanaticism that animates some workers in the prohibitionist vineyard. The more dedicated drys have indeed taken it upon themselves to teach Americans to be alcophobic, as reflected in a CSAP monograph: "One of the main points of this volume is that an essential ingredient for success is the creation of an environment in which substance use, regardless of the form it takes, is defined clearly and consistently as unacceptable." Similar desires are found in pamphlets from the tax-supported Marin Institute.

To achieve this "no use" goal, these activists advocate bans on advertising and increases in alcohol excise taxes which, as public policy analyst Doug Bandow has pointed out, results in an unethical and illegal phenomenon: "Taxpayers, most of whom drink alcohol, are underwriting what amounts to a prohibitionist campaign."

* * *

The new nutritional guidelines were not well received in the dry community. The Center for Science in the Public Interest, which is not interested in the science of moderation, greeted the guidelines with a wagging finger: "Providing information about the scientific evidence, and drawing conclusions about its utility for the general population, are two different issues.... One thing [governments] should not do is provide generalized recommendations. They should give as much attention to what the findings don't say, which is, 'Who won't benefit? And who will be harmed?'"

The same spirit holds forth among those who design and implement alcohol "awareness" programs in the public schools. When asked if the guidelines will affect school alcohol education policies, Bill Modzeleski, director of the Department of Education's Safe and Drug Free Schools program, which supports programs in 97 percent of the nation's school districts, said, "Probably not. For our population, alcohol is an illegal substance." He thoroughly disagrees with the idea that children are receiving mixed messages from the government on drinking, with schools saying alcohol is bad and the guidelines saying it can prolong life. "Our population doesn't drink for its health effects," he says.

Nor do the youngsters listen to health warnings. "Many students are heavily into binge drinking," Modzeleski says. Drinking remains "pretty steady" and has been "high right along." Maryland officials say that 70.1 percent of seniors in Shannon Eierman's school district reported having a drink within the past twelve months, and nationwide surveys reflect similar consumption patterns.

Schools will, of course, accommodate some of their charges' "inappropriate" behaviors, even to the point of showing them how to don condoms (probably not a revelation to many). Perhaps young tipplers should argue that they're going to drink anyway, so the schools should provide cab fare. In any event, the practice has been to reject any curriculum suggesting there is such a thing as responsible drinking. Instead, students are taught that drinking alcohol in any amount is yet another form of drug use, which has caused more than one family unnecessary friction at the cocktail hour.

* * *

Children are not the only Americans shielded from the moderate drinking message. While the latest health guidelines carry a reasoned message, few Americans are familiar with them. In the one place such a message would be seen by the greatest number of interested parties—the labels on alcoholic beverages—the good news about moderation suffers blackout.

Currently, the Bureau of Alcohol, Tobacco and Firearms, which oversees the labeling process, is considering three attempts to add health messages to the bottles which, by law, must continue to carry the Surgeon General's warnings about alcohol-related health and safety problems. The mildest proposal comes from the Wine Institute, which has petitioned to force labels to suggest that drinkers write off for the nutritional guidelines. The Competitive Enterprise Institute (CEI) is campaigning for a label that reads, "There is significant evidence that moderate consumption of alcoholic beverages may reduce the risk of heart disease." These will not strike many consumers as excessive claims, but ATF is in no hurry to allow changes on bottle labels. Paternalism comes first.

"The Wine Institute and others want to put forth a positive attitude about their product," says the highly personable Bill Earle, deputy associate director for regulatory programs at ATF. "They want to move up to the next level. But we're going to be very cautious. A short message could be misleading if it only communicates partial information. Remember, the dietary guide lines refer to good and bad effects of drink."

Because the bottles already contain a health warning, a suggestion of benefits could balance the picture. Yet Earle responds, "Our position with the industry is that the best place to conduct dialogue is in the free press, not necessarily in labeling or advertising by wine companies." In the meantime, he notes, "Dietary guidelines disconnected the language of 'alcohol and other drugs,' which HHS and others have used for years. That's a subtle but telling observation about the changing view."

Such subtlety is not good enough for CEI's Ben Lieberman, who says his organization is prepared to sue the bureau for not responding in a timely manner to its petition, which was delivered over a year ago. While fully understandable, CEI should not think that it is being singled out for the glacier treatment. Coors Brewing Company was forced to wage a court battle over the course of eight years to be allowed to include the strength of beers on its labels. The case ended last year when the Supreme Court ruled 9–0 to allow brewers to disclose the information, thus overcoming a 1935 law that was enacted after Prohibition's repeal.

That victory was not without its ironies, including the fact that not all beer manufacturers initially supported the change. "We think it is suicidal to market a product based on its alcohol content," said August A. Busch IV, vice-president of Anheuser-Busch. Strangely enough, all alcoholic beverages except beer are required to disclose their alcoholic content on their labels.

Ultimately the push to cut alcohol consumption is built on the belief that some 10 percent of American adults have what are called "drinking problems"—a figure that, like every statistic associated with alcohol, is questioned by specialists.

Researcher Joseph E. Josephson, writing in a publication for the Columbia University School of Public Health, has questioned the very idea that there is a large number of problem drinkers in America: "An objective assessment of government statistics on alcohol-related problems, many of them compiled in the Third Report to the U.S. Congress on Alcohol and Health in 1978, indicates that there is little sound basis for claims that there are upwards of 10 million problem drinkers (including alcoholics) in the adult population and that their number is increasing; that there are 1.5 to 2.25 million problem drinkers among women; that there are over 3 million problem drinkers among youth; that the heavy consumption of alcohol by pregnant women leads consistently to a cluster of birth defects ... [and] that half of all motor vehicle accident fatalities are alcohol-related.... These and other claims about the extent and consequences of alcohol use and abuse—some of them fanciful, others as yet to be supported to research—are part of the 'numbers game' which besets discussion of alcohol-related problems and policy."

Epidemiologist Harold A. Mulford, writing in the *Encyclopedic Handbook of Alcoholism,* made a similar charge:

NIAAA's [National Institute on Alcohol Abuse and Alcoholism] legislatively mandated reports to Congress contain the official prevalence and distribution data for the nation. They are the most publicized prevalence and distribution conclusions and the ones most often cited by politicians and program policy makers. Their official character, however, is not to be confused with scientific validity. Whether by design or not, the reports to Congress likely reflect a contemporary fact of life. The welfare, perhaps even the survival, of NIAAA depends on (1) the apparent magnitude of the alcohol problem, and (2) whether it is made to appear that a disease (rather than a moral or social problem) is being attacked.

Similar skepticism showed up in a ruling this year by the Supreme Court of Louisiana, which affirmed a lower court's ruling that the state's 21-year-old drinking age was unconstitutional. Among other things, the court cited earlier research by Professor Robert Gramling of the University of Southwestern Louisiana, which stated that "there is a lack of empirical evidence to support the assumption that raising the drinking age to 21 years old will result in less alcohol consumption by eighteen to twenty year olds. Dr. Gramling's affidavit further states his research strongly suggests that greater quantities of alcohol may be consumed by eighteen to twenty year olds where the drinking age is raised to twenty one. Finally, Dr. Gramling concludes raising the legal drinking age in 1986 did not significantly change the alcohol consumption of eighteen to twenty year olds in Louisiana."

The court added that "our review of the evidence reveals the State's own statistics clearly show that, in Louisiana, persons between the ages of twenty-one and twenty-three are involved in significantly higher numbers of alcohol related injury and fatality accidents than eighteen to twenty year olds." Louisiana has been warned that lowering the drinking age will cost it federal highway funds.

In recent years the government has undertaken a number of questionable public-safety campaigns, from banning lawn darts (which killed three people over the course of seventeen years) to targeting college coeds with AIDS prevention messages. And while some people should avoid drinking, alcohol's health benefits are no longer a matter of scientific debate. These benefits, presented reasonably, could do much more to enhance the lives of most Americans than all the cod liver oil-type admonitions foisted upon us by our surgeon generals. Plato would no doubt agree.

NO

Meir J. Stampfer, Eric B. Rimm, and Diana Chapman Walsh

ALCOHOL, THE HEART, AND PUBLIC POLICY

Light to moderate drinkers have substantially lower rates of cardiovascular mortality and mortality from all causes than do nondrinkers or heavy drinkers. This finding has been observed repeatedly in several dozen epidemiological studies using a variety of designs. Recent research has added further persuasive evidence to support a causal interpretation of this association.

In epidemiological studies, classification of moderate alcohol consumption ranges from half a drink per day (or less) in some studies up to six drinks a day in others. A 5-oz glass of wine, a 12-oz can of beer, or a shot (1.5 oz) of spirits contains about 13 g to 15 g of alcohol. We consider moderate drinking to be one to two drinks per day for a man and perhaps somewhat less for a woman. For most individuals, this is a safe definition. However, tolerance to alcohol depends on age, sex, body size, and cultural situation; therefore, no single global definition of "moderate" can be made. History of past consumption, rate of consumption, and proximity to meals also alter metabolism of alcohol.

In widely disparate populations, from across Europe and North America to Australia and Thailand, a consistent 20% to 40% reduction in coronary disease has been reported among moderate drinkers. This association is not in dispute. Although a causal interpretation is most plausible, a few investigators have advocated the alternative explanation that the comparison group of nondrinkers is at higher risk of coronary disease because that category includes covert alcohol abusers and those who quit drinking because of ill health.

Work from our group and from others strongly refutes these theories. We compared estimated average alcohol intake from our questionnaire with actual intake from 14 days of diet records. We found, in both men and women, a correlation of approximately .9 between alcohol consumption estimated from the questionnaire and that measure from diet records. Furthermore, we found highly significant correlations between reported alcohol intake and high-density lipoprotein cholesterol in both groups.

From Meir J. Stampfer, Eric B. Rimm, and Diana Chapman Walsh, "Alcohol, the Heart, and Public Policy," *American Journal of Public Health* (June 1993). Copyright © 1993 by The American Public Health Association. Reprinted by permission. References omitted.

For the heaviest alcohol users, a questionnaire or interview may not provide valid information. However, alcohol abusers are far less likely than others to participate in epidemiological studies and therefore the purported presence of heavy drinkers in the nondrinker category is an untenable explanation for the inverse association.

In large and detailed studies, one also may compare moderate alcohol consumption with very light consumption. In our analyses of 87,000 nurses and 51,000 male health professionals we found a significant inverse association with increasing alcohol consumption even with total abstainers excluded. In our two large cohorts we also tested the second, related, noncausal explanation, that men and women with preexisting disease abstain from alcohol. If true, this would tend to produce an artifactual association between abstinence and higher risk of coronary disease.

In most prospective studies, participants with diagnosed coronary disease are excluded at the start of follow-up. However, those with risk factors such as diabetes, hypertension, or hypercholesterolemia are usually not excluded. As expected, we did find a higher prevalence of these conditions among the abstainers in our cohorts. However, in alternative analyses excluding participants with those risk factors, we still found a strong inverse association between alcohol and coronary disease.

Other prospective studies have reported similar findings. Although Shaper originally did not find a similar association after excluding men with preexisting disease in the British Regional Heart Study, with additional follow-up a reduction in ischemic heart disease was found even among men free of existing disease.

Overall mortality was not reduced, but this could be explained in part by the categorization of those reporting from one half up to six drinks per day as "moderate" drinkers. Further, in this population of 7,735 men, the strong correlation between drinking and smoking makes it difficult to obtain precise estimates of the independent effect of drinking. The data from 276,802 men enrolled in the American Cancer Society prospective study provide much more convincing evidence. They show a maximal reduction in total mortality at one to two drinks per day among all participants, both before and after excluding those who were ill at baseline.

In the Kaiser-Permanente study of over 120,000 persons, Klatsky and Armstrong reported reduced coronary mortality among drinkers compared with lifelong nondrinkers. This important finding tends to refute the hypothesis that the protective effect is an artifact caused by the inclusion in the nondrinker group of moderate drinkers who quit because of disease. Similarly, in our cohorts, we excluded men and women with a marked decrease in alcohol intake over the previous 10 years; in those analyses the substantial reduction in risk among the moderate drinkers remained apparent.

Recently, attention has focused on the possible differences in the effect of different alcoholic beverages, particularly the purported special benefits of red wine. The epidemiological evidence suggests that all alcoholic beverages are similarly protective. Some studies find wine more protective; others, beer or spirits. For example, in the Health Professionals Follow-Up Study, men consuming two drinks per day of spirits were at slightly lower risk than those who consumed alcohol from other sources. In the Nurses'

Health Study, wine was found to be a bit more protective, and in an earlier prospective study, Yano et al. reported the lowest risk for moderate beer drinkers. Frankel et al. reported on specific components of red wine that may act as antioxidants to reduce atherosclerosis. However, in a recent update from the large Kaiser cohort, Klatsky and Armstrong found that white wine drinkers had a slight advantage over red wine drinkers, though both groups were at reduced risk compared with nondrinkers.

The best documented mechanism of the cardioprotective effect of alcohol is that it raises the concentration of high-density lipoprotein (HDL). At one time, it was believed that alcohol raised only the HDL-3 subfraction and that only the HDL-2 subfraction was protective. Both of these beliefs are incorrect. Alcohol increases both subfractions, but it raises HDL-3 more than it does HDL-2. Both subfractions are associated with decreased risk, and fractionating high-density lipoprotein provides little or no additional information about risk beyond that derived from total high-density lipoprotein.

Other mechanisms are likely. Alcohol intake decreases platelet aggregability and causes a marked short-term increase in tissue-type plasminogen activator. Both effects point toward an acute reduction of clot formation and hence a decrease in risk. These mechanisms are consistent with a recent case-control study that found a short-term protective effect of alcohol consumption in addition to a benefit of habitual moderate intake.

A protective effect of moderate alcohol consumption is well established from epidemiological data and plausible biological mechanisms. What are the public health implications of this finding? In a 1979 editorial, Castelli concluded that although two drinks per day appear to be protective, "with 17 million alcoholics in this country we perhaps have a message for which this country is not yet ready."

Is this a message for which the country ought to ready itself? If the medical and health establishments were to advocate regular drinking of small amounts of alcohol, would the risk of increased problem drinking outweigh the benefit of healthier hearts? Whose risk would increase and who would benefit? Can clinicians correctly identify patients from whom such advice would be contraindicated?

People—and not only alcoholics—often experience unpleasantness, and occasionally very much worse, as a result of their drinking. What we see far less clearly is how various factors combine to produce these bad outcomes—what the risk (and protective) factors are that explain why in some circumstances some people get into trouble with alcohol whereas others escape. Roughly half of American men who qualify as heavy drinkers never experience problems in connection with their alcohol use. Of those whose episodic abuse does lead to serious trouble, about half are not habitual heavy drinkers.

Studies have identified markers of substance abuse in adolescents: early trial and initiation; strong peer influences; nonconformity and rebelliousness; low achievement in school; lack of family limit-setting, involvement, and support. Among adults, being male, being younger than 30 years, having lower income, being in the working class, and coming from a family with a history of alcoholism increase the risk of heavy drinking, alcohol abuse, and alcoholism. Paradoxically, some of the same high-risk groups have higher proportions of abstainers and would, as a consequence, be particular targets of the pro-drinking message. Numerous theories —genetic, metabolic, psychological, social, cultural, and addiction-based—have been advanced to explain the onset and uneven course of problem drinking, alcohol abuse, or alcoholism. But no theory or combination of theories adequately explains what many scholars now believe are diverse phenomena. Meanwhile, numerous studies have demonstrated that physicians frequently miss the diagnosis even of severe alcoholism.

In the United States, less than 10% of the population reports drinking more than two drinks per day, the cutoff for "heavy drinking" in national survey research. This means that "moderate" drinkers, because of their much greater numbers, probably account for well over half of all alcohol problems, a finding that led researchers at the Institute of Medicine to observe in a groundbreaking report that "if all the clinically diagnosed alcoholics were to stop drinking tomorrow, a substantial fraction of what we understand as alcohol problems would still remain." The statement heralded a conceptual watershed in the way the world thinks about alcohol control, diverting the focus from treating alcoholics toward what was termed a new "public health" approach. Two key assumptions behind that approach are especially pertinent here.

First, public health thinking implies a systems approach, the object of which is to mobilize a range of change strategies—education, moral suasion, and formal rules and laws—in an integrated program of controls aimed at host, agent, and environment. In this approach, a united front and the absence of mixed messages become very important, because the hope is to create a constancy of messages and policies. The possibility that a daily dose of alcohol might be cardioprotective is a perturbation that threatens to complicate or dilute messages designed to alert drinkers to risks.

The second important assumption behind the public health approach to alcohol control is that it seeks to move the whole consumption curve toward lower per capita consumption overall. The hope is that alcohol problems will, as a consequence, abate. Again, the emergence of scientific evidence that alcohol may be salutary seems to fly in the face of this goal. It suggests that health risks increase at both tails of the consumption curve, so that wholesale shifting of the curve could put a subgroup of underconsumers at risk for heart disease.

Should we therefore promote the consumption of small amounts of alcohol? In theory, this would increase the "social availability" of alcohol—the perception among the public that drinking is normative. We simply do not know what the effect might be on overall consumption rates and on alcohol-related problems. But we do have fairly robust evidence that problems decrease with reductions in the physical and economic availability of alcoholic beverages. Problem indicators decline when sales of alcohol are sharply curtailed or prohibited and increase again when restrictions on access are relaxed. Raising the taxes on alcohol reduces consumption, even among heavy drinkers, and at least some associated injuries and deaths. Increasing the minimum legal drinking age seems to reduce highway crashes.

The public health response to alcohol abuse is far from optimal. Both the reach and the range of alcohol treatment strategies need to be expanded. We need more inventive strategies to get people with nascent problems to notice them earlier and avail themselves of low-intensity interventions and supports, which must be made more diverse.

We also need to develop innovative programs to reach people where they study, live, and work and through the mass media. The focus of such efforts should be to change public awareness and behavior concerning alcohol-associated risk. The messages should promote norms that would presumably be protective against alcohol problems:

- It is always acceptable to decline a drink.
- It is never acceptable to become really intoxicated.
- It is never acceptable to drink in situations in which alcohol is associated with significant risk—during pregnancy, while taking medications, before driving a car or using other dangerous machinery, at work, or while engaged in other pursuits that demand coordination and full possession of one's faculties.

It is impossible to predict with confidence what the public health impact might be of an effort to promote the regular consumption of small amounts of alcohol. Large longitudinal studies would be required before we could safely say who might be at risk of progressing to heavier or hazardous drinking. Resources for such research have not been available. Comprehensive cost-benefit analyses are needed to sort out the benefits and risks to individuals and to society. Research is needed, too, to clarify whether the protective effect of alcohol is general or whether the message should apply only to a subgroup. Even with better risk-factor models, we would still be hard pressed to foresee situations, which unfortunately are not uncommon, in which episodes of alcohol abuse among usually moderate drinkers might result in the injury or death of the drinker or someone else.

If a prodrinking campaign were to be mounted, it should certainly seek to avoid communicating the message to certain groups: anyone with a family history of alcoholism, people younger than age 21, and pregnant women. It should also address *all* risk factors for cardiovascular disease, since the others—such as smoking and hypertension—can be reduced by individuals without putting the health of others at risk. But our society is so lacking in effective social controls on alcohol abuse and pays such a heavy price for its inadequate response that, although a policy opposing moderate alcohol consumption may be inadvisable, the thought of a public policy promoting alcohol consumption runs strongly against the grain, however much it might capture at lease some hearts.

POSTSCRIPT

Should Moderate Use of Alcohol Be Recommended?

A recent article in the *Journal of the American Medical Association* estimates that although excessive drinking causes more than 100,000 deaths a year, if Americans stopped drinking altogether, an additional 81,000 people a year would die of heart disease. Alcohol's potential health benefits may have an impact on public policy issues, including excise taxes and advertising. Alcohol producers currently enjoy major influence on Capitol Hill. According to the Center for Responsive Politics, a Washington-based campaign watchdog group, the contributions from the alcohol industry were nearly $4.4 million in 1994.

Alcohol trade groups have promoted positive information about the benefits of moderate drinking to government agencies, the media, and trade groups with good results. The National Institute on Alcohol Abuse and Alcoholism is spending $2 million to study the health effects of moderate alcohol consumption. In 1995 the Department of Agriculture revised the alcohol section of its dietary guidelines for Americans to state, "Current evidence suggests that moderate drinking, defined as up to two drinks a day for men and one for women, is associated with a lower risk of coronary heart disease in some individuals." The guidelines still claim that heavy drinking can increase the risk of health problems and even moderate consumption poses a risk for pregnant women and alcoholics, but alcohol use is indirectly being promoted. Some trade groups are even suing the government to allow alcohol advertisements and labels to carry information about the potential health benefits of drinking!

Although the positive effects of moderate drinking have been demonstrated, there are many issues to be considered. Alcohol in moderation can be beneficial for some people because it reduces their risk of cardiovascular disease. For others, alcohol, even in moderation, can be a health risk. If alcohol was promoted as a healthful beverage, would abstainers be inclined to take up drinking? And would individuals predisposed to alcoholism become alcoholic? For an overview of addiction to drugs and alcohol see "How We Get Addicted," *Time* (May 5, 1997) and "What is Addiction?" *Consumer Reports on Health* (April 1996). For additional readings on the benefits and risks of alcohol consumption see "Drink to Your Heart's Content" and "Alcoholism: Character or Genetics?" *Insight* (March 3, 1997); "The Hazards of Alcohol," *Current Health* (January 1996); "Alcohol: Spirit of Health?" *Consumer Reports on Health* (April 1996); and "Uncorking the Facts About Alcohol and Your Health," *Tufts University Diet and Nutrition Letter* (August 1995).

ISSUE 9

Is Marijuana Dangerous and Addictive?

YES: Eric A. Voth, from "Should Marijuana Be Legalized as a Medicine? No, It's Dangerous and Addictive," *The World and I* (June 1994)

NO: Ethan A. Nadelmann, from "Reefer Madness 1997: The New Bag of Scare Tactics," *Rolling Stone* (February 20, 1997)

ISSUE SUMMARY

YES: Eric A. Voth, medical director of Chemical Dependency Services at St. Francis Hospital in Topeka, Kansas, argues that marijuana produces many adverse effects and that its effectiveness as a medicine is supported only by anecdotes.

NO: Ethan A. Nadelmann, director of the Lindesmith Center, a New York drug policy research institute, claims that government officials continue to promote the myth that marijuana is harmful and leads to the use of hard drugs; he states that the war on marijuana is being fought for purely political, not health, reasons.

At one time there were no laws in the United States regulating the use or sale of drugs including marijuana. Rather than by legislation, their use was regulated by religious teaching and social custom. As society grew more complex and more heterogeneous, the need for more formal regulation of drug sales, production, and use developed.

Attempts at regulating patent medications through legislation began in the early 1900s. In 1920 Congress, under pressure from temperance organizations, passed an amendment prohibiting the manufacture and sale of all alcoholic beverages. From 1920 until 1933, the demand for alcohol was met by organized crime, who either manufactured it illicitly or smuggled it into the United States. The government's inability to enforce the law and increasing violence finally led to the repeal of Prohibition in 1933.

Many years later, in the 1960s, drug usage again began to worry many Americans. Heroin abuse had become epidemic in urban areas, and many middle-class young adults had begun to experiment with marijuana and LSD by the end of the decade. Cocaine also became popular first among the middle class and later among inner-city residents. Today, crack houses, babies born with drug addictions, and drug-related crimes and shootings are the images of a new epidemic of drug abuse.

Many of those who believe illicit drugs are a major problem in this country, however, are usually referring to hard drugs such as cocaine and heroin. Soft drugs like marijuana, though not legal, are not often perceived as a major threat to the safety and well-being of our citizens. Millions of Americans have tried marijuana and did not become addicted. The drug has also been used illegally by those suffering from AIDS, glaucoma, and cancer to alleviate their symptoms and to stimulate their appetites. Should marijuana be legalized as a medicine, or is it too addictive and dangerous? In California, Proposition 215 passed in the November 1996 ballot. A similar measure passed in Arizona. These initiatives convinced voters to relax current laws against marijuana use for medical and humane reasons.

Opponents of these recent measures argue that marijuana use has been steadily rising among teenagers and this may lead to experimentation with hard drugs. There is concern that if marijuana is legal via a doctor's prescription, the drug will be more readily available. There is also concern that the health benefits of smoking marijuana are overrated. For instance, among glaucoma sufferers, in order to achieve benefits from the drug, patients would literally have to be stoned all the time. Marijuana appears to be beneficial for combating the weight loss and wasting associated with AIDS and some cancers by stimulating the appetite and controlling nausea. There are, however, legal, effective prescription drugs on the market that stimulate the appetite and control nausea. Unfortunately, the efficacy of marijuana is unclear since, as an illicit drug, studies to adequately test it have been thwarted by drug control agencies.

If marijuana's effectiveness in treating the symptoms of disease is unclear, is it actually dangerous and addictive? Scientists claim that the drug can negatively affect cognition and motor function. It can also have an impact on short-term memory and can interfere with perception and learning. Physical health effects include lung damage. Until recently, scientists had little evidence that marijuana was actually addictive. Whereas heavy users did not seem to experience actual withdrawal symptoms, studies with laboratory animals given large doses of THC, the active ingredient in marijuana, suffered withdrawal symptoms similar to those characteristics of rodents withdrawing from opiates.

Not all researchers agree, however, that marijuana is dangerous and addictive. The absence of well-designed, long-term studies on the effects of marijuana use further complicates the issue, as does the current potency of the drug. Growers have become more skilled about developing strains of marijuana with high concentrations of THC. Today's varieties may be 3 to 5 times more potent than the pot of the 1960s. Much of the data are unclear, but what is known is that young users of the drug are likely to have problems learning. In addition, some users are at risk for developing dependence.

In the following selections, Eric Voth argues that marijuana causes many physical and psychological effects, including potential addiction. Ethan Nadelmann claims that there are no proven studies to support the views that marijuana is more dangerous than previously thought or that it is a gateway to more dangerous drugs.

YES

Eric A. Voth

SHOULD MARIJUANA BE LEGALIZED AS A MEDICINE? NO, IT'S DANGEROUS AND ADDICTIVE

To best understand the problems associated with legalizing marijuana, it is useful to examine drug legalization in general and then to discuss the specific pitfalls of legal marijuana.

Advocates generally argue that crime would decrease under legalization, that dealers would be driven out of the market by lower prices, that legalization works in other countries, that government would benefit from the sales tax on drugs, that Prohibition did not work, and that the "war on drugs" has failed.

Examining currently legal drugs provides an insight as to the possible effect of legalizing other drugs. First, alcohol is responsible for approximately 100,000 deaths every year and 11 million cases of alcoholism. Virtually every bodily system is adversely affected by alcoholism. While Prohibition was an unfortunately violent time, many of the hardships of that era were really the result of the Depression. Prohibition did decrease the rate of alcohol consumption; alcohol-related deaths climbed steadily after Prohibition was repealed.

Tobacco use is responsible for 400,000 premature deaths per year. It causes emphysema, chronic bronchitis, heart disease, lung cancer, head and neck cancers, vascular disease, and hypertension, to name a few disorders. The taxes on tobacco come nowhere close to paying for the health problems caused by the drug.

The argument that legalization would decrease crime exemplifies a great lack of understanding of drug abuse. Most drug-associated crime is committed to acquire drugs or under the influence of drugs. The Netherlands has often been heralded by the drug culture as a country where decriminalization has worked. In fact, drug-related holdups and shootings have increased 60 percent and 40 percent, respectively, since decriminalization. This has caused the government to start enforcing the drug laws more strictly.

Because of its powerful drug lobby, the Netherlands has never been able to mount a taxation campaign against its legal drugs. We suffer a similar phenomenon in the United States in that the tobacco lobby has successfully defeated most taxation initiatives against tobacco.

The argument that drug dealers would be driven out of the market by lower prices ignores the fact that legalization will probably result in as many as 250,000 to over two million new addicts. Broader markets, even with lower prices, certainly will not drive dealers out of the market. Our overburdened medical system will not be able to handle the drastic increase in the number of addicts.

MEDICAL MARIJUANA

Richard Cowan, national director of the National Organization for the Reform of Marijuana Laws (NORML), has stated that acceptance of medicinal uses of marijuana is pivotal for its legalization.

In 1972, the drug culture petitioned the Drug Enforcement Administration (DEA) to reschedule marijuana from a Schedule I drug (unable to be prescribed, high potential for abuse, not currently accepted for medicinal use, unsafe) to a Schedule II drug (high potential for abuse, currently accepted for medical use, potential for abuse, but prescribable).

This rescheduling petition was initiated by NORML, the Alliance for Cannabis Therapeutics (ACT), and the Cannabis Corporation of America. Of note is the fact that none of these drug-culture organizations has a recognized medical or scientific background, nor do they represent any accredited medical entity.

After substantial legal maneuvering by the drug culture, the DEA carefully documented the case against the rescheduling of marijuana and denied the petition. To examine the potential for therapeutic uses of marijuana, the DEA turned to testimony from nationally recognized experts who rejected the medical use of marijuana (published in the *Federal Register*, December 29, 1989, and March 26, 1992).

In the face of this expert testimony, the drug lobby could only produce anecdotes and the testimony of a handful of physicians with limited or absent clinical experience with marijuana. (Marijuana has not been accepted as a medicine by the AMA, the National Multiple Sclerosis Society, the American Glaucoma Society, the American Academy of Ophthalmology, and the American Cancer Society.)

The drug culture organizations appealed the DEA's decision. Recently, the U.S. Court of Appeals for the District of Columbia denied their petition to reschedule marijuana. This important decision also sets forth the new guideline that only rigorous scientific standards can satisfy the requirement of "currently accepted medical use." These preconditions are:

1. The drug has a known and reproducible chemistry;
2. Adequate safety studies;
3. Adequate and well-controlled studies proving efficacy; and
4. Qualified experts accept the drug.

In addition, the decision stated, "The administrator reasonably accorded more weight to the opinions of the experts than to the laymen and doctors on which the petitioners relied."

In his 1993 book *Marihuana: The Forbidden Medicine*, the psychiatrist Dr. Lester

Grinspoon assembled a group of anecdotes to justify the rescheduling of marijuana. Similar to the promarijuana lobby during rescheduling hearings, Grinspoon asserts that marijuana should be used to help relieve nausea (during cancer chemotherapy), glaucoma, wasting in AIDS, depression, menstrual cramps, pain, and virtually unlimited ailments. His anecdotes have no controls, no standardization of dose, no quality control, and no independent medical evaluation for efficacy or toxicity.

ONLY ANECDOTES PROVE ITS EFFICACY

The historical uses of marijuana in such cultures as India, Asia, the Middle East, South Africa, and South America are cited by Grinspoon as evidence of appropriate medical uses of the drug. One of Grinspoon's references is an 1860 assertion that marijuana had supposed beneficial effects "without interfering with the actions of the internal organs" (this is inaccurate). Let us not forget that medicine in earlier years was fraught with potions and remedies. Many of these were absolutely useless or even harmful to unsuspecting subjects. This is when our current FDA [Food and Drug Administration] and drug scheduling processes evolved, which should not be undermined.

The medical marijuana campaign gained momentum in February 1990, when a student project, initiated by Rick Doblin, published interpretations of a questionnaire that he had sent to oncologists. Doblin is closely associated with the Multidisciplinary Association for Psychedelic Studies, a drug-culture lobbying organization. This group strongly supports the legalization and medical uses of the street drugs LSD and MDMA (Ecstasy). Doblins' staff sponsor at Harvard, Mark Kleiman, voiced his support for the legalization of marijuana in his recent book *Against Excess*. Neither author has a medical background, nor do they disclose their intrinsic bias toward the legalization of marijuana.

By manipulation of the statistics, the authors contend that 48 percent of their respondents would prescribe marijuana if legal and 54 percent feel it should be available by prescription. But the researchers fail to relate that the respondents account for only 9 percent of practicing oncologists. Only 6 percent of those surveyed feel that marijuana was effective in 50 percent or more of their patients.

Only 18 percent of the surveyed group believe marijuana to be safe and efficacious. Five percent of those surveyed favor making marijuana available by prescription. These numbers become less significant if compared to the number of all practicing oncologists. Furthermore, this survey was conducted before the release for use of the medication ondansetron (Zofran®), which is extremely effective to relieve the nausea associated with chemotherapy.

Unfortunately, the "results" of this unscientific but well-publicized study incorrectly give the impression that oncologists want marijuana available as medicine. But researchers neither asked if the oncologists had systematically examined their patients for negative effects of marijuana use nor if the oncologists were familiar with the myriad of health consequences of marijuana use. Furthermore, they did not ask oncologists if their attitudes about marijuana were affected by their own current or past marijuana use.

Contrary to the findings of Doblin and Kleiman, Dr. Richard Schwartz determined through a survey of practicing oncologists that THC (the major active ingredient of marijuana) ranked ninth in their preference for the treatment of mild nausea and sixth for the treatment of severe nausea. Only 6 percent had prescribed THC (by prescription or marijuana) for more than 50 patients. It was found that nausea was relieved in only 50 percent of the patients who received THC and that 25 percent had adverse side effects.

COMPLICATIONS OF MARIJUANA USE

According to the 1992 National Household Survey on Drug Abuse, 48 percent of young adults have used marijuana and 11 percent continue to use it. In 1992, 8.2 percent of young adults age 26 to 34 admitted having used marijuana in the last month, a figure that was up from 7.0 percent in 1991. Marijuana remains the most frequently used illegal drug. The chronic use of marijuana has now been demonstrated to lead to higher utilization of the health-care system, a long-suspected phenomenon.

Mental, affective, and behavioral changes are the most easily recognized consequences of marijuana use. Concentration, motor coordination, and memory are adversely impacted. For example, the ability to perform complex tasks such as flying is impaired even 24 hours after the acute intoxication phase. The association of marijuana use with trauma and intoxicated motor vehicle operation is also well established.

Memory is impaired for several months after cessation of use. After chronic use, marijuana addicts admit that their motivation to succeed lessens. Several biochemical models have demonstrated abnormal changes in brain cells, brain blood flow, and brain waves. Pathologic behavior such as psychosis is also associated with marijuana use. The more chronic the use, as would be necessary for treating diseases such as glaucoma, the higher the risk of mental problems.

Despite arguments from the drug culture to the contrary, marijuana is addictive. This addiction has been well described by users. It consists of both a physical dependence (tolerance and subsequent withdrawal) and a psychological habituation. Strangely, in the course of the rescheduling hearings, prodrug organizations admitted that "marijuana has a high potential for abuse and that abuse of the marijuana plant may lead to severe psychological or physical dependence," points that they now publicly deny. Unlike those addicted to many other drugs, the marijuana addict is exceptionally slow to recognize the addiction.

The gateway effect of marijuana is also well established in research. Use of alcohol, tobacco, and marijuana are major risk factors for subsequent addiction and more extensive drug use.

Smoked marijuana contains double to triple the concentrations of tar, carbon monoxide, and carcinogens found in cigarette smoke. Marijuana adversely impairs lung function by causing abnormalities in the cells lining the airways of the upper and lower respiratory tract and in the airspaces deep within the lung. It has been linked to head and neck cancer.

Contaminants of marijuana smoke include certain forms of bacteria and fungi. Users with impaired immunity are at particular risk for disease and infection when they inhale these substances.

Adverse effects of marijuana on the unborn were suspected after studies in Rhesus monkeys demonstrated spontaneous abortion. When exposed to marijuana during gestation, humans demonstrate changes in size and weight as well as neurologic abnormalities. A very alarming association also exists between maternal marijuana use and certain forms of cancer in offspring. Additionally, hormonal function in both male and female children is disrupted.

One of the earliest findings was the negative effect of marijuana on various immune functions, including cellular immunity and pulmonary immunity. Impaired ability to fight infection is now documented in humans who use marijuana. They have been shown to exhibit an inability to fight herpes infections and a blunted response to therapy for genital warts. The potential for these complications exists in all forms of administration of marijuana.

It should be clear that use of the drug bears substantial health risks. In populations at high risk for infection and immune suppression (AIDS and cancer chemotherapy patients), the risks are unacceptable.

SUMMARY

The unfortunate reality is that the drug culture is exploiting the unwitting public and the suffering of patients with chronic illnesses for its own benefit. Under the false and dangerous claims that smoking marijuana is a harmless recreational activity and that it offers significant benefits to those suffering from a variety of tragic ailments, the drug culture seeks to use bogus information to gain public acceptance for the legalization of marijuana.

NO

Ethan A. Nadelmann

REEFER MADNESS 1997: THE NEW BAG OF SCARE TACTICS

The war on drugs is really a war on marijuana," says professor Lynn Zimmer, a sociologist at Queens College, in New York, who is widely regarded as one of the nation's leading analysts of drug policy. Marijuana, says Zimmer, is the leading justification for drug testing in the workplace, the main target of anti-drug efforts in the schools and the media, and the principal preoccupation of drug warriors in and out of government today. The drug warriors' tactics include—along with arrests, seizures, incarceration and the intimidation of doctors who would prescribe pot for the terminally ill—a more sinister approach. Spokesmen are quoted by journalists and appear on the evening news and on talk shows, making frightening claims about marijuana's harmful effects, spinning unproven theories and, in some cases, distorting the known truth in an effort to demonize even casual users of pot.

It's no wonder that the warriors find themselves in a quandary. They're essentially fighting a war against the 70 million Americans who have tried marijuana, including half of all Americans aged 18–35 and more than a quarter of everyone older than 35. Polls have indicated that a fourth of all adult Americans favor legalizing pot, which, after alcohol, tobacco and caffeine, is the fourth most popular psychoactive drug in the world.

"You can't scare middle-class parents with a war on heroin and cocaine," says Zimmer." These drugs are too removed, too remote. Marijuana brings it home."

Bill Clinton's administration, desperate not to appear soft on drugs, has indulged in its share of scare tactics. Clinton's newly appointed drug czar, Gen. Barry McCaffrey, has set the tone for the federal government's new stance, threatening sanctions against medical doctors in California and Arizona (RS 750/751), where citizens voted in November to allow the medicinal use of cannabis. More typical, however, is the approach taken by Secretary of Health and Human Services Donna Shalala, who disingenuously told reporters last December [1996], "All available research has concluded that marijuana is dangerous to our health."

Is pot dangerous? Is there any scientific research to back up Shalala's claim? There are, of course, reasons to be concerned about marijuana. It is, like alcohol, a powerful psychoactive drug. Used irresponsibly, it contributes to accidents on the roads and in the workplace. During the period of intoxication, short-term memory is impaired. Heavy pot smokers face some of the same risks as cigarette smokers. And some people become dependent upon marijuana, using it as a crutch to avoid dealing with relationships and responsibilities.

Among kids, especially, it is the daily use of marijuana, not experimental or occasional use, that merits concern. According to the latest annual survey of drug use among high-school students, the percentage of eighth-graders who admit to daily pot smoking increased from 0.2 percent in 1991 to 1.5 percent in 1996. Among 10th-graders, there was an increase from 0.8 percent to 3.5 percent; among seniors, an increase from 2 percent to nearly 5 percent. Of course, smoking marijuana every day would contribute to a teenager's problems in school and socially, but more likely it is an indicator of something else that is basically wrong.

On the other hand, there is ample evidence that the majority of the 70 million Americans who have tried marijuana are doing just fine. Since the early 1970s, the government has funded studies that have ended up proving that pot is not harmful, then disavowed the findings. In 1988, following an extensive review of the scientific evidence on marijuana, the Drug Enforcement Administration's own administrative-law judge, Francis Young, concluded that marijuana "in its natural form is one of the safest therapeutically active substances known to man." Virtually every independent commission assigned to examine the evidence on marijuana and marijuana policy —including the Shafer Commission appointed by President Richard Nixon, a National Academy of Sciences committee in the early 1980s, and numerous others both in the U.S. and abroad—have concluded that marijuana poses fewer dangers to individuals and society than either alcohol or tobacco and should be decriminalized.

And there is little reason to expect anything different from the Clinton administration's January [1997] announcement that it will spend $1 million to review all the evidence on the medical benefits of marijuana. The problem is that no Congress or president has ever had the guts to follow through on the recommendations of independent commissions assigned to balance the risks and harms of marijuana with the risks and harms of marijuana policies. It's still impossible, for instance, for any government official to speak out publicly about the difference between responsible and irresponsible use of marijuana, as they would with alcohol. All marijuana use is defined as drug abuse—notwithstanding extensive evidence that most marijuana users suffer little if any harm. That position may be intellectually and scientifically indefensible, but those in government regard it as politically and legally obligatory.

So the government resorts to scare tactics and misinformation, relying increasingly on three claims: that today's marijuana is much more potent than the version that kids' parents smoked a decade or two ago; that new research has shown the drug to be more dangerous to our health than previously thought; and that marijuana use is a gateway to more dangerous drugs.

Are these claims true? Is today's marijuana much more potent? Is marijuana much more dangerous than previously believed? Is marijuana a "gateway drug"?

Most marijuana researchers depend on government grants to finance their studies. This poses two problems. First, the government tends to encourage and fund only those research proposals that seek to identify harmful effects of marijuana. There are few incentives to investigate the benefits of marijuana, medicinal or otherwise, and little interest in determining either the safety margins of occasional use or ways of reducing the harms of marijuana use. Studies that identify marijuana as harmful are well publicized by the governments' public-affairs officers. Findings that fail to confirm any harms are ignored.

Second, few marijuana researchers dare publicly challenge the government's anti-marijuana campaign. Scientists know that the grant-review process can be both scientifically objective and politically subjective. If too many studies fail to identify and emphasize the harms of marijuana, subsequent research proposals may not fare well in grant competitions. It takes a lot of courage for a scientist—dependent upon government grants for his or her livelihood—to raise questions about government policies and statements regarding marijuana. Not many scientists are that brave.

Fortunately, there are a few researchers who maintain their independence. Zimmer, the sociologist at Queens College, and Dr. John P. Morgan, a physician and pharmacologist who teaches at the City University Medical School, in New York, don't rely on government funding. They have recently completed a book, *Marijuana Myths, Marijuana Facts: A Review of the Scientific Evidence*, that systematically analyzes and dissects hundreds of studies on marijuana, including virtually all of those cited by government officials and other anti-drug crusaders to justify the war on marijuana. The result is the most comprehensive and objective review of the scientific evidence on marijuana since the National Institute of Medicine's report in 1982—one that both debunks many of the myths propagated by drug warriors and tells the truth about what is actually known of marijuana's harms and margins of safety. What follows is drawn largely from their work.

THE POTENCY QUESTION

No claim has taken hold so well as the charge that marijuana is much more potent than in the past. "If people... confessing to marijuana use in the late '60s... sucked in on one of today's marijuana cigarettes, they'd fall down backward," said William Bennett, President George Bush's first drug czar, in 1990. "Marijuana is 40 times more potent today... than 10, 15, 20 years ago," another drug czar, Lee Brown, claimed, in 1995. And from the ranking Democrat of the Senate Judiciary Committee, Joseph Biden, in 1996: "It's like comparing buckshot in a shot-gun shell to a laser-guided missile."

Is any of this true? No. Although high-potency marijuana may be more available today than previously, the pharmacological experience of smoking marijuana today is the same as in the 1960s and 1970s. The only data on marijuana potency over time comes from the government-funded Potency Monitoring Project at the University of Mississippi. Since 1981, the average THC (tetrahydrocannabinol, marijuana's principal psychoactive chemical) content of PMP samples—all of which come from drug seizures by U.S. police agencies—has fluctuated between 2.28 percent and 3.82 percent. The project's findings during the 1970s were substantially lower, possibly because the samples were improperly stored (which can cause degradation of THC) and partly due to an overdependence on low-grade Mexican "kilobricks." Independent analyses of marijuana during the 1970s, which included samples from sources other than police agencies, reported much higher THC levels, ranging from 2 percent to 5 percent, with some samples as high as 14 percent.

Marijuana of less than 0.5 percent potency has almost no psychoactivity; in fact, in laboratory studies, subjects are often unable to distinguish a placebo from marijuana with less than 1 percent THC. It's not very likely that marijuana would have become so popular during the 1970s if the average THC content had been so low. Today, some regular marijuana users may have access to expensive, high-potency marijuana, often grown indoors under artificial light by small-scale, low-volume growers. But the potency of the "commercial grade" marijuana smoked by most Americans is not much different than it was 10, 15 or 20 years ago.

Even if marijuana potency had increased, that would not mean the drug has necessarily become more dangerous. It is impossible to consume a lethal dose of marijuana, regardless of its THC content. And in laboratory studies, smokers often fail to distinguish variations in potency of up to 100 percent. Increases of 200 percent to 300 percent in potency result in only 35 percent to 40 percent increases in smokers' "subjective high" ratings. "Bad trips" and other adverse psychoactive reactions typically have little to do with marijuana potency. Moreover, when potency increases, smokers tend to smoke less, thus causing less damage to their lungs.

The bottom line is this: If parents want to know what their kids are smoking today, they need only recall their own experiences. Neither marijuana nor the experience of smoking marijuana has changed much.

SEX, HEALTH AND MEMORY

Claims of increased THC potency aside, much of the new war on marijuana relies on claims of new scientific research that shows marijuana to be far more dangerous than previously thought.

There are tons of anecdotal reports that marijuana enhances sex. And there are repeated claims that marijuana interferes with male and female sex hormones, can cause infertility, and produces feminine characteristics in males and masculine characteristics in females. Speaking at Framingham High School, in Massachusetts, in late 1994, President Clinton spoke about "the danger of using marijuana, especially to young women, and what might happen to their childbearing capacity in the future."

What's the truth? Some animal studies indicate that high doses of THC diminish the production of some sex hormones and may impair reproduction. In human studies, however, scientists typically find no impact on sex-hormone levels. In the few studies that do show some impact, such as lower sperm counts and sperm motility, the effects are modest, temporary and of no apparent consequence for reproductive capacity. A real-life example: Jamaica's Rastafarians, who smoke large amounts of the sacred herb, appear to have no problem making babies.

In 1972, a letter to the *New England Journal of Medicine* described three cases of breast enlargement in men who had smoked marijuana. In 1980, a letter to the *Journal of Pediatrics* described a 16-year-old marijuana smoker who had failed to progress to puberty. Both reports received substantial publicity, but neither has been confirmed through research. But studies involving larger numbers of marijuana users and non-users have found no evidence that marijuana distorts or delays sexual development, masculinizes females or feminizes males. There may be good reasons for telling kids not to smoke marijuana, but the president's warnings were based on myth, not fact.

Now that thousands of people with AIDS are smoking marijuana to stimulate their appetites and promote weight gain, opponents keep insisting that marijuana's damaging effects on the immune system negate any potential benefits. Here again, the claims are based almost entirely on studies in which laboratory animals are given extremely large doses of THC. There's no evidence that marijuana users have higher rates of infectious disease than non-users. That's not to say that there are no dangers. For people with compromised immune systems, smoking can cause lung infections. There is also a risk for AIDS patients that they will contract a pulmonary disease called aspergillosis caused by fungal spores sometimes found on improperly stored marijuana. One solution to this problem would be careful screening of marijuana supplies, a role for the government or pharmaceutical companies. And that is another reason to prescribe legal, controlled marijuana to more than the eight Americans who are now entitled to receive it.

Everyone knows that marijuana—like other psychoactive drugs consumed in sufficient doses—screws up short-term memory. Kids who get high (or drunk) before going to class are less likely to learn what their teachers are trying to teach them. Their minds are more likely to wander. People under the influence of marijuana can remember things they learned previously, but their capacity to learn and recall new information is diminished. Although some find marijuana useful for problem solving and creative tasks, there is little question that marijuana is not conducive to learning in school and other highly structured environments.

The question of whether marijuana use permanently impairs memory and other cognitive functions is a separate issue. During the '70s, the U.S. government funded three comprehensive field studies in Jamaica, Greece and Costa Rica, in which long-term heavy cannabis users and non-users were subjected to a battery of standardized tests of their cognitive functions. The researchers found virtually no differences between the two groups.

More recently, two studies funded by the National Institute on Drug Abuse reported evidence of cognitive harm in high-dose marijuana users. The first, published in *Psychopharmacology*, in 1993, found that heavy marijuana users— who reported seven or more uses per week for an average of 6.5 years— scored lower than non-users on math and verbal tests. But the researchers also found that "intermediate" users—those smoking marijuana five to six times per week—were indistinguishable from non-users.

The second study, published in the *Journal of the American Medical Association,* in 1996, found differences between daily marijuana users and those who smoked fewer than 10 times per month, but the differences were minor. The light smokers performed slightly better on two memory tests and one card-sorting test—while no differences were found on tests of attention, verbal fluency and complex drawing.

What we know now, based on existing research, is that if heavy marijuana use produces cognitive impairment, it is relatively minor—and may have little or no practical significance.

Gateway Drugs?

The "gateway theory," formerly known as the "steppingstone hypothesis," has long been a staple of anti-marijuana campaigns. Marijuana use, it is claimed, leads inexorably to the use of more dangerous drugs like cocaine, heroin and LSD. If we can stop kids from trying marijuana, we can win the drug war.

The most recent, and oft-repeated, version of the gateway theory—an analysis conducted by the National Center on Addiction and Substance Abuse at Columbia University—asserts that youthful marijuana users are 85 times more likely than non-users to use cocaine. To obtain this figure, the proportion of marijuana users who had ever tried cocaine (17 percent) was divided by the proportion of cocaine users who had never used marijuana (0.2 percent). The "risk factor" is large not because so many marijuana users experiment with cocaine—only a minority actually do—but because

people who use cocaine, a relatively unpopular drug, are likely to have also used the more popular drug marijuana. Similarly, marijuana users are more likely than non-users to have had previous experience with legal drugs like alcohol, tobacco and caffeine.

Alcohol, tobacco and caffeine do not cause people to use marijuana. And marijuana does not cause people to use cocaine, heroin or LSD. There is no pharmacological basis for the gateway theory, since marijuana does not change brain chemistry in a way that causes drug-seeking, drug-taking behavior. In fact, there is no theory here at all—just a description of the typical sequence in which people who use many drugs begin by using ones that are more common.

The relationship between marijuana use and the use of other drugs is constantly changing. In some societies, marijuana use follows, rather than precedes, use of heroin and other drugs. Among American high-school seniors, the proportion of marijuana users who have tried cocaine decreased from a high of 33 percent, in 1986, to 14 percent, in 1995. Americans who smoke pot may be more likely to try other illegal drugs than those who don't smoke it. But for a large majority of marijuana users, marijuana is a terminus rather than a gateway drug.

"Now we're putting the research into the hands of parents," Donna Shalala claimed at a recent press conference, renewing the government's war against marijuana. But if it's the truth that Shalala wants to distribute, Zimmer and Morgan's *Marijuana Myths, Marijuana Facts* is a better source.

POSTSCRIPT

Is Marijuana Dangerous and Addictive?

Recent initiatives in California and Arizona that bring marijuana closer to being legal are making many people nervous. The propositions in those states would allow the drug to be prescribed by physicians for medicinal purposes. The majority of Americans are against making marijuana completely legal. A compromise would be to decriminalize marijuana, making it neither strictly legal nor illegal. If decriminalized, there would be no penalty for personal or medical use or possession, although there would continue to be criminal penalties for sale for profit and distribution to minors. Marijuana has been decriminalized in a few states, but it is illegal in most of the country.

Decriminalization appeals to attorney Peter Riga, in "The Drug War Is a Crime: Let's Try Decriminalization," *Commonweal* (July 16, 1993); editor Marcia Angell, in "Alcohol and Other Drugs: Toward a More Rational and Consistent Policy," *The New England Journal of Medicine* (August 25, 1994); and journalist Robert Hough, in "Reefer Sadness," *Toronto Globe and Mail* (November 9, 1991). Eric Schlosser, in "Reefer Madness," *The Atlantic Monthly* (August, 1994), argues that there are far too many people in jails for marijuana offenses.

In early 1992, the Drug Enforcement Administration published a document claiming that the federal government was justified in its continued prohibition of marijuana for medicinal purposes. The report indicated that too many questions surrounded the effectiveness of medicinal marijuana. See "Medical Marijuana: To Prescribe or Not to Prescribe, That is the Question," *Journal of Addictive Diseases* (vol. 14, 1995). The effectiveness of marijuana as therapy for cancer and AIDS patients continues to be debated, but the Center on Addiction and Substance Abuse of Columbia University maintains that recent research suggests that the drug is addictive and can wreck the lives of users, particularly teenagers. They argue that legalizing marijuana would undermine the impact of drug education and increase usage.

Other articles that debate the safety and legality of marijuana include the following: "Does Heavy Marijuana Use Impair Human Cognition?" *JAMA* (February 21, 1996); "The Return of Reefer Madness," *The Progressive* (May 1996); "Smoke Alarm," *Reason* (May 1996); "Pot Luck," *National Review* (November 11, 1996); "The Battle for Medical Marijuana," *The Nation* (January 6, 1997); "Federal Foolishness and Marijuana," *The New England Journal of Medicine* (January 30, 1997); "The War Over Weed," *Newsweek* (February 3, 1997); and "Prescription Drugs," *Reason* (February 1997).

On the Internet . . .

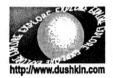

Women's Health Interactive
Women's Health Interactive offers topics relating to women's health, including a personal nutritional analysis for women. *http://www.women's-health.com*

The National Alliance of Breast Cancer Organizations
For current information on breast cancer, the National Alliance of Breast Cancer Organizations' Web site supplies information on ongoing studies. *http://www.nabco.org*

HIV Positive.com: Your Comprehensive Resource to Improved Quality of Life
AIDS Assistance is a site aimed at improving the quality of life for anyone touched by the disease. It offers everything from nutrition information to financial advice and drug advisories. *http://www.HIVpositive.com*

The Men's Issues Page
The Men's Issues page has an alphabetical subject index as a source of men's issues, including fatherhood, physical health, and related topics. This site provides a variety of men's health, social, and psychological concerns. *http://www.vix.com/pub/men/index.html*

PART 4

Sexuality and Gender Issues

Few issues could be of greater controversy than those concerning gender and sexuality. Recent generations of Americans have rejected "traditional" sexual roles and values, which has resulted in a significant increase in babies born out of wedlock, the spread of sexually transmitted diseases, and the rise of legal abortions. This section debates the health risks of breast implants, the morality of abortion, the gender gap in health care, and the risk of contracting AIDS for non-drug-abusing heterosexuals.

■ Are Silicone Breast Implants a Health Risk to Women?

■ Does Health Care Delivery and Research Benefit Men at the Expense of Women?

■ Is AIDS a Major Threat to the Heterosexual, Non-Drug-Abusing Population?

■ Can Abortion Be a Morally Acceptable Choice?

ISSUE 10

Are Silicone Breast Implants a Health Risk to Women?

YES: Jennifer Washburn, from "Reality Check: Can 400,000 Women Be Wrong?" *Ms.* (March/April 1996)

NO: Michael Fumento, from "A Confederacy of Boobs," *Reason* (October 1995)

ISSUE SUMMARY

YES: Reporter Jennifer Washburn challenges two studies that claim silicone gel implants do no harm and finds over 10 percent of the women who received implants are ill.

NO: Journalist Michael Fumento claims that special interests and the press have conspired to ban implants despite the fact that no scientific study has linked them to cancer or other diseases.

From 1979 to 1992, the peak years for breast implant surgery in the United States, nearly 150,000 women had their breasts enlarged or reconstructed. By 1994 breast augmentation was the third most common cosmetic operation in this country despite the 1992 ban by the Food and Drug Administration (FDA). Overall, approximately 1 million women have had the surgery. Because of health concerns, the FDA banned silicone gel, which was replaced with implants filled with sterile salt water. Initially, silicone appeared to be a perfect substance to enlarge breasts (or other body parts); but it became apparent that injecting any foreign substance into the body causes an inflammatory response. When silicone was initially used to enlarge breasts, it was injected directly into the body, but this caused pain and infection. Dow Corning, in 1962, developed a silicone-filled prosthesis that adhered to the chest muscles. The device prevented the silicone from migrating to other body parts, reducing the risk of inflammation.

In 1992 Dr. David Kessler, the FDA director, banned silicone breast implants after responding to mounting concerns that they caused autoimmune and connective tissue damage and disease. Specifically, the autoimmune disorders included cancer, lupus, rheumatoid arthritis, scleroderma, and polymyalgia. The ban resulted in a flood of lawsuits, as women by the thousands sued the manufacturers of the implants. Juries sympathetic to the women's plight awarded huge damages. In April 1994, in a class action settlement, the major manufacturers agreed to pay over $4 billion to women with breast implants, $1 billion of which was set aside for the attorneys.

Do breast implants actually cause these diseases? Interestingly, there were almost no reliable scientific studies published by the time of the 1992 ban. Since then, several have been published. In investigations conducted by the Mayo Clinic and Harvard University, no connection was found between implants and connective tissue disease. As other studies are added to the evidence, however, absolute proof of the relationship between implants and autoimmune disease is lacking, though some women did experience surgical complications (as with any surgery, complications, including infection and hemorrhage, can occur). In addition, some women experienced scar tissue formation around the breasts and, in some cases, the implant ruptured, releasing silicone gel into the surrounding tissues and flattening the breast.

How then, in the absence of proof from well-designed studies, did the idea of autoimmune disease risk develop in the first place, and why did women with implants win in court? Probably from a mixture of anecdotes and speculation. As isolated reports became the basis of litigation and the publicity in the media grew, more women came forward with similar symptoms. Since the ban, women with implants who have these symptoms are more likely to come to light because of the heightened awareness of the situation. This extra attention may increase the impression that there is a *proven* link even if there is not. Also, some physicians who are sympathetic and believe in a relationship between implants and disease tend to draw these women to their practice. As a result, studying these women does not answer the question of whether implants actually increase the risk of autoimmune disease.

Many scientific organizations, including the American Medical Association, the FDA advisory panel on General and Plastic Surgery Devices, and committees commissioned by the British, Canadian, and French governments, have all agreed that there is no proof that silicone implants cause autoimmune diseases or systemwide harm. Evidence from studies completed at the Mayo Clinic and Harvard University have shown that although implants may cause localized problems such as swelling, there is no proof to support the litigation. Why, then, were the courts, the media, and the public so certain that breast implants were dangerous?

According to Dr. Marcia Angell, executive editor of the *New England Journal of Medicine*, the answer to this question is in the way science, the public, and the law regard evidence. As our society becomes more dependent on science and technology, there are bound to be further misconceptions about scientific evidence that could become a danger to the public. In the following selections, Jennifer Washburn disagrees. She asserts that the major studies disputing a relationship between implants and autoimmune disease are full of holes and should be discounted. Michael Fumento agrees with Angell. He claims that the attack and litigation involving silicone breast implants is nothing more than a campaign of misinformation.

YES

Jennifer Washburn

REALITY CHECK: CAN 400,000 WOMEN BE WRONG?

In September 1993, Charlotte Mahlum, a waitress from Elko, Nevada, and the mother of two children, sued the Dow Corning Corporation and one of its parent companies, the Dow Chemical Company, alleging that silicone breast implants manufactured by Dow Corning had made her sick. Mahlum, 44 years old, had had the implants put in after a double mastectomy in 1985. Six years later, she developed joint and muscle aches, full-body rashes, and chronic fatigue. Soon afterward, she began to suffer tremors and seizures, and was diagnosed with axonal polyneuropathy, a condition that prevents brain signals from reaching the outermost nerves. At times she suffered fits of uncontrollable shaking, and she eventually lost control of her bowels.

When Mahlum had her implants taken out in 1993, silicone breast implants had been off the market for a year (for all but mastectomy patients), removed by the Food and Drug Administration (FDA), whose commissioner, David Kessler, said at the time, "We know more about the life span of automobile tires than we do about the longevity of breast implants." When Mahlum's surgeon opened up her chest, he discovered that one implant had ruptured, but he was unable to remove all of the gel that had seeped into surrounding tissue. Today, Charlotte Mahlum is still extremely ill.

In May 1995, Dow Corning declared bankruptcy, placing itself beyond the reach of the trial courts. The bankruptcy was announced days after the collapse of the Breast Implant Global Settlement, in which implant manufacturers had agreed to compensate the members of a class action suit who claimed to have—or feared the development of—illnesses associated with silicone implants. At least 400,000 women had signed up for the suit, and their numbers were growing.

Mahlum proceeded with her case against Dow Chemical, which owns 50 percent of Dow Corning's stock. Although Dow Chemical never manufactured silicone breast implants, it performed much of the original research and testing on liquid silicone, which makes up 80 to 85 percent of the gel used in Dow Corning implants. On October 30, 1995, a Nevada jury ruled in Mahlum's favor, awarding $14.1 million to her and her husband, $10 million of it in punitive damages. It was one of the highest awards ever granted in a breast implant case. Dow Chemical plans to appeal this ruling.

Although the Mahlum jury had reviewed internal documents that showed that both companies knew liquid silicone was dangerous inside the body, the verdict outraged implant manufacturers, who insist that there is no proven link between silicone implants and disease. It also sparked an outpouring of criticism in the media. "It's the judges' fault," blasted a Wall *Street Journal* editorial, lamenting that breast implant companies are "paying billions in damages despite a mountain of evidence they didn't do anything wrong." Even advocates of legal reform got into the act, insisting that the case proved that the U.S. legal system is in desperate need of fixing.

More than 100,000 of the approximately one million U.S. women who have received silicone breast implants are currently ill. But the companies and many commentators insist that the autoimmune diseases thousands of women suffer from don't exist. For proof they point to two studies published in the *New England Journal of Medicine*. The first, by the Mayo Clinic, appeared in 1994. The second came out a year later, reporting on research performed by Harvard University and Brigham and Women's Hospital, which is affiliated with Harvard's medical school. Both say there is no link between silicone breast implants and autoimmune diseases. The studies have been held up as proof that lawyers like Mahlum's are using "junk science" to win large awards at the expense of innocent corporations.

Is that true? Or could two such respected institutions as the Mayo Clinic and Harvard University actually be guilty of practicing shoddy science themselves? *Ms.* [magazine] has found, through speaking with doctors, researchers, plaintiffs' lawyers, and the two institutions as well, that there is a great deal wrong with these studies.

Although plastic surgeons have been promising their patients that silicone breast implants are perfectly safe ever since the products became available in 1963, implants were put on the market without long-term testing. But that doesn't mean that no testing was done at all. In a letter to the *New York Times*, Fredric Ellis and Ernest Hornsby, lawyers for Charlotte Mahlum, stated that "Dow Chemical found out in the 1960s that liquid silicone affected the immune system and central nervous system and could even be effective as an insecticide. Instead of disclosing this research to the scientific community, Dow Chemical concealed the results and entered into secret development agreements with Dow Corning to develop silicone as a drug and as an insecticide." When Dow Corning did report the results of research, it was often far from truthful. In a 1973 article in *Medical Instrumentation*, Dow reported on a study of four dogs that had been implanted with miniature silicone breast implants. The article only reported the six-month results—that the dogs had suffered some inflammation, but no other adverse effects—since Dow said the results at the end of the study's full two years were the same. But in fact, lawyers for a woman who was suing Dow proved in court that after two years, one dog had died and the others suffered from severe chronic inflammation, thyroiditis, autoimmune response, and spots on the spleen.

Doctors soon began seeing the effects of Dow's decision not to fully disclose the results of silicone testing. Women came to them describing debilitating pain, often in the chest and shoulder. As we now know, within two to four years of receiving a silicone implant, nearly 70 percent of patients suffer capsular contracture, a hardening of the scar tissue around the implant, which squeezes the implant into a hard disk. But as painful and disfiguring as capsular contracture can be, it is not nearly as serious as the danger women face when silicone enters their bodies, either through leakage or implant rupture. In its early literature, Dow Corning said that the implants would last a lifetime, but in reality, many don't make it past 15 years. A study published in *Annals of Plastic Surgery* in 1994 reported that among women surveyed who had implants for five years or less, 93 percent of the implants were intact. But only 30 percent of implants that were six to 15 years old remained intact. And in 1995, the same journal reported on a study of 300 breast implant patients: 71.3 percent of them had experienced rupture or severe silicone leakage.

Dow Corning knew that gel could leak from its implants and that they had a high rupture rate. In a 1983 company memo, a researcher points out that the safety of implants is based upon the assumption that "ruptures do not occur or are removed quickly when they do occur by additional surgery. Experience has shown this latter assumption to not be accurate... some physicians have noted ruptures... that may go undetected for unknown time periods."

Yet Dow Corning failed to investigate the long-term health consequences of liquid silicone leaking into the body. Other researchers have, and although their research is still in progress, there are some things we do know. Doctors have found proof that silicone can travel to internal organs and can settle there. Dr. Douglas Shanklin, a professor of medicine at the University of Tennessee, who has been studying what he believes to be silicone-related disorders for ten years, says he recently saw an implant patient with silicone fluid in her brain and spinal fluid. This woman cannot feel where her feet and hands are, has lost her memory, and cannot keep her balance because her nerve sensors are impaired. "They have been grounded out, just like an electrical wire," says Dr. Shanklin.

* * *

According to Shanklin, silicone leaking into the body causes a "cellular immune reaction," which shows up initially as inflammation. "The body's immune system is trying to get rid of this stuff, but it can't. We can't metabolize silicone." Our immune system doesn't know that and keeps on fighting. "Eventually, after 10, 12, or 14 years, this primary attack... is exhausted. Then the body begins attacking its own cell tissue and organs," resulting in autoimmune disease, says Shanklin. Traditional autoimmune, or connective tissue, diseases include rheumatoid arthritis and lupus.

But Dr. Shanklin and the majority of doctors treating women with implants have found that the women primarily suffer not from traditional autoimmune diseases, but from a specific constellation of problems—including joint pains, skin rashes, numbness, and fatigue—that medicine has never before seen grouped together in this way. Rather than analyze and define what this new syndrome might be, most large-scale studies have concentrated on looking for previously identified diseases—and have rarely found them.

The Harvard/Brigham study, also known as the "Nurses' Study," and the Mayo Clinic study should have changed all that. Considering how much was riding on this research, it is surprising to discover that both studies are full of holes—thanks to problems in design as well as to conflicts of interest.

* * *

Neither the Mayo nor the Harvard/Brigham study focused on "atypical" symptoms. The Mayo Clinic looked at 14 isolated symptoms, although researchers believe it is the clustering of these symptoms that indicates silicone disease. The researchers relied on information on medical charts, where symptoms like skin rashes are less likely to have been noted than are firm disease diagnoses. Women in the study were never examined or interviewed by Mayo's researchers, and no attempt was made to inquire about symptoms that weren't on the charts.

The Harvard/Brigham study claims to have looked at a broad range of atypical symptoms, but only women who reported being diagnosed with a *traditional* connective-tissue disease were given the questionnaire on atypical symptoms. Many women who are severely ill would inevitably have been excluded with this method. (The final count included only 32 women with implants *and* connective tissue disease.) During questioning under oath, the study's authors admitted that, despite earlier claims, they had, in fact, only examined traditional diseases.

"We're dealing with atypical disorders. Anyone who read the literature going back to the 1970s would have known that you need to look beyond classical diseases," says Dr. Gary Solomon, who is the associate director of rheumatology at the

Hospital for Joint Diseases Orthopaedic Institute in New York City. "It is frankly disturbing that these medical studies did not consider this. One can only suspect that this was intentional."

Critics also say that the studies look at too few women to find an increased risk of even the traditional diseases that they were looking for. The Mayo Clinic studied the health records of 749 women with implants (and 1,498 controls). The Harvard researchers chose 1,183 women with implants (876 of them silicone) for their study. But since a traditional autoimmune disease like scleroderma —a fibrotic thickening of skin and vital organs—occurs in only .02 to .04 percent of the population, "to detect even a doubling of the baseline rate of scleroderma, you would need to have at least 30,000 women in your study," explains Dr. Solomon.

And neither study considered a long enough "latency period." Doctors estimate that the average length of time it takes for a woman with implants to begin showing symptoms of illness is eight to ten years. In the Mayo study, women were tracked for a mean of 7.8 years after implantation. The Harvard researchers interviewed women who had had implants for a mean of 9.9 years, but they included women whose implants were only 30 days old. (Even more astonishing, the researchers included one woman who said she'd had her silicone implants nearly 40 years, even though the first implants were not available until 1963—29 years before the study began.) "This is not unlike R. J. Reynolds funding a study that examines people in their thirties, and finding no increased risk of lung cancer," says Dr. Shanna Swan, an epidemiologist at the University of California at Berkeley's School of Public Health. Many doctors believe it may take decades for the full effects of silicone poisoning to appear.

* * *

Both studies have also been plagued with conflict of interest charges. Dr. Matthew Liang, for instance, a coauthor of the Harvard study, was paid $2,525 by law firms representing Dow Corning and other manufacturers, for consulting work. Meanwhile, the Mayo study was funded by the National Institutes of Health (NIH) and the Plastic Surgery Educational Foundation (PSEF), which receives funding from implant manufacturers. Part of the $174,000 that PSEF gave the Mayo Clinic came from Dow Corning and two other manufacturers, McGhan Medical and Bristol-Meyers Squibb. The companies say this isn't a problem, that they have "no input on what research the foundation chooses to fund." But documents show that they do influence which studies get money, and sometimes they oversee research. In an August 31, 1990, letter to Abt Associates, a research firm that was hoping to study atypical diseases, foundation president Barrett Noone wrote: "The manufacturer's group in general and Dow Corning in specific were disinclined to behave in a collaborative manner.... My colleagues and I are disappointed by their decision not to fund your study." On November 24, 1992, the vice president for research and development at Mentor Corporation, also an implant manufacturer, wrote to the foundation concerning a different study, one the company did want to fund: "We are in direct contact with these authors and discussing the various aspects of these study plan[s]. As the protocols are finalized, these authors will directly send the final protocol to your organization."

Dow Corning may have had an even more direct hand in the Harvard study. Three months before a questionnaire was sent to participants, researcher Dr. Jorge Sanchez Guerrero provided a copy of the questionnaire to Dow Corning epidemiologists. At press time, Matthew Liang had refused to release information to the courts that could reveal whether the questionnaire was altered to suit Dow Corning.

Given the problems with these studies, is there any research that can clarify the relation between silicone implants and disease? There are, in fact, hundreds of peer-reviewed medical studies that have found that silicone breast implants and their components are dangerous to human health. But these studies, like those of Harvard and Mayo, are not definitive. Nevertheless, they point to areas for concern. At an NIH workshop a year ago, several studies showed evidence of autoimmune problems linked to silicone. One, by Dr. Michael Potter of the National Cancer Institute, found that after being injected with silicone gel, as many as 80 per cent of mice developed the equivalent of multiple myeloma, a rare cancer that attacks immune system cells.

Another study (not presented at the NIH workshop) that has caused concern is one led by Dr. Shanklin at the University of Tennessee, and a colleague, Dr. David Smalley. Their research indicates that children born to symptomatic women with silicone implants sometimes have the same silicone-specific cellular immune activity as their mothers—i.e., their bodies are fighting a foreign substance that appears to be silicone.

The NIH is finally putting together a large-scale investigation of "atypical disease symptoms," using 18,000 women, 13,000 of whom have implants. In addition, a "Silicone-Related Syndrome Study Group" has been created by members of the American College of Rheumatology (ACR) to define and describe the diseases that some women with implants are suffering from. (The ACR itself is caught in a battle over silicone. At the college's annual meeting in October 1995, its directors announced that implants do not cause rheumatic diseases, claiming that the courts that had ruled in favor of women with implants were relying on "anecdotal evidence." Members of the ACR were furious and demanded that the directors retract their statement, pointing out that 16 out of 18 studies presented at the conference indicated links between implants and certain diseases.)

Some doctors are pinning their hopes on Harvard's "Women's Health Cohort Study," of nearly 400,000 women, but others worry that Dow Corning has also funded this study—to the tune of its full $6.8 million. As it turns out, interim findings from the cohort study (that were leaked to the press in 1995) indicate a 45 to 49 percent increased risk of rheumatoid arthritis among women with silicone implants. Despite these findings, which admittedly could change when the data are fully analyzed, Matthew Liang publicly insists that implants are safe.

* * *

Meanwhile, claiming that Americans sue each other too much, the Republican Congress seeks to make it more difficult for the women who have yet to go to court to win their cases against silicone implant manufacturers. Advocates claim they are trying to curb a litigation explosion that is burdening the courts. Yet, according to the National Center for State Courts, tort suits (cases concerning injury or damages) are just 9 percent of all state court filings, and product liability suits are only 4 percent of that. To many analysts, today's tort reform is another case of corporations using their political clout to escape potential liability. And liability is certainly a big issue for both Dow Chemical and Dow Corning.

The Manhattan Institute, a conservative think tank and long-time lobbyer for tort reform, held a conference in Washington last June, featuring Dow Corning's CEO, Richard Hazleton, who took the opportunity to deliver Dow's wish list on reform. First came the "exclusion of biomaterials suppliers from litigation brought against medical device manufacturers." Dow, of course, is a supplier to many implant manufacturers. Next was a cap on punitive damages; under the cap proposed by the Republicans, Charlotte Mahlum—who will be sick for the rest of her life—would not have received much more than $250,000.

Despite Dow's obvious interest in legal reform, much of the media has bought into the company's analysis of the implant crisis. Marcia Angell, the executive editor of the *New England Journal of Medicine*, wrote an article' in *The New Republic* last year in which she blasted "rapacious attorneys," "well-paid doctors who stretch the science and ethical limits of their profession," and "healthy women" for "responding to the lure of big financial awards."

The *New York Times* also promotes this interpretation. Gina Kolata, a *Times* science reporter, pronounced the Harvard study "so compelling . . . that some leading rheumatologists contend that the issue of whether implants cause these diseases can now be considered closed." What about the women who have been diagnosed with illnesses? Kolata told *Ms.*

that some of them might be responding to "the power of suggestion."

We have been down this road before. Women in real pain going to doctors and being told that it is all in their heads. Women being encouraged to use medical devices that don't function properly and being told these devices are perfectly safe when they aren't. What we haven't had before, certainly not on this scale, is tens of thousands of women who were perfectly healthy being given something that has jeopardized their health. At the same time, women who are in the midst of fighting one devastating disease—breast cancer—are being asked to risk other illnesses. And the time bomb is still ticking. Only about 300,000 women have passed the latency period (half of all women who have received breast implants got them after 1988). There are approximately 700,000 more women who, if they are not sick yet, must wait and watch to see if they will be.

NO

Michael Fumento

A CONFEDERACY OF BOOBS

"Not only are they abusing the judicial system, but they are emotionally abusing the women." That's what one silicone breast implant recipient told the *Boston Herald* following the decision of Dow Corning to file for bankruptcy. Dow Corning had contributed about half of a $4.2 billion settlement—the biggest ever—for women claiming to suffer various illnesses from their implants.

[In 1995], however, it became clear that there were far more women trying to get a piece of the pie than there were slices. Plaintiffs' attorneys were saying that $74 billion might be needed to satisfy just the first set of claims against the companies. Rather than close its doors forever, Dow Corning chose to try to limit its losses.

Financially, it's unclear where the bankruptcy leaves implant claimants. But what has become more and more certain since the settlement was reached back in 1993 is that while both the judicial system and silicone implant recipients have been terribly abused, the villain isn't Dow Corning or any other implant maker.

Indeed, women with breast implants have been nothing more than pawns in a bizarre game involving lawyers, feminists, headline hounds, and super-inflated bureaucratic egos. The stakes, however, go beyond the physical and mental health of women with implants to include the future health of millions of Americans who will need insertable medical devices. Indeed, the multimillion-dollar awards against silicone implant manufacturers have already triggered a wave of suits against medical implants made of solid silicone and even some containing no silicone at all.

"We have great concerns that any medical device with silicone in it will not survive," says Elizabeth Connell, a professor of gynecology and obstetrics at Emory University and head of two Food and Drug Administration [FDA] silicone breast implant panels that unsuccessfully recommended leaving the devices on the market. Since June 1992, most uses of silicone breast implants have been banned by the FDA. Annually, some 1.5 million patients receive silicone eye lenses; another 670,000 get artificial silicone joints. All told, about 7.5 million medical devices are implanted in Americans each year. Many of

From Michael Fumento, "A Confederacy of Boobs," *Reason* (October 1995). Copyright © 1995 by The Reason Foundation. Reprinted by permission.

these devices—such as pacemakers, heart valves, and shunts which draw fluid off the brain—are life savers.

Hence, the misinformed campaign against silicone breast implants raises issues that go far beyond the not insignificant question of whether women should be able to change their appearance as they see fit. A strange alliance of diverse interests, including FDA bureaucrats interested in broadening their powers, feminists who equate boob jobs with mutilation, and reporters more interested in good copy than relevant medical research, worked together to take implants off the market. The anti-implant campaign is nothing less than a case study in how medical public policy is often driven by anecdotal rather than epidemiological evidence, formulated by ideologues who have little regard for what individuals might value, and discussed in a consistently one-sided manner.

The use of silicone implants to enlarge the size of the breast dates back to 1963. Somewhere around one million American women have received them. Implants may be used either for "augmentation"—making a healthy breast or pair of breasts larger—or to replace a breast removed during mastectomy. It appears that about 60 percent of breast implants have been used for augmentation.

While there has been mention of possible disease caused by implants as far back as 1978, the kick-off point of the scare that ultimately prompted the FDA to ban silicone implants may have been the airing of an implant feature on CBS's *Face to Face with Connie Chung* in 1990. Chung's graphic imagery—she called silicone gel "an ooze of slimy gelatin that could be poisoning" women —spurred one stampede of women to

have their implants removed and another to file suits against implant makers.

As Chung herself later put it, the show "unleashed a torrent of protests and investigations around the country." Soon, women were bombarded with such stories as "Toxic Breasts," "The Hazards of Silicone," and "Time Bombs in the Breasts." The height of hysteria may have been reached when, after the FDA moratorium, two women removed their own implants with razor blades. They said they had no success in getting doctors to remove them.

A new front opened up in December 1991, when a California jury awarded a Marin County woman, Mariann Hopkins, $7.3 million from Dow Corning. She alleged aches, pains, and fatigue caused by her implants without citing any illness more specific than autoimmune disease, a catchall phrase for a variety of connective-tissue diseases such as rheumatoid arthritis, scleroderma, lupus, Sjogren's Syndrome, fibromyalgia, and Raynaud's Disease.

In January 1992, the FDA declared a voluntary (but strongly recommended) moratorium on the sale and use of silicone breast implants pending review of additional information, saying, "physicians should cease using them and manufacturers should stop shipping them." Four months later, the FDA essentially converted this to a ban, although the agency did allow continued use of the implants for women who had suffered mastectomies and permitted a small number of women who wanted implants for cosmetic purposes to enroll in long-term studies.

*   *   *

Like many health scares, the one over silicone implants is primarily American.

Only a few countries besides the United States forbid the devices within their borders. One is Canada, even though the Canadian Independent Advisory Committee review showed no causal link between silicone breast implants and serious illness. While most countries haven't even seriously considered removing silicone implants from use, some, such as the United Kingdom, have reviewed the evidence and affirmatively stated that implants should remain available. In June 1994, the 20-member European Committee on Quality Assurance and Medical Devices in Plastic Surgery declared it "does not support any restriction on the use of silicone-gel filled implants."

Because of the ban in the United States, American women have gone to other countries, including the United Kingdom, Mexico, France, and Germany, to get implants. One popular package mixing implantation in an English hospital with a trip to Shakespeare's birthplace is called "Boobs n' Bard." Having to go abroad for implants, of course, prices some women out of the market. Women who do travel for implants face different problems: If something goes wrong with the surgery, the doctor is thousands of miles away. And malpractice suits are difficult to pursue in much of the world and virtually impossible in South and Central America.

The FDA seriously considered pulling saline-filled implants off the market as well. But in late 1994, it decided to allow their continued use pending approval applications due in 1998. Silicone is generally preferred to saline because it gives the breast a more natural feel. To keep saline-filled breasts from swishing like a waterbed, it is necessary to pack them tight with the solution. In breasts that are quite small to begin with, wrinkles or ripples in the implant surface are more easily visible through the skin and the breast may not move or hang as naturally as it would with silicone implants.

Whatever goes into the implant of the future, the silicone implants of today are in the bodies of a million or more women who need to know what risk, if any, these devices pose.

There are two ways that women can be exposed to silicone from an implant. One is when microscopic droplets of silicone fluid "bleed" through the envelope of a gel-filled implant. "Low-bleed" implants have been available since the early 1980s and have reduced the amount of silicone that escapes from the implant. In any event, because scar tissue quickly forms around the implant, the gel usually goes no further than one or two millimeters beyond the implant wall.

The other way women can be exposed is through rupture. According to the FDA, about 4 percent to 6 percent of silicone implants have ruptured, though studies in progress indicate this figure is probably too low.

Nonetheless, again the scar "capsule" that invariably grows around the implant tends to hold any silicone even if it breaks, which explains why so many ruptures are outwardly undetectable. While the gel has gone beyond the pouch, it still usually remains in place, although it has been found in the lymphatic system of some women.

That implants can cause physical problems is beyond doubt. It has long been known, for instance, that the scar capsule can harden and constrict, sometimes painfully so. This hardening can make necessary follow-up treatment to remove the scar tissue. Makers of later model implants claim to have reduced this problem, but it's too early to say what success they may have had.

But when critics warn of the dangers of silicone implants, this usually minor problem is seldom what they're talking about. According to Jack Fisher, a San Diego plastic surgeon and outspoken defender of implants, more than 50 symptoms are alleged to be caused by implants, including memory loss, dry mouth, cancer, bladder problems, difficulty swallowing, joint pain, decreased sex drive, and a host of autoimmune diseases. Some have referred to this broad constellation of symptoms as "silicone-gel syndrome." But if it is a syndrome it appears the proper definition would have to be any illness that any woman with implants ever contracts.

To sympathetic observers, such a wide array of symptoms must seem alarming. But a general rule of epidemiology is that the more diverse the symptoms allegedly related to a single cause are, the less likely it is that the suspected cause is real. This basic precept is, in a sense, the mirror image of snake-oil cures that promise to remedy all sorts of unrelated symptoms. Many of the most commonly cited symptoms of silicone exposure—such as fatigue, headaches, and difficulty swallowing—can be brought on by suggestion. As a result, people who hear that implants may cause certain problems may then develop them. These are the same "side effects" described by participants in drug studies who are actually receiving placebos.

And, in fact, most of the evidence against implants is anecdotal: It is based on reports from women who are sick and have implants and claim the two conditions are related. Thus, if a woman with implants ever develops symptoms that

doctors can't readily explain, everyone simply assumes that silicone is the cause. Sometimes this sort of reasoning is expressed in the very titles (of the implant scare articles. Consider the headline for the *San Francisco Chronicle's* article about Mariann Hopkins: "After Breast Implant, Horror Began."

While such a loose correlation may be appealing to people looking for quick and easy answers, it is essentially the same logical fallacy that blames black cats for inexplicable illness. Yet, in some cases, the silicone-gel symptoms actually predate the implants. Indeed, such a curious time frame appears to have been the case even in the first big implant settlement.

One of Mariann Hopkins's treating physicians testified that, although her diagnosis of mixed connective-tissue disease did not come until after the implants were put in, she had already displayed symptoms of connective-tissue disease as early as two years before receiving implants. The doctor even testified that another physician was so concerned that he subjected her to a battery of tests for one type of connective-tissue illness called systemic rheumatic disease. Those came back negative, but they were not tests specifically for mixed connective-tissue disease. Had they been and had they come back positive, it's unlikely Hopkins would have ever received the $7.3 million award.

But then again, the jury did not seem overly influenced by those most knowledgeable of Hopkins's medical history. At the time of trial, Hopkins was basically free of symptoms, thanks to a low dose of medicine. And none of Hopkins's treating physicians testified at the trial that they believed her illness to be related to the implants.

Instead, the jury made its finding on the basis of outside testimony that implants could cause such disease, testimony from professional anti-implant witnesses such as Tampa, Florida, physician Frank Vasey, who makes his living by treating women he says are sick from their implants.

Perhaps the most serious charge against silicone implants is also the weakest—that they may cause breast cancer. Although such influential groups as Sidney Wolfe's Public Citizen (founded by Ralph Nader) have made the claim, repeated studies have shown no such link. The only cancers ever plausibly attributed to silicone—in a study released over 40 years ago—were connective-tissue sarcomas that appeared in strains of rodents especially susceptible to cancer.

* * *

The simple truth is that no epidemiological studies have linked cancer in people to implants. The largest study is also the most recent: After looking at a group of almost 11,000 women from the Alberta, Canada, area, the Alberta Cancer Board concluded, "The incidence of breast cancer among the women who had breast augmentation could not be said to be either significantly higher or lower than that among the general population.

Polyurethane implants, which make up about 10 percent of implants currently in use, are a special case. Manufactured by Surgitek Inc., a subsidiary (of Bristol-Myers Squibb Co., these implants featured a gel-filled pouch with a layer of polyurethane foam coating the silicone envelope. The implants were a special target of Connie Chung's *Face to Face* report. Under such heat, Surgitek felt it had no choice but to remove them from the market in 1991. (Nevertheless, a *USA To-*

day illustration in May 1995 accompanying an anti-implant editorial depicted a polyurethane-coated implant.)

The purpose of the foam was to reduce the chance of scar tissue contracting around the implant. But when the foam breaks down chemically, it produces a substance called 2-toluene diamine (TDA) that is considered a probable animal carcinogen and a possible human one. Although that would seem to be an obvious source of trouble, it turns out that, like all the other serious accusations against breast implants, the charges against polyurethane implants don't hold up under epidemiological scrutiny. The only difference is that in this case the FDA has admitted it.

In late June, Bristol-Myers Squibb concluded an FDA-solicited study to determine how much TDA really ended up in the system of women with polyurethane implants. The amount (when any was found at all) was so small that even assuming it is a *definite* human carcinogen—using the FDA's own rating system—the risk of cancer was one in a million. Since only about 110,000 women have had such implants, the FDA stated in a position paper, "FDA estimates it is unlikely that exposure to TDA will cause cancer in even one of the women with these implants." The agency added, "The health risk connected with surgical removal of the implants is far greater than the risk of developing cancer."

There's another, deeper irony in the whole polyurethane controversy, one the FDA obviously couldn't state: that a product designed to alleviate the only absolutely certain health problem clearly linked to implants was forced off the market because of worries over other unproven health effects.

Since silicone gel from implants is most commonly accused of causing autoimmune disease, or connective-tissue disease, it isn't surprising that a large number of studies on both animals and humans have looked for a link between silicone exposure and autoimmune/connective-tissue disease. When the British Department of Health undertook a review of these studies earlier this year, it found approximately 270 papers published after 1971 alone.

The animal studies, the department concluded, "provide no immunological reason for concern over the use of silicone gels in implants." The report went even further, however: "None of these studies demonstrated that the coexistence of connective-tissue disease with silicone breast implants is any more prevalent than would be expected by chance."

The largest study of connective-tissue disease to date appeared in the *New England Journal of Medicine* [in] June [1995]. Conducted by the Harvard School of Public Health and the Brigham and Women's Hospital in Boston, the study looked for evidence of 41 types of connective-tissue disease among 87,501 nurses, of whom 1,183 had implants.

* * *

The results were unambiguous. The researchers found no "association between silicone breast implants and connective-tissue diseases, defined according to a variety of standardized criteria." Already anticipating the charge that they knew would be forthcoming from plaintiffs' lawyers—that silicone implants cause a special kind of autoimmune disease that doesn't show up with standardized criteria—the authors added, "or signs or symptoms of these diseases." In fact, they reported that women with silicone implants were significantly less likely to relate symptoms of these diseases or to complain of symptoms or signs of illness resembling connective-tissue disease.

For many health professionals, the *NEJM* study, added on top of all the others, was the final piece of proof needed. "I think we have enough data to end the moratorium," George E. Erlich, a Philadelphia rheumatologist and head of the FDA arthritis advisory committee, told *The New York Times.* Erlich emphasized he was speaking for himself and not the FDA committee, but he added that the International League of the Associations of Rheumatology also agreed unanimously there was no evidence linking implants to connective-tissue disease. And long before that, the American College of Rheumatology had already issued its own statement, saying, "There is no convincing evidence that these implants cause any generalized disease."

If the evidence against silicone implants is so weak—and has always been so—why have they inspired such commotion and fear? The chief reason has to do with the federal bureaucrat whose various power-grabbing machinations would embarrass a villain from Central Casting: David Kessler, commissioner of the FDA.

In December 1991, Kessler called together a panel of physicians, self-styled consumer representatives, and the like to evaluate the evidence of potential harm caused by implants. The verdict of the panel, though by no means unanimous, was that the devices should remain on the market pending collection of further data from studies already underway.

That, however, did not please Kessler, who ordered FDA staffers to solicit case histories from doctors of implant recipients who later claimed to have suffered ills as a possible result. Since lawyers had already begun soliciting women with complaints and sending them on to specially chosen doctors, finding such case histories was probably not difficult. In any event, case histories reveal little because they don't allow for comparison groups. That's what the epidemiological studies were, but Kessler couldn't wait for them.

In January 1992, Kessler implemented the moratorium, citing the case studies as the reason (and glossing over the fact that he himself solicited them). The next month, he reconvened the panel to ply them with his new "evidence." The panel didn't budge and Kessler once again ignored its advice.

"We still saw no clear evidence of danger, though there were a number of unanswered questions," says Emory's Connell, who served as the chair of both panels. "We felt breast implants should stay available to women who, with informed consent, wanted to use them." Three and a half years after the first panel voted to recommend keeping the implants available, Connell says she would clearly do so again. "I think the difference is we could say it this time with a great deal more assurance."

"A whole new literature has been developed since that time," she explains. "We were operating on anecdotal evidence and case history. Now the evidence has been gathered by good people in well-designed studies so it's an entirely different situation."

So why did the FDA ban silicone implants despite the lack of evidence that they are harmful? Pressure came from repeated anecdotal reports in both print and television media. The moratorium that became a ban occurred after more than a year of intense media pressure, including Connie Chung's inflammatory show, which was repeated a year later.

Congressional pressure, in the form of the late Rep. Ted Weiss (D-N.Y.), also came down on the FDA. Weiss, who chaired the House committee with jurisdiction over the FDA, accused Dow Corning of possible misconduct in its effort to document the safety of silicone implants and called for both the Justice Department and the FDA to investigate the company. ([In] May [1995], the Justice Department dropped the investigation for lack of evidence.) He also accused the FDA of dragging its feet over the polyurethane-implant issue.

To be sure, there was pressure to keep implants available, too. It came from the American Medical Association, implant makers, plastic surgeons, and breast-cancer groups. But this was not the sort of public pressure that can embarrass an agency, and the breast cancer groups' objections were dealt with by allowing continued use of silicone implants for breast reconstruction following mastectomy.

The decision to ban implants was just the sort of thing one would expect from a regulatory body that puts so much emphasis on safety that it can't take anything else into account. *New England Journal of Medicine* Editor Marcia Angell has said that the FDA probably acted the way it did because implants are cosmetic and are therefore of only subjective worth. Such worth, says Angell, can't be plugged into Kessler's cost-benefit analysis.

In an *NEJM* editorial, Angell noted that nobody questions allowing the use of automobiles, even though they kill over 40,000 Americans a year, because we all have a common understanding of the worth of cars. "In the case of breast implants" though, wrote Angell, "the benefit has to do with the personal judgments about the quality of life, which are subjective and unique to each woman." But given "the difficulty of assessing the benefits, the FDA has acted as though there were none—at least when implants are used for augmentation." The result, said Angell, "is that [FDA Commissioner Kessler] may be holding breast implants to an impossibly high standard: Since there are no benefits, there should be no risks."

* * *

The FDA's pseudo-scientific approach lends support to the more obviously ideological attack on breast implants from feminists. To many of the most vocal and influential feminists, a preference for big breasts represents female oppression. Susan K. Brownmiller, in her landmark 1984 book *Femininity*, opined that "[e]nlarging one's breasts to suit male fantasies" represents the exploitation of women. "Big breasts are one of many factors that have slowed women down in the competitive race of life," she said. "Symbolically, in the conservative Fifties, when American women were encouraged to stay at home, the heavily inflated bosom was celebrated and fetishized as the feminine ideal. In decades of spirited feminist activity such as the Twenties and the present when women advance into untraditional jobs, small, streamlined breasts are glorified in fashion."

If large breasts signal oppression, say these feminists, then the implants used to enlarge one's breasts are tools of oppression. Scarsdale psychologist Rita Freedman, writing in *Beauty Bound*, claims, "Having been taught that feminine beauty means having full, softly rounded breasts, women judge them-

selves against this standard. Missing the mark, they put on padded bras or suffer silicone implants." Naomi Wolf, in her 1991 bestseller *The Beauty Myth* , states, "Breast surgery, in its mangling of erotic feeling, is a form of sexual mutilation."

Having gone this far with imagery, it's s small step to start blaming implants for physical ills. This is precisely what happened after anecdotes began to appear linking implants to disease. Susan Faludi, in her popular book *Backlash: The War Against Women*, wrote matter-of-factly that leaking implants "could cause toxicity, lupus, rheumatoid arthritis, and autoimmune diseases such as scleroderma."

To such polemicists, it doesn't matter that the evidence for negative effects was weak. It was just too fitting that something in their minds so harmful to women as a class should be harmful to them as individuals.

Two women on the FDA panel translated such thoughts into direct action. Vivian Snyder, the panel's "consumer representative," told Kessler in a letter that "[t]he federal government now has the power to deliver a profoundly important message to the American public involving basic values, concepts of beauty and health," adding, "it would really be wonderful if the FDA could address such attitude-impacting mental health issues as what is really healthy and normal and maybe even beautiful...."

The other panelist was *Beauty Bound* author Rita Freedman. She sent a letter to Kessler decrying that implants "perpetuate the myth of Barbie Doll's Body" and asked whether breast augmentation will become, "like rhinoplasty [nose surgery], a rite of passage for affluent teens."

Such feminist participation in the anti-implant crusade has proven ironic, since the FDA's virtual ban has denied what feminists have always proclaimed as their goal—a woman's right to choose for herself. Faludi herself acknowledges that at one time the leading feminist journal, *Ms.*, "deemed plastic surgery a way of 'reinventing yourself—a strategy for women who dare to take control of their lives.' "

Writing in *NEJM*, Angell says, "It is possible to deplore the pressures that women feel to conform to a stereotyped standard of beauty, while at the same time defending their right to make their own decisions." If anything, says Angell, the act of withdrawing implants could be viewed as sexist because "people are regularly permitted to take risks that are probably much greater than the likely risk from breast implants," citing cigarette smoking and excess alcohol consumption.

* * *

When the FDA slapped the moratorium on implants, the impact went far beyond prohibiting a single surgical technique. "The widespread fear—and the multimillion-dollar lawsuits—have dated largely from the FDA's removal of breast implants from the market," says Angell.

One study comparing the attitudes of women with implants before and after the FDA moratorium found that after the moratorium the level of satisfaction dropped markedly, from 98 percent satisfied to 71–79 percent satisfied. The study authors said their findings were similar to those of the American Society for Plastic and Reconstructive Surgery in another poll.

As for prompting the "multimillion-dollar lawsuits," one need look no further for evidence than so many of the attorney advertisements soliciting silicone implant recipients. "THE FDA WARNS THAT SILICONE GEL-FILLED BREAST IMPLANTS PRESENT HEALTH RISKS" blared a typical ad of this sort in the Newark, New Jersey, *Star-Ledger*. Implant critics often cite money as the only concern of Dow Corning and other manufacturers. But few notice that the group which stands to gain the most from liability cases—trial lawyers—has a love of filthy lucre. In a single case involving three women complaining of implant-related illness, a jury in 1994 awarded $33.5 million, although the judgment was later reversed by an appeals court and then settled. Thirty-three percent of a multi million-dollar award—lawyers typically take a third off the top—can be a powerful incentive for a law firm.

It's hardly surprising, then, that the American Trial Lawyers Association conducts regular seminars for implant plaintiffs' attorneys. It does so using selected data provided by Sidney Wolfe of Public Citizen, the group most identified with criticism of implants. For $750, Public Citizen will also provide trial lawyers a list of medical experts and consultants, FDA reviews and FDA panel testimony, and a variety of other litigation documents. It will also refer clients to those lawyers.

Suing implant manufacturers has become a boom industry in the United States, with lawyers out to convince women that even though they may feel just fine they are really sick and must be properly compensated. With so much money to spread around, it also isn't difficult to get doctors to find patients.

"I get calls from women who say, 'I have implants. Where do I pick up the money?' " says Sandy Finestone of the Women's Implant Information Center in Irvine, California. The center disseminates information on implant safety. "You dangle $4 billion in front of them and it certainly gets their attention." Finestone has two polyurethane-coated implants that she makes clear will not be the subject of litigation.

Indeed, attorneys have not only ignored scientists, they've attacked them. After Mayo Clinic rheumatologist Sherine E. Gabriel published a study in *NEJM* in June 1994, a lawyer claiming to represent 2,000–3,000 implant recipients began filing legal demands against her. "The magnitude of the demands is staggering; the burden is staggering," she told *The New York Times.* "They want over 800 transcripts from researchers that were here, they want hundreds of data bases, dozens of file cabinets and the entire medical records of all Olmsted County [Michigan] women, whether or lot they were in the study."

Not surprisingly, Gabriel says the demands have "severely compromised" her ability to do research and made colleagues of hers back off from doing their own implant research, for fear their findings would also infuriate plaintiffs' lawyers. "Some," she says. "determined that the price in terms of their own research careers is too high to pay."

The widespread association of silicone implants with various illnesses is largely the result of unsophisticated reporting on the topic. "The media may be portraying a closer link between implants and autoimmune disease that is actually merited because younger women tend to he more prone to autoimmune disease than other groups," explains David Leffell, associate professor of dermatology at the Yale School of Medicine. But the real question, says Leffel, is whether women with silicone implants are getting these diseases at levels higher than expected. All signs point to no.

With silicone implants, the media have managed to make news as much as report it. Clearly, they have had a significant impact on public perceptions, which then fueled both litigation and contributed to the FDA moratorium. This in turn fueled more litigation.

Whatever role sheer confusion—and ignorance of scientific data and principles —played on the part of the media, it is disturbing to realize that opportunities to present the other side were often ignored. In 1991, for instance, CBS reran the Connie Chung show that did so much to kick off the implant scare. But at the last minute, the network yanked a Dow Corning rebuttal to the program's charges. CBS didn't explain its decision. Apparently it felt its viewers would not benefit from an airing of both sides of the issue.

Unfortunately, the anti–silicone implant crusade has given women something very tangible to fear. Because of the negative publicity, as early as 1991 insurance companies were already denying or restricting medical coverage to women with implants. Now, because some doctors and lawyers have tied various illnesses to implants, women with implants who do eventually get any of those illnesses may find themselves without medical coverage. The founder of the Washington, D.C., chapter of the Y-ME National Breast Cancer Organization told a congressional panel, "In some instances, it is easier for a cancer patient to obtain insurance than one who has implants."

* * *

In early June, even before the *NEJM* connective-tissue disease study, Y-ME Executive Director Sharon Green wrote to Kessler asking him to "make a public statement regarding the most recent epidemiological studies...to stop the current frenzy." The only statement he issued that month was a response to the *NEJM* study saying yet more evidence was needed.

Emory's Connell says the FDA's actions and the legal profession's high-tech ambulance chasing are "costing us not only what we [already] have but the chance for new and better products in the future. I think we're in a worse mess in American medicine than we've ever been in. Instead of leading the world, we're now a third-rate country in terms of our ability to develop new drugs and devices."

Indeed, J. Donald Hill, chairman of cardiovascular surgery at California Pacific Medical Center, worries that the anti-implant crusade will broaden into an attack against a wide variety of medical aids already on the market. The first device to go down the tubes may be the Norplant contraceptive, which after implantation into the arm releases a tiny amount of silicone into the system. While no suits have yet been filed, lawyers are encouraging women with the devices who have any sort of illness to contact them. Trial lawyer seminars are already being held, using some of the same instructors and same self-styled medical experts who torpedoed breast implants.

In a country so heavily dependent on science to improve the quality of our lives, to defend our shores, to feed our growing population, to prevent and cure illness, the resoundingly anti-scientific and successful crusade against silicone implants portends problems that right now cannot even be guessed.

POSTSCRIPT

Are Silicone Breast Implants a Health Risk to Women?

Why have so many women had silicone sacs surgically implanted in their chests? Some who have breasts removed due to cancer have opted for breast reconstruction, but the most common reason has been that healthy women wished to achieve better body proportions. They often claim that the devices have enhanced their self-confidence and the quality of their life. Overall, about 90 percent of these women are satisfied with their implants. Others, however, feel very strongly that women who have the implants have been victimized by society and men; that breast enlargement through surgery was something that had been thrust upon them by a society obsessed with unnatural ideas of female attractiveness. The editors of *Ms.*, in a March/April 1996 editorial, claimed that the idea of unnaturally large breasts as perfect begins in childhood when little girls play with Barbie dolls. "Keeping us in a constant state of insecurity about our looks not only fuels the multibillion-dollar beauty and fashion industries and the boon in cosmetic surgery, but it also helps maintain the status quo." To many feminists, a preference for large breasts represents female oppression. In her book *Femininity* (Fawcett, 1985), Susan K. Brownmiller contended that enlarging breasts to please male fantasies represents the exploitation of women.

For whatever reasons women opt for breast implants, the safety issue remains. Pathologist Nir Kossovsky believes silicone breast implants can negatively affect a woman's immune system and has testified in court to that effect. See "Silicone in the System," *Discover* (December 1995). Other publications that question the safety of silicone implants include "How Silicone Ended Up in Women's Breasts," *Ms.* (March/April 1996). "Assessing Breast Implant Complications," *The New England Journal of Medicine* (March 1997) discusses a study that investigated 749 women who received implants between 1964 and 1991. Nearly 24 percent had had localized complications including infection and scar tissue formation. The study did not assess autoimmune complications. In *Science on Trial: The Clash of Medical Evidence and the Law in the Breast Implant Case* (W. W. Norton, 1996), executive editor of the *New England Journal of Medicine* Marcia Angell discusses the lack of scientific rigor used in the breast implant litigation. Dr. Angell asserts that public opinion and media, not valid data, determined the outcome of the $4 billion lawsuit. She also maintains that although localized problems have occurred among women with implants, evidence does not show that systemic conditions including cancer and autoimmune diseases result from silicone breast implants.

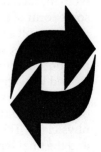

ISSUE 11

Does Health Care Delivery and Research Benefit Men at the Expense of Women?

YES: Leslie Laurence and Beth Weinhouse, from *Outrageous Practices: The Alarming Truth About How Medicine Mistreats Women* (Fawcett Columbine, 1994)

NO: Andrew G. Kadar, from "The Sex-Bias Myth in Medicine," *The Atlantic Monthly* (August 1994)

ISSUE SUMMARY

YES: Health and medical reporters Leslie Laurence and Beth Weinhouse claim that women have been excluded from most research on new drugs, medical treatments, and surgical techniques that are routinely offered to men.

NO: Physician Andrew G. Kadar argues that women actually receive more medical care and benefit more from medical research than do men, which explains why women generally live longer than men.

According to many researchers, women appear to respond differently from men to a varied array of medications and diseases. For instance, although heart disease is the leading killer of both men and women, women are less likely to survive heart attacks and heart surgery. Since the most influential studies of heart disease have studied only men, scientists and researchers are unable to explain the gender differences. Women activists claim that medical research has focused on men for too long and now it is time to change this pattern.

Heart disease, the leading killer of both men and women, has long been considered a male condition by both physicians and the public. This is probably because men develop the affliction at an earlier age than do women. But women catch up after menopause. By age 65 about one-third of women have some form of heart disease, high blood pressure, and/or stroke.

As a result of this perception, doctors tended to ignore womens' complaints of chest pains and other symptoms of heart disease or considered them to be psychosomatic. When women *were* treated for heart disease, they were often treated less aggressively than men with similar symptoms.

In 1989 Harvard University reported that taking an aspirin tablet every other day could prevent heart disease based on a study involving 22,000 male physicians. The findings were generalized to include both men and women, and the final reports claimed that aspirin, which helps prevent blood clotting, would be useful to all adults. Dr. Suzanne Oparil, president of the American Heart Association, however, believes that aspirin might not be beneficial to women because they have generally faster rates of blood clotting than men.

Why were women excluded in the Harvard aspirin study or in other research that might help prevent their premature deaths or disabilities? The answer goes back to 1975, when the National Commission for the Protection of Human Subjects of Biomedical and Behavioral Research issued guidelines limiting research on pregnant women. This ban on using women stemmed from fears following the thalidomide crisis in the late 1950s.

In 1985 the National Institutes of Health (NIH) issued a statement urging researchers to include women in their studies. In 1990 it was reported, however, that women were still excluded in major federally funded clinical studies and that the NIH was not enforcing its policy of including women.

Things began to change, beginning with the 1991 launching of the *Women's Health Initiative*, a 14-year study of women's health. And in 1993 the FDA lifted its ban on using women in drug trials.

A relatively recent concern pertains to AIDS and HIV-related conditions. In particular, AIDS research has a proportionately higher number of men participating in drug and other scientific trials. What is known about HIV and AIDS seems to have been acquired from research on men only.

Despite concerns that health care and research in the United States benefit men at the expense of women, there is ample evidence to the contrary: Department of Health and Human Services studies show that women see their physicians more frequently, have more surgery, and are admitted to hospitals more often than men. Currently, two out of three medical dollars are spent by women.

Women have benefitted from medical research involving high-tech procedures. Laparoscopic surgery and ultrasound are two advanced techniques that were first developed for use on women's bodies (these procedures were later adapted for men). Women's diseases have also been the recipient of research dollars. Breast cancer, the second leading cancer killer of women, has received more funding than any other tumor research. In 1993 the National Cancer Institute spent over $213 million dollars on breast cancer and $51 million dollars on prostate cancer. Although one-third more women die of breast cancer than men of prostate cancer, research into breast cancer received more than four times the funding of prostate cancer research.

In the following selections, Leslie Laurence and Beth Weinhouse argue that women have been shortchanged with regard to health care and medical research. Andrew G. Kadar disagrees, claiming that though it is often believed that women do not get the same consideration in medical care and research as men, the truth appears to be exactly the opposite.

YES

**Leslie Laurence and
Beth Weinhouse**

OUTRAGEOUS PRACTICES: THE ALARMING TRUTH ABOUT HOW MEDICINE MISTREATS WOMEN

There is unfortunately a clear path from the ignorant attitudes about women's bodies prevalent in the last century to the ignorant attitudes that exist today. A century ago physicians removed women's ovaries to treat a variety of unrelated complaints. They believed women's reproductive organs were responsible for almost everything that can and did go wrong with the human body. How much has changed? Recent medical students say that, during anatomy lectures on the female reproductive system, lecturers take pains to describe the female reproductive system as inefficient, badly designed, and prone to problems....

We may be horrified by the "ovariotomies" and "clitoridectomies" of the nineteenth century, but what of the hundreds of thousands of unnecessary hysterectomies being performed today?...

Nearly 550,000 hysterectomies are performed in the United States each year, making hysterectomy one of the most common operations of all. Yet the vast majority of these operations are elective, not lifesaving. When the American College of Obstetricians and Gynecologists recently announced its wish for ob-gyns to become the primary-care physicians for postmenopausal women, one woman doctor retorted, "If they want to do that, they're going to have to leave some organs in first."

How far have we really come from the days when women were told their psychological symptoms were due to physical problems and their reproductive organs were removed as a cure? Today women are frequently told that their very real physical symptoms—chest pains, menstrual problems, endometriosis, gastrointestinal pain—are psychological, and are handed a prescription for antidepressants or tranquilizers.

The medical textbooks of the 1800s may seem laughably ignorant today, but as recently as the 1970s physicians were being taught that morning sickness was caused by a woman's resentment at being a mother, PMS [premenstrual syndrome] was also a psychological disorder, and menopause represented the end of a woman's usefulness in life. And the doctors who were trained with those textbooks are still practicing medicine.

Instead of putting today's inequities in perspective, the examples of past abuses of women serve only to show that we haven't come as far as we thought. . . .

THE RESEARCH GAP

In June 1990, American women got a rude shock. For all the complaints women leveled against the health care system —most having to do with insensitive male doctors and dissatisfaction with gynecological and obstetric care—the majority of women still assumed that at least they were included in America's state-of-the-art medical research. But they were wrong. For at least the past several decades women in this country had been systematically excluded from the vast majority of research to develop new drugs, medical treatments, and surgical techniques.

It was on June 18, 1990, that the government's General Accounting Office (GAO) released its report of an audit of the National Institutes of Health (NIH). The audit found that although NIH had formulated a policy in 1986 for including women as research subjects, little had been done to implement or monitor that policy. In fact, most researchers applying for NIH grants were not even aware that they were supposed to include women, since the NIH grant-application book contained no mention of the policy. Because the 1986 policy urged rather than required attention to gender bias, most institutes, and most researchers, had simply decided to ignore it altogether or pay it only slight heed: "It used to be

enough for a researcher to say, 'Women and minorities will not be excluded from this study,'" explains one woman in NIH's Division of Research Grants. But not excluding women is very different from actively recruiting and including them. . . .

The GAO found that women were being underrepresented in studies of diseases affecting both men and women. In the fifty applications reviewed, one-fifth made no mention of gender and over one-third said the subjects would include both sexes, but did not give percentages. Some all-male studies gave no rationale for their exclusivity. "The [NIH] may win the Nobel Prize, but I'd like to see them get the *Good Housekeeping* seal of approval," said Congresswoman Barbara Mikulski (D-Md.), voicing her hopes that the behemoth medical institution could be made more woman-friendly.

As if medical research were some kind of exclusive male club, some of the biggest and most important medical studies of recent years had failed to enroll a single woman:

• The Baltimore Longitudinal Study, one of the largest studies to examine the natural process of aging, began in 1958 and included no women for its first twenty years because, according to Gene Cohen, then deputy director of the National Institute on Aging (NIA), the facility in which the study was conducted had only one toilet. The study's 1984 report, entitled "Normal Human Aging," contained no data on women. (Currently 40 percent of the participants in this study are women . . . although 60 percent of the population over age sixty-five is female.)

• The by-now-infamous Physicians' Health Study, which concluded in 1988 that taking an aspirin a day might reduce the risk of heart disease, included 22,000 men and no women.

- The 1982 Multiple Risk Factor Intervention Trial, known as Mr. Fit, a long-term study of lifestyle factors related to cholesterol and heart disease, included 13,000 men and no women. To this day no definitive answer exists on whether dietary change and exercise can benefit women in preventing heart disease.
- A Harvard School of Public Health study investigating the possible link between caffeine consumption and heart disease involved over 45,000 men and no women.
- Perhaps most unbelievably, a pilot project at Rockefeller University to study how obesity affected breast and uterine cancer was conducted solely on men. Said Congresswoman Olympia Snowe (R-Me.) upon hearing of this study, "Somehow, I find it hard to believe that the male-dominated medical community would tolerate a study of prostate cancer that used only women as research subjects." ...

Protection or Paternalism?

The objection to women's participation in health research that is most difficult to counter is the concern over exposing a fetus to a drug or treatment that might be dangerous, or at least has not been proven safe. Recent history makes it impossible to dismiss these fears. In the 1950s the drug thalidomide, given to European women to combat nausea during pregnancy, caused thousands of children to be born with severe deformities. In this country the drug diethylstilbestrol (DES) was widely prescribed to pregnant women during the 1940s and 1950s to prevent miscarriage, but has led to gynecological cancers and other medical problems in the offspring of the women who took it.

But in their effort to expose the fetus to "zero risk," scientists have shied away from including not just pregnant women in their studies, but any woman who could potentially become pregnant.

Translated into research practice, that meant that no woman between the ages of fifteen and fifty could participate in the earliest stages of new drug research unless she had been surgically sterilized or had a hysterectomy. (And since many studies have an upper age limit of sixty-five, that leaves a narrow window of opportunity for women to participate.) Exceptions were made only in the case of extremely severe or life-threatening illnesses.

While policies to protect unborn children seem to make sense on first reading, upon closer examination they represent protectionism run amok. An increasing number of studies are showing that exposure to chemicals and environmental toxins can affect *sperm*, yet no one is suggesting that men be excluded from research in order to protect their unborn children. When Proscar, a drug used to treat enlarged prostate glands, was found to cause birth defects in the offspring of male animals given the drug, men in the drug trials simply had to sign a consent form saying they would use condoms. Women weren't given the option of using contraception during the trial. By grouping together all women between the ages of fifteen and fifty as potentially pregnant, researchers were implying that women have no control over their reproductive lives. ...

WOMEN'S HEARTS: THE DEADLY DIFFERENCE

Kathy O'Brien (not her real name), a forty-two-year-old smoker, had been experiencing chest pains on and off for about a year. Her father and two of her uncles had died of heart attacks when young. She went to a clinic in the rural area of northwest New Jersey where she lived, and there the local doctors told her she probably had gallstones. When the pain got worse, she went back to the clinic, where they told her she'd have to have a sonogram of her gallbladder. She left without having it done. Instead Kathy went home, collapsed from chest pain, and nearly died. She had suffered a massive heart attack and gone into cardiac arrest. Technically dead, she had to be defibrillated with electrical shocks on the way to the hospital. The following day she was transferred to a larger, teaching hospital, where doctors did an angiogram and found a blockage in a major blood vessel. After bypass surgery she recovered well. But why, wondered the cardiologists at the larger hospital, didn't anyone recognize heart disease in a heavy smoker with chest pain and a serious family history of death from heart attack?

Though it has been the leading cause of death in American women since 1908, heart disease is one of the best-kept secrets of women's health. It wasn't until 1964 that the American Heart Association [AHA] sponsored its first conference on women and heart disease.…

The real topic of this conference wasn't women and heart disease, however. It was how women could take care of their *husbands'* hearts. "Hearts and Husbands: The First Women's Conference on Coronary Heart Disease" explained to women the important role they played in keeping their spouses healthy. "The conference was a symposium on how to take care of your *man:* how to feed him and make sure he didn't get heart disease, and how to take care of him if he did," explains Mary Ann Malloy, M.D., a cardiologist at Loyola University Medical Center in Chicago, and head of the AHA's local Women and Heart Disease committee. The conference organizers prepared an educational pamphlet called "Eight Questions Wives Ask." There was no discussion at all of ways for women to recognize their own symptoms or to prevent the disease that was killing more of them than any other, no mention of how women could look after their own heart health. And no one objected, including women, because, for the medical profession and the public, heart disease was an exclusively male problem.

Both physicians and the public still harbor the misconception that women do not suffer from heart disease. Yet many more women die from cardiovascular disease—478,000 in 1993—than from all forms of cancer combined, which are responsible for 237,000 deaths. Although women seem to fear breast cancer more, only one in eight women will develop it (and not all of them will die of it), while one in two will develop cardiovascular disease. And for those who persist in thinking of heart disease as a male province, in 1992 (the most recent statistics available), more women than men died of cardiovascular disease. Among women, 46 percent of all deaths are due to cardiovascular disease; in men it's 40 percent. Because heart disease tends to be an illness of older, postmenopausal women, the incidence of heart disease, and the number of deaths, have been rising as women's life expectancies have increased. "Women didn't die of heart disease when the median age of death was the fifties or sixties," says Nanette K. Wenger, M.D., professor of medicine (cardiology) at Emory University School of Medicine in Atlanta.

Yet despite these ominous numbers, the vast majority of research into coronary artery disease, the type of heart disease that causes most heart attacks, has been done on middle-aged men. "We're very much in an infancy in terms of understanding heart disease in women," says Irma L. Mebane-Sims, Ph.D., an epidemiologist at the National Heart, Lung and Blood Institute. Compared with men's hearts, women's hearts are still largely a mystery. . . .

"IT'S ALL IN YOUR HEAD": MISUNDERSTANDING WOMEN'S COMPLAINTS

Just as the physical diseases of women are poorly understood, so, too, are a panoply of psychosomatic disorders, extremely controversial diagnoses in which emotional distresses are transferred into physical symptoms for which people then seek treatment. Somatization, as this process is known, has existed for centuries and is, to this day, remarkably common: Some 80 percent of healthy adults are believed to have psychogenic symptoms in any given week—for instance a stomachache that coincides with an important deadline or a headache that comes on after a fight with the boss. . . .

Such a dynamic has a great bearing on women: they make up the majority of people suffering from such psychosomatic disorders as chronic fatigue syndrome, fibromyalgia, irritable bowel syndrome, and chronic pelvic pain (which can also be the result of an organic disorder such as endometriosis). The hidden scandal is that there is no shortage of doctors who will treat women's psychogenic complaints as if they're organic in origin, often leading to a chamber of medical horrors, including an array of unnecessary surgeries instead of the treatment women may really need: help in understanding the emotional reasons for their disease.

Of course women are willing participants in their mistreatment. Resisting psychological consultation, they embark on a medical odyssey, dragging their strange array of symptoms from specialist to specialist until they find someone who will give them the one thing they desperately need: a diagnosis. "These are very beleaguered patients," says Nortin Hadler, M.D., a North Carolina rheumatologist with a particular interest in somatization. "The worst thing to happen to any patient is not to be believed. You can't get better if you can't prove you're ill."

The corollary is that, because women suffer from psychosomatic illness disproportionately and express their medical problems in a more open and emotional style compared with men, their complaints frequently *aren't* listened to—even when they're directly related to an organic disease. "The perception among many physicians is that women tend to complain a lot, so you shouldn't pay too much attention to them," says Donna Stewart, head of women's health at Toronto Hospital, a teaching hospital affiliated with the University of Toronto. As a result, many of women's *legitimate* physical ailments are not attended to, sometimes with serious consequences. . . .

WOMEN AND DOCTORS: A TROUBLED RELATIONSHIP

Most women who visit physicians aren't aware of the lack of research into women's health, the difficulties in diagnosing women with cardiac disease, or the discrimination against women in medical school. What they *are* aware of is dissatisfaction with their physicians and with their health care in general. They base these opinions on what goes on in the doctor's office and the respect—or lack of it—they receive there. "The usual experience for a woman going to a gynecologist includes humiliation, depersonalization, even pain, and too seldom does she come away with her needs having been met," asserts gynecologist John M. Smith, M.D., author of *Women and Doctors*. And gynecologists are certainly not the only physicians guilty of this mistreatment.

Marianne J. Legato, M.D., associate director of the Center for Women's Health at Columbia–Presbyterian Medical Center, has toured the country talking with women about their experiences as patients. "The general mood is anger," she says. Women complained to her that their physicians were insensitive, uninterested, rushed, arrogant, and uncommunicative. Because women's health care is fragmented, with women seeing a gynecologist for reproductive health, an internist for a general physical, and other specialists for more specific problems, one woman told her she felt "like a salami, with a slice in every doctor's office in town."

None of this surprises Dr. Legato, who says that medicine is a mirror of the rest of society and its values. "Women, the old, the poor, children, and minority groups as a whole who haven't achieved economic power are taken less seriously and held in less regard ... which kind of leaves the emphasis on white males."

Many physicians interact with their women patients based on a view of the female sex that was already archaic decades ago. "If she's premenopausal, she is dismissed as suffering from PMS; if she's postmenopausal, then she obviously needs hormone replacement therapy; if she's a homemaker, she has too much time on her hands; if she's a business executive, then the pressure of her job is too much for her. She just can't win," writes Isadore Rosenfeld, M.D.

Medical school textbooks from only two decades ago portray women not much differently from the "walking wombs" that physicians treated in the 1800s. In this century gynecologists embraced the idea that hormones were the long-suspected link between the uterus and the brain. This theory led them to believe that a pelvic exam could help diagnose mental problems. Conditions such as painful or irregular periods, excessive morning sickness or labor pain, and infertility became indications that a woman was battling her femininity. One 1947 obstetrics textbook, still on a practicing physician's shelf, introduces a chapter on such pregnancy problems as heartburn, nausea and vomiting, constipation, backache, varicose veins, and hemorrhoids with the sentence "Women with satisfactory self-control and more than average intelligence have fewer complaints than do other women."

Things still hadn't improved by the 1970s. A 1973 study of how women were portrayed in gynecology textbooks found that most textbooks were more concerned with the well-being of a woman's husband than with the woman herself. Wrote the authors, "Women are consistently described as anatomically destined to reproduce, nurture, and keep their husbands happy." A popular 1971 ob-gyn textbook portrayed women as helpless, childlike creatures who couldn't survive sex, pregnancy, delivery, or child raising without their doctors and added, "The traits that compose the core of the female personality are feminine narcissism, masochism, and passivity."

While current textbooks seem generally more sensitive and realistic, the physicians who trained on the older books are still in practice. When *JAMA*, a leading medical journal, ran an article in 1991 about gender disparities in medical care, they received a letter from a physician in Ohio who wrote that perhaps women's "overanxiousness" about their health and their greater use of health services "may be due to temperamental differences in gender-mediated clinical features of depression, which are manifested by women's less active, more ruminative responses that are linked to dysfunction of the right frontal cortex in which the metabolic rate is higher in females." In other words women are more anxious about their health because they are somehow brain-damaged. With doctors like this, no wonder women are unhappy.

Women as Patients

Surveys show that women are more dissatisfied with their physicians than men are. And the dissatisfaction is not necessarily due to the quality of the medical care women receive, but to the lack of communication and respect they perceive in the encounter. In a 1993 Commonwealth Fund survey of twenty-five hundred women and a thousand men on the subject of women's health, women reported greater communication problems with their physicians, and were more likely to change doctors because of their dissatisfaction. One out of four women said she had been "talked down to" or treated like a child by a physician. Nearly one out of five women had been told that a reported medical condition was "all in your head."

The perception nationwide is that doctors and patients just don't understand each other. A study of one thousand complaints from dissatisfied patients at a large Michigan health maintenance organization found that more than 90 percent of the problems involved communication. "The most common complaints had to do with a lack of compassion on the physician's part," says Richard M. Frankel, Ph.D., associate professor of medicine at the University of Rochester School of Medicine and Dentistry. "Patients would complain their physician never looked at them during the entire encounter, made them feel humiliated or used medical jargon that left them confused." ...

"Women are patronized and treated like little girls," says Ann R. Turkel, M.D., assistant clinical professor of psychiatry, Columbia University College of Physicians and Surgeons. "They're even referred to as girls. Male physicians will call female patients by their first names, but they are always called 'Doctor.' They don't do that with men. Women are patted on the head, called 'dear' or 'honey.' And doctors tell them things like, 'Don't you worry your pretty little head about it. That's not for you to worry about; that's for me to worry about.' Then they're surprised when women see these statements and reactions as degrading and insulting." ...

There is also a perception among women that physicians don't take women's time seriously. How else to explain what happened to Roberta, a busy magazine editor who was on a tight deadline schedule the day of her doctor's appointment. "My office was just one city block from the doctor's office, so I called them five minutes before my appointment time to see if the doctor was running on schedule," she recalls. The receptionist assured her he was, so Roberta left her office and arrived at her appointment on time—only to be kept waiting for nearly an hour. "When I finally saw the doctor, I was practically shaking with rage, and my blood pressure was sky high," she says. Even though the doctor apologized and spent a lot of time talking with her after the checkup, Roberta decided to find another doctor.

"I think women are kept waiting longer for an appointment than men are," says Dr. Turkel. "I wouldn't go to a gynecologist who kept me waiting in the waiting room for an hour and a half, but I hear these stories all the time from women patients about their gynecologist's office."

Advice columnist Ann Landers even gave a rare interview to *JAMA* to let physicians know how dissatisfied women are with their doctors. "I can't say too often how angry women are about having to wait in the doctor's office," she said. "And, who do they complain to? The office manager, who is also a woman. Then, when the male doctor finally sees them—an hour later —the woman is so glad to see him that she soft-pedals the inconvenience. She wants to see the doctor as a 'knight in shining armor.' This should change. The doctor's time is no more important than the patient's and, while I can understand special circumstances, I can't understand why a doctor is *always* running late."

Doctors may treat women as if they are inferior patients, but studies show that they are anything but. Women tend to ask more questions—and receive more information because of their inquisitiveness. Women also show more emotion during office visits and are more likely to confide a personal problem that may have a bearing on their health to their physicians. Men, on the other hand, ask fewer questions of their physicians, give less information to the doctor, and display less emotion. During a typical fifteen-minute office visit, women ask an average of six questions. Men don't ask any. . . .

Although physicians should be thrilled to have patients who are interested in their health, ask questions, and volunteer personal information, women's concerns are often dismissed as symptoms of anxiety, their questions brushed aside. In business, successful executives are often seen as having forceful, take-charge personalities, while women with similar attributes are described as aggressive or bitchy. In medicine, male patients seem to describe symptoms, while women complain. Instead of valuing women as active, informed patients, doctors are more likely to prefer patients who don't ask questions, don't interrupt, don't question their judgment, and—perhaps most important—get in and out of the office as quickly as possible. Researchers have actually found that physicians *like* male patients better than female ones, even when factors such as age, education, income, and occupation are controlled for.

Perhaps because of these attitudes, women often feel frustrated when they try to ask questions and receive explanations. One study reported that women received significantly more explanations than men—but not significantly more explaining *time*. Wrote the authors, "It is possible that many of the explanations they received were brief and perfunctory. Or, put differently, the men may have received fewer but fuller explanations than the women." The study also found that women were less likely than men to receive explanations that matched the level of technicality of the questions they asked. Doctors tended to talk down to women when answering their questions....

Miscommunication or Mistreatment?
Far more serious than patronizing attitudes and lack of consideration for women's time are the myths about women patients' complaints that jeopardize women's health care.

"Physician folklore says that women are more demanding patients," says Karen Carlson, M.D., an internist at Massachusetts General Hospital in Boston. "From my experience women are interested in health and prevention, desire to be listed to and treated with respect, want the opportunity to present and explain their agenda, and want their symptoms and concerns taken seriously."

But all too often women's symptoms are not taken seriously because physicians erroneously believe that these symptoms have no physical basis and that women's complaints are simply a sign of their demanding natures.

A 1979 study compared the medical records of fifty-two married couples to see how they had been treated for five common problems: back pain, headache, dizziness, chest pain, and fatigue. "The physicians' workups were significantly more extensive for the men than they were for women," reported the authors. "These data tend to support the argument

that male physicians take medical illness more seriously in men than in women."

Another study found that women were shortchanged even in general checkups. Men's visits are more likely to include vision and hearing tests, chest X rays, ECGs, blood tests, rectal examinations, and urinalyses.

Dr. Carlson, speaking to a roomful of women physicians at an annual meeting of the American Medical Women's Association, cited evidence to show that women may actually complain *less* than men. "The myth is that women complain more, but studies show another truth," she says. Carlson cited studies showing that, compared with men, women with colon cancer are more likely to delay care and experience diagnostic delay. That women with chronic joint symptoms and arthritis are less likely to report pain. That women have more severe and frequent colds, but men are more likely to overrate their symptoms. That women delay seeking help for chest pain or symptoms of a heart attack. These studies point to women as being more stoic, yet when they finally do show up in the doctor's office, they are apt to be met with skepticism.

Betsy Murphy (not her real name) had been seeing the same doctor for years. "We had a perfectly fine relationship as long as I just went for my yearly checkups and didn't ask a lot of questions," she recalls. "But then I got my first yeast infection and had to go see him for a prescription—the medicine wasn't available over-the-counter then." Betsy told her doctor what she thought she had—she had talked to enough friends and read enough magazine articles to recognize the distinctive cottage-cheeselike discharge, yeasty odor, and intense itching. "But he ignored me when I told him what I thought was wrong. After he took a culture and examined it under the microscope, he sneeringly said, 'Well, Ms. Murphy, it seems as if your diagnosis is correct.'" Although he diagnosed the problem and prescribed the medication, Betsy left his office feeling insulted and patronized.

At a recent workshop on the patient-physician partnership, an auditorium full of physicians was asked how they would handle a "problem" patient. One of these "problems" was the patient who comes in and announces his or her own diagnosis. The physicians, almost unanimously, ridiculed the patient for daring to speculate what was wrong. They preferred that someone just present a description of symptoms, as specifically and articulately as possible. "It's no help for someone to come to me and say, "I have a cold and I just need some medicine,'" said a participating doctor to a journalist in the audience. "Instead the patient should describe how they feel as specifically as possible. And obviously some people are more articulate and some less; that's where the doctor's skill comes in." In other words, a patient should show up for an appointment and tell the doctor, "I have a stuffy nose and I keep sneezing," and then wait for the doctor, in his infinite wisdom, to pronounce, "You have a cold." For a patient, male or female, who is reasonably certain what is wrong, the suggestion seems ludicrous.

Women's dissatisfaction with their medical care can lead to serious health consequences. They may switch doctors so frequently that they receive no continuity of care. Or they may simply avoid seeing doctors altogether because they find the experience humiliating. When men without a regular source of health care are asked why they don't have one, they tend to reply that they don't need a doctor. But women are more apt to say that they cannot find the right doctor, or that they have recently moved, or that their previous doctor is no longer available. In the Commonwealth Fund poll, 41 percent of women (compared with 27 percent of men) said they had switched doctors in the past because they were dissatisfied. "If you brought your car in to be fixed and the person who fixed it did an okay but not great job, but was nasty, wouldn't you go to another mechanic? The same is true of physicians," says Frankel.

Physicians seem to realize there's a problem, but many of their efforts to remedy it are laughable. One 1993 article in the medical newspaper *American Medical News* advised doctors that if they wanted to make their practice "women-friendly," they should "create an atmosphere similar to that of a living room. This includes the seating, lighting and wall decorations." Yet it's difficult to imagine any woman listing "ugly wallpaper" as a reason for being dissatisfied with her health care. It's not the decor women are complaining about when they complain about doctors' offices.

Ob-gyn John Smith lists padded stirrups and speculum warmers as among the improvements women have gotten their doctors to make since the 1960s. But even those superficial improvements are not enough. What women really want are doctors who will listen to them, talk to them, and treat their medical questions and problems with respect and empathy....

THE FUTURE OF WOMEN'S HEALTH

... Despite helter-skelter improvements in the care of women, the move toward special centers, nurse-run practices, and medical school curricula in women's health suggests a larger trend: the feminization of medicine. More women than ever are entering medical school. By the year 2010 the AMA estimates that one-third of all doctors will be women.... Not surprisingly these women are bringing a feminine, and sometimes feminist, sensibility to the practice of medicine.

"Feminism is about empowering all our patients—men, women, and children —and treating them with respect," says Laura Helfman, M.D., an emergency room doctor in North Carolina. "We're doctors, we're not gods up on high." To Helfman this means taking the opportunity to do "a gentle and warm pelvic exam so I can reeducate the person receiving it that it doesn't have to be awful." To a gynecologist friend of hers it means making sure the patients never have to wait and that they always get to speak with the doctor. To a surgeon friend it means holding the patient's hand in the recovery room....

These practitioners are putting the rest of the health care system on notice. Women, both as physicians and as patients, are primed to transform the way medicine is practiced in this country. And so we celebrate the new female norm: the 60-kilogram woman. She has breasts and a uterus and a heart and lungs and kidneys. But she's much more than that. No longer a metaphor for disease, she's the model for health.... The time is right for a new woman-centered health care movement. It's the least women should demand.

NO

Andrew G. Kadar

THE SEX-BIAS MYTH IN MEDICINE

"When it comes to health-care research and delivery, women can no longer be treated as second-class citizens." So said the President of the United States on October 18, 1993.

He and the First Lady had just hosted a reception for the National Breast Cancer Coalition, an advocacy group, after receiving a petition containing 2.6 million signatures which demanded increased funding for breast-cancer prevention and treatment. While the Clintons met with leaders of the group in the East Room of the White House, a thousand demonstrators rallied across the street in support. The President echoed their call, decrying the neglect of medical care for women.

Two years earlier Bernadine Healy, then the director of the National Institutes of Health [NIH], charged that "women have all too often been treated less than equally in... health care." More recently Representative Pat Schroeder, a co-chair of the Congressional Caucus for Women's Issues, sponsored legislation to "ensure that biomedical research does not once again overlook women and their health." Newspaper articles expressed similar sentiments.

The list of accusations is long and startling. Women's-health-care advocates indict "sex-biased" doctors for stereotyping women as hysterical hypochondriacs, for taking women's complaints less seriously than men's, and for giving them less thorough diagnostic workups. A study conducted at the University of California at San Diego in 1979 concluded that men's complaints of back pain, chest pain, dizziness, fatigue, and headache more often resulted in extensive workups than did similar complaints from women. Hard scientific evidence therefore seemed to confirm women's anecdotal reports.

Men more often than women undergo angiographies and coronary-artery-bypass-graft operations. Even though heart disease is the No. 1 killer of women as well as men, this sophisticated, state-of-the-art technology, critics contend, is selectively denied to women.

The problem is said to be repeated in medical research: women, critics argue, are routinely ignored in favor of men. When the NIH inventoried all the research it had funded in 1987, the money spent on studying diseases unique to women amounted to only 13.5 percent of the total research budget.

Perhaps the most emotionally charged disease for women is breast cancer. If a tumor devastated men on a similar scale, critics say, we would declare a state of national emergency and launch a no-cost-barred Apollo Project–style program to cure it. In the words of Matilda Cuomo, the wife of the governor of New York, "If we can send a woman to the moon, we can surely find a cure for breast cancer." The neglect of breast-cancer research, we have been told, is both sexist and a national disgrace.

Nearly all heart-disease research is said to be conducted on men, with the conclusions blindly generalized to women. In July of 1989 researchers from the Harvard Medical School reported the results of a five-year study on the effects of aspirin in preventing cardiovascular disease in 22,071 male physicians. Thousands of men were studied, but not one woman: women's health, critics charge, was obviously not considered important enough to explore similarly. Here, they say, we have definite, smoking-gun evidence of the neglect of women in medical research —only one example of a widespread, dangerous phenomenon.

Still another difference: pharmaceutical companies make a policy of giving new drugs to men first, while women wait to benefit from the advances. And even then the medicines are often inadequately tested on women.

To remedy all this neglect, we need to devote preferential attention and funds, in the words of the *Journal of the American Medical Women's Association*, to "the greatest resource this country will ever have, namely, the health of its women."

Discrimination on such a large scale cries out for restitution—if the charges are true.

In fact one sex does appear to be favored in the amount of attention devoted to its medical needs. In the United States it is estimated that one sex spends twice as much money on health care as the other does. The NIH also spends twice as much money on research into the diseases specific to one sex as it does on research into those specific to the other, and only one sex has a section of the NIH devoted entirely to the study of disease afflicting it. That sex is not men, however. It is women.

* * *

In the United States women seek out and consequently receive more medical care than men. This is true even if pregnancy-related care is excluded. Department of Health and Human Services surveys show that women visit doctors more often than men, are hospitalized more often, and undergo more operations. Women are more likely than men to visit a doctor for a general physical exam when they are feeling well, and complain of symptoms more often. Thus two out of every three health-care dollars are spent by women.

Quantity, of course, does not guarantee quality. Do women receive second-rate diagnostic workups?

The 1979 San Diego study, which concluded that men's complaints more often led to extensive workups than did women's, used the charts of 104 men and women (fifty-two married couples) as data. This small-scale regional survey prompted a more extensive national review of 46,868 office visits. The results, reported in 1981, were quite different from those of the San Diego study.

In this larger, more representative sample, the care received by men and women was similar about two thirds of the time. When the care was different, women overall received more diagnostic tests and treatment—more lab tests, blood-pressure checks, drug prescriptions, and return appointments.

Several other, small-scale studies have weighed in on both sides of this issue. The San Diego researchers looked at another 200 men and women in 1984, and this time found "no significant differences in the extent and content" of workups. Some women's-health-care advocates have chosen to ignore data from the second San Diego study and the national survey while touting the first study as evidence that doctors, to quote once again from the *Journal of the American Medical Women's Association*, do "not take complaints as seriously" when they come from women: "an example of a double standard influencing diagnostic workups."

When prescribing care for heart disease, doctors consider such factors as age, other medical problems, and the likelihood that the patient will benefit from testing and surgery. Coronary-artery disease afflicts men at a much younger age, killing them three times as often as women until age sixty-five. Younger patients have fewer additional medical problems that preclude aggressive, high-risk procedures. And smaller patients have smaller coronary arteries, which become obstructed more often after surgery. Whereas this is true for both sexes, obviously more women fit into the smaller-patient category. When these differences are factored in, sex divergence in cardiac care begins to fade away.

To the extent that divergence remains, women may be getting better treatment.

At least that was the conclusion of a University of North Carolina/Duke University study that looked at the records of 5,795 patients treated from 1969 to 1984. The most symptomatic and severely diseased men and women were equally likely to be referred for bypass surgery. Among the patients with less-severe disease—the ones to whom surgery offers little or no survival benefit over medical therapy—women were less likely to be scheduled for bypass surgery. This seems proper in light of the greater risk of surgical complications, owing to women's smaller coronary arteries. In fact, the researchers questioned the wisdom of surgery in the less symptomatic men and suggested that "the effect of gender on treatment selection may have led to more appropriate treatment of women."

As for sophisticated, pioneering technology selectively designed for the benefit of one sex, laparoscopic surgery was largely confined to gynecology for more than twenty years. Using viewing and manipulating instruments that can be inserted into the abdomen through keyhole-sized incisions, doctors are able to diagnose and repair, sparing the patient a larger incision and a longer, more painful recuperation. Laparoscopic tubal sterilization, first performed in 1936, became common practice in the late 1960s. Over time the development of more-versatile instruments and of fiber-optic video capability made possible the performance of more-complex operations. The laparoscopic removal of ectopic pregnancy was reported in 1973. Finally, in 1987, the same technology was applied in gallbladder surgery, and men began to enjoy its benefits too.

Years after ultrasound instruments were designed to look inside the uterus, the same technology was adapted to search for tumors in the prostate. Other pioneering developments conceived to improve the health care of women include mammography, bone-density testing for osteoporosis, surgery to alleviate bladder incontinence, hormone therapy to relieve the symptoms of menopause, and a host of procedures, including in vitro fertilization, developed to facilitate impregnation. Perhaps so many new developments occur in women's health care because one branch of medicine and a group of doctors, gynecologists, are explicitly concerned with the health of women. No corresponding group of doctors is dedicated to the care of men.

So women receive more care than men, sometimes receive better care than men, and benefit more than men do from some developing technologies. This hardly looks like proof that women's health is viewed as secondary in importance to men's health.

* * *

The 1987 NIH inventory did indeed find that only 13.5 percent of the NIH research budget was devoted to studying diseases unique to women. But 80 percent of the budget went into research for the benefit of both sexes, including basic research in fields such as genetics and immunology and also research into diseases such as lymphoma, arthritis, and sickle-cell anemia. Both men and women suffer from these ailments, and both sexes served as study subjects. The remaining 6.5 percent of NIH research funds were devoted to afflictions unique to men. Oddly, the women's 13.5 percent has been cited as evidence of neglect. The much smaller men's share of the budget is rarely mentioned in these references.

As for breast cancer, the second most lethal malignancy in females, investiga-

tion in that field has long received more funding from the National Cancer Institute [NCI] than any other tumor research, though lung cancer heads the list of fatal tumors for both sexes. The second most lethal malignancy in males is also a sex-specific tumor: prostate cancer. Last year approximately 46,000 women succumbed to breast cancer and 35,000 men to prostate cancer; the NCI spent $213.7 million on breast-cancer research and $51.1 million on study of the prostate. Thus although about a third more women died of breast cancer than men of prostate cancer, breast-cancer research received more than four times the funding. More than three times as much money per fatality was spent on the women's disease. Breast cancer accounted for 8.8 percent of cancer fatalities in the United States and for 13 percent of the NCI research budget; the corresponding figures for prostate cancer were 6.7 percent of fatalities and three percent of the funding. The spending for breast-cancer research is projected to increase by 23 percent this year, to $262.9 million; prostate-research spending will increase by 7.6 percent, to $55 million.

The female cancers of the cervix and the uterus accounted for 10,100 deaths and $48.5 million in research last year, and ovarian cancer accounted for 13,300 deaths and $32.5 million in research. Thus the research funding for all female-specific cancers is substantially larger per fatality than the funding for prostate cancer.

Is this level of spending on women's health just a recent development, needed to make up for years of prior neglect? The NCI is divided into sections dealing with issues such as cancer biology and diagnosis, prevention and control, etiology, and treatment. Until funding allocations for sex-specific concerns became a political issue, in the mid-1980s, the NCI did not track organ-specific spending data. The earliest information now available was reconstructed retroactively to 1981. Nevertheless, these early data provide a window on spending patterns in the era before political pressure began to intensify for more research on women. Each year from 1981 to 1985 funding for breast-cancer research exceeded funding for prostate cancer by a ratio of roughly five to one. A rational, nonpolitical explanation for this is that breast cancer attacks a larger number of patients, at a younger age. In any event, the data failed to support claims that women were neglected in that era.

Again, most medical research is conducted on diseases that afflict both sexes. Women's-health advocates charge that we collect data from studies of men and then extrapolate to women. A look at the actual data reveals a different reality.

The best-known and most ambitious study of cardiovascular health over time began in the town of Framingham, Massachusetts, in 1948. Researchers started with 2,336 men and 2,873 women aged thirty to sixty-two, and have followed the survivors of this group with biennial physical exams and lab tests for more than forty-five years. In this and many other observational studies women have been well represented.

With respect to the aspirin study, the researchers at Harvard Medical School did not focus exclusively on men. Both sexes were studied nearly concurrently. The men's study was more rigorous, because it was placebo-controlled (that is, some subjects were randomly assigned to receive placebos instead of aspirin); the women's study was based on responses to questionnaires sent to nurses and a review of medical records. The women's study, however, followed nearly four times as many subjects as the men's study (87,678 versus 22,071), and it followed its subjects for a year longer (six versus five) than the men's study did. The results of the men's study were reported in the *New England Journal of Medicine* in July of 1989 and prompted charges of sexism in medical research. The women's-study results were printed in the *Journal of the American Medical Association* in July of 1991, and were generally ignored by the nonmedical press.

Most studies on the prevention of "premature" (occurring in people under age sixty-five) coronary-artery disease have, in fact, been conducted on men. Since middle-aged women have a much lower incidence of this illness than their male counterparts (they provide less than a third as many cases), documenting the preventive effect of a given treatment in these women is much more difficult. More experiments were conducted on men not because women were considered less important but because women suffer less from this disease. Older women do develop coronary disease (albeit at a lower rate than older men), but the experiments were not performed on older men either. At most the data suggest an emphasis on the prevention of disease in younger people.

Incidentally, all clinical breast-cancer research currently funded by the NCI is being conducted on women, even though 300 men a year die of this tumor. Do studies on the prevention of breast cancer with specifically exclude males signify a neglect of men's health? Or should a disease be studied in the group most at risk? Obviously, the coronary-disease research situation and the breast-cancer research situation are not equivalent, but together they do serve to illustrate a point: diseases are most often studied in the highest-risk group, regardless of sex.

What about all the new drug tests that exclude women? Don't they prove the pharmaceutical industry's insensitivity to and disregard for females?

The Food and Drug Administration [FDA] divides human testing of new medicines into three stages. Phase 1 studies are done on a small number of volunteers over a brief period of time, primarily to test safety. Phase 2 studies typically involve a few hundred patients and are designed to look more closely at safety and effectiveness. Phase 3 tests precede approval for commercial release and generally include several thousand patients.

In 1977 the FDA issued guidelines that specifically excluded women with "childbearing potential" from phase 1 and early phase 2 studies; they were to be included in late phase 2 and phase 3 trials in proportion to their expected use of the medication. FDA surveys conducted in 1983 and 1988 showed that the two sexes had been proportionally represented in clinical trials by the time drugs were approved for release.

The 1977 guidelines codified a policy already informally in effect since the thalidomide tragedy shocked the world in 1962. The births of armless or otherwise deformed babies in that era dramatically highlighted the special risks incurred when fertile women ingest drugs. So the policy of excluding such women from the early phases of drug testing arose out of concern, not out of disregard, for them. The policy was changed last year, as a consequence of political protest and recognition that early studies in both sexes might better direct testing.

* * *

Throughout human history from antiquity until the beginning of this century men, on the average, lived slightly longer than women. By 1920 women's life expectancy in the United States was one year greater than men's (54.6 years versus 53.6). After that the gap increased steadily, to 3.5 years in 1930, 4.4 years in 1940, 5.5 in 1950, 6.5 in 1960, and 7.7 in 1970. For the past quarter of a century the gap has remained relatively steady: around seven years. In 1990 the figure was seven years (78.8 versus 71.8).

Thus in the latter part of the twentieth century women live about 10 percent longer than men. A significant part of the reason for this is medical care.

In past centuries complications during childbirth were a major cause of traumatic death in women. Medical advances have dramatically eliminated most of this risk. Infections such as smallpox, cholera, and tuberculosis killed large numbers of men and women at similar ages. The elimination of infection as the dominant cause of death has boosted the prominence of diseases that selectively afflict men earlier in life.

Age-adjusted mortality rates for men are higher for all twelve leading causes of death, including heart disease, stroke, cancer, lung disease (emphysema and pneumonia), liver disease (cirrhosis), suicide, and homicide. We have come to accept women's longer life span as natural, the consequence of their greater biological fitness. Yet this greater fitness never manifested itself in all the millennia of human history that preceded the present era and its medical-care system—the same system that women's-health advocates accuse of neglecting the female sex.

To remedy the alleged neglect, an Office of Research on Women's Health was established by the NIH in 1990. In 1991 the NIH launched its largest epidemiological project ever, the Women's Health Initiative. Costing more than $600 million, this fifteen-year program will study the effects of estrogen therapy, diet, dietary supplements, and exercise on heart disease, breast cancer, colon cancer, osteoporosis, and other diseases in 160,000 postmenopausal women. The study is ambitious in scope and may well result in many advances in the care of older women.

What it will not do is close the "medical gender gap," the difference in the quality of care given the two sexes. The reason is that the gap does not favor men. As we have seen, women receive more medical care and benefit more from medical research. The net result is the most important gap of all: seven years, 10 percent of life.

POSTSCRIPT

Does Health Care Delivery and Research Benefit Men at the Expense of Women?

"Nobody was paying attention to women's health," says Phyllis Greenberger, executive director of the Society for the Advancement of Women's Health Research in Washington, D.C. "For years, women's health issues were ignored because the men who were making the decisions didn't think they were important." This situation may be turning around. In 1987 only 14 percent of the $5.7 billion National Institutes of Health (NIH) budget was spent on women's health research. In 1994 the NIH spent over $1.4 billion dollars on health research related to women's diseases in hopes of finding treatments and cures for osteoporosis (bone thinning), heart disease, and breast cancer. In addition to increased funding, pressure from the Congressional Caucus for Women's Issues forced the NIH, the nation's largest research funder, to include women in all applicable clinical trials of medical treatments. The Food and Drug Administration (FDA) also issued guidelines in 1993 to include women in tests of new drugs.

These reforms, however, are not welcomed by all physicians and researchers. Professor Curtis Meinert of Johns Hopkins University doubts that the new approach will uncover significant differences between the genders either in treatment or in their responses to diseases. Meinert also feels that including women in all studies will require so many additional participants that research will become prohibitively expensive. Benjamin Wittes and Janet Wittes, employees of Statistics Collaborative, a company that designs clinical trials, echo Meinert's view in "Group Therapy," *The New Republic* (April 5, 1993). This viewpoint is also held by Marcia Angell, editor of *The New England Journal of Medicine*. Angell feels that claiming important biological differences between men and women as a rule is not plausible.

The effort to quadruple federal expenditures on breast cancer research has also been criticized. Some scientists have complained that designating so much money for one disease will be at the expense of research into cures and treatment for other illnesses. An article entitled "Equality Law Could Backfire on Researchers," *New Scientist* (August 7, 1993) argues that redressing past inequities by including women and minorities more often in research could backfire.

The claim that women with chest pains or other symptoms of heart disease are treated less aggressively than men has also been disputed. A study reported in "Absence of Sex Bias in the Referral of Patients for Cardiac Catheterization," *The New England Journal of Medicine* (April 21, 1994) found that women were treated as appropriately as men for their specific conditions and that gender was not a significant factor in doctors' deciding on a course of treatment. In "Why Do Women Last Longer Than Men?" *New Scientist* (October 23, 1993), the reasons behind males' shorter life spans are discussed. Life span and longevity are also addressed in "Survey Shows Women May Live Longer, but Not Healthier Than Men," *Nation's Health* (August 1993).

Many articles, in both the popular press and the scientific literature, maintain that there is a gender bias in medicine. These include the following: "What Doctors Don't Know About Women's Bodies," *Ladies Home Journal* (February 1997); "Men, Women, and Health Insurance," *The New England Journal of Medicine*, (January 16, 1997); "Are Women the Weaker Sex?" *American Health* (July/August 1996); "Did You Know That Women Continue to Get Shockingly Substandard Medical Care?" *Health Confidential* (January 1995); "Women's Health Falls Through the Cracks," *Shape* (April 1994); "The Neglected Sex," *American Health* (December 1993); "The High Cost of Being a Woman," *Working Woman* (November 1993); "The Identity Politics of Biomedical Research," *Siecus Report* (October/November 1993); "Gender Bias in Biomedical Research," *Journal of the American Medical Women's Association* (September 1993); "Gender Bias in Health Care," *Women Lawyers' Journal* (September 1993); "Survey Shows Poor State of Health Care Offered to Black Women in U.S.," *Jet* (August 9, 1993); and "The Gender Agenda," *Economist* (March 20, 1993).

For an overview on women's health, see "Women's Health Issues," *CQ Researcher* (May 13, 1994), which addresses such topics as hormone therapy debates, whether or not women's health should be a separate medical specialty, breast cancer, hysterectomies, and leading causes of death for men and women. See also "Women in the New World Order: Where Old Values Command New Respect," *Journal of the American Dietetics Association* (May 1997). Two books on gender bias in women's health are *Women and Health Research: Ethical and Legal Issue of Including Women in Clinical Studies* by Anna Mastroianni et al. (National Academy Press, 1994) and *Unequal Treatment: What You Don't Know About How Women Are Mistreated by the Medical Community* by Eileen Nechas and Denise Foley (Simon & Schuster, 1994).

ISSUE 12

Is AIDS a Major Threat to the Heterosexual, Non-Drug-Abusing Population?

YES: William B. Johnston and Kevin R. Hopkins, from *The Catastrophe Ahead* (Praeger, 1990)

NO: David R. Boldt, from "Aiding AIDS: The Story of a Media Virus," *Media Critic* (April 1997)

ISSUE SUMMARY

YES: William B. Johnston, a senior research fellow and the vice president of the Hudson Institute, and Kevin R. Hopkins, an adjunct senior fellow of the Hudson Institute, describe the rise of AIDS cases among heterosexuals and warn that unless people make a serious attempt to alter behaviors that put them at risk for the disease, this population will be facing an AIDS epidemic.

NO: Columnist for the *Philadelphia Inquirer* David R. Boldt claims that public health officials with the help of the media have exaggerated the risk of heterosexual AIDS.

AIDS has been called the world's most serious health concern since the bubonic plague killed off one-third of the population of Europe in the fourteenth century. Unless there is a major breakthrough, every person with AIDS will ultimately die (unlike the plague, which some survived). Currently, there is no vaccine or cure for the disease.

It is not clear if AIDS is a "new" disease or one that has been around and has only recently begun to spread. As early as 1977 medical journals carried articles reporting on a pneumonia-like disease that affected mostly young, homosexual males. The disease, first called the "gay plague," was ultimately called "acquired immunodeficiency syndrome," or AIDS. In 1983 scientists isolated the virus responsible for the disease, which eventually became known as the human immunodeficiency virus (HIV). This virus attacks and destroys white blood cells (T-lymphocytes), which are integral to the body's immune system, and damages the body's ability to fight other diseases. Without a functioning immune system to ward off other germs, the HIV-infected person becomes vulnerable to harmful organisms that may cause life-threatening diseases, such as pneumonia.

Although HIV initially appeared to affect mostly male homosexuals, it soon began to spread to intravenous (IV) drug users, persons receiving infected blood products, and the sexual partners of HIV-infected individuals. The virus can also be transmitted to children born to infected mothers. Persons who are infected may not have symptoms of AIDS, but they are still capable of passing the virus on to others.

In the early 1980s about 150 cases of AIDS were reported in the United States. By early 1997 over 450,000 cases and approximately 270,000 deaths from AIDS were identified by the Centers for Disease Control. AIDS is currently the leading cause of death among people in the 25–44 years age group. AIDS has spread throughout the world. In Africa over 1 million persons are thought to be infected, and whole villages have fallen victim to the disease. Thousands of Europeans, South Americans, and Asians also are infected with AIDS.

In Africa the disease appears to be transmitted mostly through heterosexual intercourse. In the United States, the reported number of AIDS cases spread in this manner is low; the vast majority of cases is still confined to bi- or homosexual men and IV drug users. Currently, approximately 83 percent of AIDS cases are linked to either IV drug use or male homosexual behavior. The majority of cases identified as heterosexual are attributed to persons having sex with IV drug users.

Though the proportion of cases attributed to heterosexual contact rose from 9.2 percent in 1993 to 10.3 percent in 1994, there is a belief that the rapid spread of AIDS among heterosexuals is a myth spread by the media. In 1987 the *New York Times* claimed "AIDS May Dwarf the Plague," and *US News and World Report* wrote "the disease of *them* suddenly is the disease of *us*." In February 1993 the *New York Times* reported on a National Research Council study: "The AIDS epidemic will have little impact on the lives of most Americans or the way society functions." The council declared that AIDS continued to be concentrated among bi- and homosexuals, drug users, the poor, and the undereducated.

Not everyone agrees with this analysis. In the following selections, William B. Johnston and Kevin R. Hopkins claim that heterosexually transmitted AIDS is the second stage of the epidemic and that by not feeling susceptible, many heterosexuals will be at risk, having not taken appropriate precautions. They argue that heterosexual transmission of HIV is now greater than that for homosexual and bisexual men and that they should be made aware of the dangers. Columnist David Boldt disagrees. He claims the media and the Centers for Disease Control greatly exaggerated the threat of heterosexual AIDS.

YES

William B. Johnston and Kevin R. Hopkins

AIDS IS A SERIOUS PROBLEM FOR HETEROSEXUALS

It is distressing to note that the number of new AIDS [acquired immuno-deficiency syndrome] cases in the heterosexual transmission category is now growing more rapidly than the number of AIDS cases among gay and bisexual men. The fact that AIDS cases represent infections that took place five or ten years earlier implies that, even as early as 1980, the number of new infections transmitted among heterosexuals was growing faster than new infections transmitted among gays. It is not certain that the virus will continue to spread as fully through the heterosexual community as it has among gays. What is clear is that the spread of new infections has been proceeding at a faster pace among heterosexuals than it has among gay and bisexual men for at least the last several years.

In addition, it has become apparent recently that the incubation period of HIV [human immunodeficiency virus] may be much longer than originally thought—and thus that the AIDS case data reveal even less about the current state of the epidemic than previously acknowledged. Early reports indicated that most people infected with the virus who were going to contract AIDS would do so within four or five years, with the remainder escaping the debilitating end-state of the disease. Such a long latency period would have caused enough serious complications in using AIDS case data for planning public policy. But more recent findings are even more troublesome. Long-term studies of both homosexual men and heterosexuals infected during transfusion now place the average incubation period at nine years or more, with some people remaining free of symptoms for as long as fifteen years. Hence, people infected today might not show up on the CDC [Centers for Disease Control] AIDS register until the turn of the century, giving them well over a decade to transmit the disease to others....

SOBERING RESULTS

In addition to knowing how many people are now infected with the AIDS virus, it is important to know the distribution of infection among the

From William B. Johnston and Kevin R. Hopkins, *The Catastrophe Ahead* (Praeger, 1990), pp. 51–63. Copyright © 1990 by William B. Johnston and Kevin R. Hopkins. Reprinted by permission of Greenwood Publishing Group, Inc., Westport, CT.

various population subgroups and the rate at which the disease is spreading within these groups. The government's official position, as stated by the CDC, is that HIV infection "remains largely confined to the populations at recognized risk," including gay men, IV [intravenous] drug users, and heterosexual partners of people known to be infected with the virus.

In the absence of repeated, nationally representative sero-prevalence studies, it is impossible to say definitely whether this optimism is warranted. But there are ways to test the thesis that AIDS and HIV infection are not much of a heterosexual problem—and the results are both surprising and sobering....

The CDC breaks down AIDS case data by sex, race, age, sexual orientation, and presumed means of contracting the virus. Extreme care must be taken in using this disaggregated data, however, particularly with regard to the means by which the AIDS victim is supposed to have contracted the disease. The CDC employs a hierarchical assignment scale that places homosexual contact and drug use at the highest levels. That is, any male AIDS victim who has ever had sex with another man, even once, is generally regarded as having contracted the disease homosexually, and any person who has recently used IV drugs, even once, is generally regarded as having been infected through the IV drug route —regardless of the extent and riskiness of that person's heterosexual activities.

As a result, at least some of those people assigned by the CDC to the gay and IV drug use transmission categories actually may have received the virus through heterosexual contact. While the potential number of such misidentified cases is not large, neither is it trivial. As of mid-1988,

as many as 3.5 percent of AIDS cases attributed to other factors (i.e., gay sex or IV drug abuse) theoretically could have resulted from heterosexual intercourse— a figure, if all cases were misclassified, that would be as high as the entire category of officially recognized heterosexual transmission cases. And even this is a minimum estimate, since the CDC's risk category for "heterosexual contact" is not identical to engagement in heterosexual activity. Rather, the CDC's category includes sex only with AIDS patients or those "at risk" for AIDS (e.g., IV drug users or persons from countries with a high incidence of AIDS)—a very small share of possible heterosexual partners. The category makes no allowance for an AIDS victim's heterosexual contact with people who did not fall into these tightly defined "risk groups," even though these other people also may have been infected and may have been transmitting the virus. Thus, the CDC heterosexual contact category is a rock-bottom estimate of heterosexual transmissions that lead to AIDS. It may understate true heterosexual transmissions by a considerable degree, perhaps by as much as half or more.

A second and more frequently noted source of error in accounting for heterosexual transmissions lies in the "undetermined" group of AIDS cases. This category "includes patients on whom risk information is incomplete (due to death, refusal to be interviewed, or inability to follow up), patients still under investigation, men reported only to have had heterosexual contact with a prostitute, and interviewed patients for whom no specific risk was identified." Most of these people may have been infected by routes other than heterosexual contact, although outside experts estimate that as many as one-sixth to one-third actually were the result of heterosexual intercourse. In any case, it is fair to say that, in assessing the heterosexual dimensions of the epidemic, the CDC has taken the most cautious course possible, excluding virtually everyone from the overtly labeled heterosexual category who possibly could have been infected otherwise—and even excluding those for whom no other obvious infection route could be identified.

HETEROSEXUALS WITH AIDS

But there is a much larger issue, one that is less often recognized. Even if correctly calculated, the number of heterosexually *transmitted* AIDS cases (i.e., people who contracted the disease through heterosexual contact) is not the same thing as the number of heterosexuals *with* AIDS (those people whose primary sexual outlet is heterosexual regardless of how they received the virus). In fact, excluding gay men, who constituted some 63 percent of AIDS cases reported as of mid-1989, the vast majority of the remaining AIDS patients (IV drug abusers, hemophiliacs, transfusion cases as well as heterosexual contact cases) were heterosexuals. And at least some of those men classed as having received the disease through homosexual contacts were predominantly heterosexual in practice. Taking these factors into account, and adjusting the AIDS data for delays in reporting, reveals a sizable heterosexual HIV problem: among the adjusted total of AIDS cases diagnosed through the end of 1988, nearly one-third were heterosexuals. While only about 17 percent of total AIDS cases among whites were heterosexuals, more than half of all minority AIDS cases—some 57 percent of blacks and 52 percent of Hispanics—came from among heterosexuals.

The point is that these people, no matter how they contracted the disease, can pass it on to other heterosexuals. One cannot draw comfort from the small size of the CDC's "heterosexual contact" transmission category for AIDS, not only because it undercounts the number of AIDS cases actually resulting from heterosexual contact, but because it greatly understates—almost by an order of magnitude—the number of heterosexuals who *have* AIDS. William A. Haseltine of Boston's Dana-Farber Cancer Institute has observed, "The infections may not have been acquired by heterosexual sex. However, the patients themselves are heterosexual. To this must be added the statement that most of the people who currently have AIDS and who are heterosexuals have been infected for about ten years and have been transmitting the virus to their partners throughout this period." . . .

A conservative estimate shows that slightly less than half of all infections by the end of 1988 were among gay men, who accounted for some 70 percent of whites with HIV but only 24 percent of blacks and 28 percent of Hispanics. The converse of course, is also true: *about half of all HIV infections have occurred among heterosexuals, with the overwhelming share of infections among minorities taking place among heterosexuals.* Moreover, the number of new infections per year among gay men has fallen by nearly 50 percent since 1984, making theirs a rapidly declining share of the overall epidemic.

By contrast, heterosexual intravenous drug abusers are one of the fastest growing segments of the infected population. Already, as of the end of 1988, they comprised more than one-third of all infected persons. The great majority of these infected drug users were blacks and His-

Figure 1

Heterosexual Contact With Persons With, or at High Risk for, HIV Infection

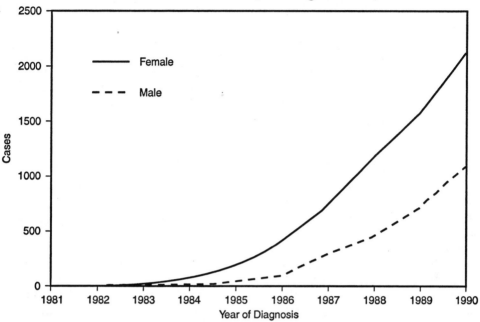

Source: Centers for Disease Control, *Morbidity and Mortality Weekly Report*, June 7, 1991.

panics, with only about a quarter being white. Still, the rate of increase in *new* infections among this group already appears to be slowing down. The number of new infections among drug users may well peak within the next few years, so this group will represent a declining share of the overall epidemic of HIV infection as well.

As serious as this pattern of infection is among gay and bisexual men and IV drug users, it is becoming even more severe among non-drug-using heterosexuals. In total, a best estimate is that there were at least 630,000 heterosexuals infected with HIV as of the end of 1988— a number several times the top-range CDC estimate, and vastly above the most frequently quoted CDC estimate of 30,000 non-hemophiliac, non-drug-

using infected heterosexuals (which is, of course, a much more restrictive measure). To be sure, most of these 630,000 or so heterosexual infections (some two-thirds) have occurred among IV drug users, although that does not change the fact that these people can transmit the disease by heterosexual contact. But the number of infections among heterosexuals who do not use IV drugs is far from minor— a best estimate of nearly 200,000 people. Some 52 percent of these heterosexuals are poor, some 67 percent minorities, and some 67 percent men.

MAINSTREAM POPULATION

These characteristics aside, a substantial number of these people—a best estimate of more than 86,000—are members of the so-called "mainstream" heterosexual population. They are not poor, and they are not IV drug users. Moreover, the number of new infections per year among all non-drug-using heterosexuals has risen by more than three times since 1983, making this group as well one of the fastest growing segments of the HIV-infected population. As Haseltine points out, "AIDS is already a heterosexual problem" in the United States.

How did the spread of HIV infection become so pervasive throughout the heterosexual community? In statistical terms, the answer is simple: as noted, a substantial share, some one-third, of already diagnosed AIDS cases are among heterosexuals, and these represent only a small number of the far larger group of heterosexuals who have been infected but who have not yet come down with AIDS. Moreover, unlike the gay and IV drug-using communities, whose numbers are relatively small, the sexually active heterosexual population is extremely large. And because of the high incidence of divorce and dissolution of other monogamous relationships, heterosexuals move frequently into and out of the pool of sexually active persons, even if they are at times insulated from the virus through celibacy or monogamy.

There also are numerous avenues by which heterosexuals can become infected. Many gay or bisexual men have sex regularly with heterosexual women as well as with men and can infect women in this way. Many otherwise sexually conventional men engage in intercourse with female prostitutes, who generally exhibit high levels of HIV infection. Infected IV drug-using heterosexuals have as sex partners other heterosexuals, many of whom are not IV drug users. Indeed, a study confirms not only that this transfer of HIV infection from drug users to non-users is occurring, but that it is taking place among the middle class as well as the poor, where the majority of drug users apparently are concentrated.

AN UNAVOIDABLE EPIDEMIC

Finally, heterosexuals have sex with other heterosexuals. As with the spread of the disease in the gay community, all that is needed for a self-perpetuating epidemic is for a sufficient number of the most sexually active members of a population to be infected and to pass the virus on to others before they become ill and die. If studies such as that by William Masters, Virginia Johnson, and Robert Kolodny are anywhere near accurate—that is, if as many as 5 to 14 percent of the most sexually active heterosexuals are carriers of the virus—then a breakout of the disease into the nonmonogamous heterosexual population is more than a theoretical possibility. It is almost unavoidable unless dramatic behavioral change or medical progress takes place soon.

NO

David R. Boldt

AIDING AIDS: THE STORY OF A MEDIA VIRUS

When Amanda Bennett became *The Wall Street Journal*'s Atlanta bureau chief in October 1995, she undertook to solve a mystery about AIDS statistics that had long perplexed her. For years, news story after news story had declared that the United States stood on the brink of an AIDS epidemic among heterosexuals. But Bennett, formerly one of the *Journal*'s principal economics writers as well as foreign correspondent based in China, knew there was no clear evidence to support this notion. Now in charge of a bureau that covered the Centers for Disease Control (CDC), the main federal agency dealing with AIDS, she recruited staff-reporter Anita Sharpe to join her in an effort to discover who was trying to fool the nation, and why.

A key moment came last December [1996] when the two journalists watched a videotape of the public service announcements that the CDC had first distributed in October 1987 as part of its "America Responds to AIDS" campaign. The spots (as well as brochures mailed to 117 million homes) featured one white face after another—a Methodist minister's son, a New York socialite, and other seemingly affluent women—repeating the campaign's mantra: "If I can get AIDS, anyone can."

Bennett and Sharpe realized that this message was extremely misleading, since members of certain identifiable groups—homosexual men, intravenous-drug users, or the sexual partners of IV-drug users—are far more at risk than others, and since heterosexuals who refrained from sexual relations with IV-drug users face little danger. The two journalists grasped that the people in the spots claiming to have AIDS almost certainly belonged to one of the at-risk groups. This, in fact, was the case. The minister's son was gay, and the socialite was married to an IV-drug user. *They* could indeed get AIDS, but that did not mean "anyone" else was equally at risk.

"It wasn't like having a revelation," Sharpe recalls. "It was more a feeling that, of course, this is where it all started."

That is, it all started at the CDC. Increasingly confident that the CDC was chiefly responsible for exaggerating the risk of heterosexual AIDS in the United States, Bennett and Sharpe found, after much sleuthing, that the agency had actually intended to hype this risk and mislead the public. The two journalists established that at a meeting at CDC headquarters in 1987, agency officials made the decision to deceive Americans into believing that AIDS is an equal-opportunity disease. "Our information came from people who were in the room," says Bennett.

The *Journal* published the discoveries of Bennett and Sharpe in a front-page article on May 1, 1996. The article explained that the CDC justified its disinformation campaign on grounds that the Reagan administration had blocked the agency's initiatives aimed at high-risk groups. The article also acknowledged the argument that exaggerating the dangers and lying to the public might have been the only way for the CDC to get national support for its programs. In a May 21 letter to the editor, CDC Director David Satcher and top official Helene Gayle did not, on a point-by-point basis, dispute the information Bennett and Sharpe provided. It was "false," the letter said, to claim that the agency had exaggerated the risk or devoted too many resources to people at little risk, but it concluded: "As you noted in your article, a number of factors historically have made targeting direct-prevention messages to those at greatest risk difficult. Even now, confronting the issues associated with preventing HIV among gay and bisexual men and injection-drug users is challenging." Unofficially—during encounters with CDC personnel in supermarket aisles—Bennett and Sharpe were told that their article was "right on."

For a daily newspaper, the Bennett-Sharpe exposé, which jumped to an entire inside page, was remarkably complete, an exemplary piece of journalism. Yet there was one major omission: The article skipped over the news media's deep complicity in aiding and abetting the heterosexual AIDS scare.

When for example, the CDC issued a release indicating that the number of heterosexuals with AIDS had doubled, the press largely failed to explain that the increase stemmed mainly from a change in CDC bookkeeping. The media also indulged the story line that women were, as one 1992 *New York Times* story put it, "the new face of AIDS," the implication being that all women were equally at risk. Seldom noted was that while the number of women with AIDS was increasing, those women getting AIDS were still largely those who were sexual partners of IV-drug users. Then, too, the media pushed the story advanced by the CDC —but for which there was never any convincing evidence—that AIDS was spreading like wild-fire among teenagers and college students.

From *The New York Times* and network news reports to *Money, Dance,* and *Skin Diver*, practically every news outlet helped propel the story onward. In perhaps the single most egregious example of over-hyping, Katie Leishman's "Heterosexuals and AIDS: The Second Stage of the Epidemic" in the February 1987 *Atlantic Monthly* made virtually no attempt to back up its alarmist contentions. News organizations even managed to distort reality by disproportionately featuring as AIDS victims individuals from low-risk groups. As a 1987 study by the Center for Media and Public Affairs found, heterosexuals were eight times more likely to appear as AIDS victims in TV news reports than they were to actually contract the disease.

Not without reason has AIDS expert Michael Fumento remarked that the basic response of the media to the CDC's view of heterosexual AIDS was "you supply the grain of truth, and we'll supply the panic."

While reporting their story, Bennett and Sharpe found that over the years the facts exposing the myth of heterosexual AIDS were indeed available. All anyone had to do, Sharpe says, was "read the fine print" in the CDC reports.

And a few reporters had in fact done that. The *Philadelphia Inquirer*'s Donald Drake and the *Chicago Tribune*'s John Crewdson spotted the exaggeration of the threat to heterosexuals and pointed it out. Drake, for example, questioned the data provided by AIDS researchers. "You would say to them, 'Well, if these people are high-risk, and these people are high-risk, then doesn't it follow that these people are low-risk?' But they wouldn't say that. They wouldn't close the circle for you." Skeptical reporters were the exceptions, however, and in retrospect they look like people standing in a river of sewage trying to reverse the flow with a canoe paddle. For their labors, these contrarian journalists endured hostility —often from within their own newsrooms. When Crewdson wrote in 1987 that the threat of heterosexual AIDS was overblown because "the numbers just didn't add up," he recalls, "I was roundly criticized."

*　*　*

Michael Fumento probably wishes he had been only "roundly criticized." A lawyer-turned-freelancer, Fumento was the first person to undertake a major treatment of the story of heterosexual AIDS. News stories about the purported "doubling" of the percentage of heterosexual AIDS cases sparked his interest. Fumento was skeptical, because he knew that heterosexual transmission still ac-

counted for only 4 percent of the total number of AIDS cases. Upon closer inspection he discovered that the increase in the number of heterosexuals with AIDS was almost entirely the result of CDC bookkeeping: In 1986, the agency had reclassified to the heterosexual category cases involving Haitians and Africans who had recently entered the United States—a move most news stories had overlooked. (Later that year, the CDC manufactured a similar increase by throwing the "undetermined" cases into the heterosexual category.)

Fumento spent the next six months writing an article for *Commentary* entitled, "AIDS: Are Heterosexuals at Risk?" Fumento's answer: not very much.

The initial response to this piece was largely favorable. *The Washington Post*'s William Raspberry wrote a complimentary column, and on NBC's *Today,* Bryant Gumbel gave Fumento a congenial grilling. "He was on my side," Fumento recalls. Meanwhile, the U.S. Civil Rights Commission, now dominated by Reagan appointees, hired Fumento to research the civil rights implications of AIDS. Encouraged by this series of events, Fumento decided to write a book.

In August 1988, *The New Republic* published "The Political Uses of an Epidemic," a cover story adapted from a chapter in his forthcoming book. The article drew the attention of his bosses at the Civil Rights Commission, and they were not amused. The problem so far as the commission was concerned was Fumento's criticism of key conservative Republicans—including Jack Kemp, William Bennett, Pat Robertson, and Gary Bauer—for endorsing the anyone-can-get-AIDS theme, apparently because it dovetailed with Republican efforts to reduce sexual promiscuity.

These social-issue conservatives also happened to support the continued existence of the embattled commission. Worried that this crucial support might erode if Fumento continued to work for the commission, officials forced him to resign.

But this experience was nothing compared to what Fumento went through after Basic Books published his *The Myth of Heterosexual AIDS* in January 1990. For starters, Fumento was fired from his new job in Denver, Colorado, as an editorial writer for the *Rocky Mountain News*. This firing, he remains convinced, was a politically motivated reaction to his book, though Vincent Carroll, editor of the editorial page, says Fumento was fired for spending too much time on phone calls connected with promotion of his book. Another editor recalls problems on Friday afternoons when the staff was pushing to get the weekend pages out and "Mike would be screaming on the phone about anal sex." But firing Fumento, this editor adds, was too stiff a penalty.

Next came the hostile reviews and personal attacks. Under the headline "Critics Say Author Twists Conclusions," a *USA Today* profile quoted AIDS activists and public health officials calling Fumento and his book "irresponsible," "mean-spirited," "myopic," "homophobic," and "sexist." A reviewer for *The Orange County Register* misquoted the book as saying some minority groups were genetically predisposed to AIDS (it says the opposite), and then accused Fumento of "pure and simple racism." The *Village Voice* contended that the book was built on a "foundation of lies."

Science, one of the most prestigious scientific magazines in the country, assigned the book for review to a professor of post-structuralist linguistics, Paula Treichler, rather than to a scientist. While unable to deconstruct the facts on which Fumento's book was based, she tore into him for political incorrectness. "Fumento's political agenda is never... very far from his science," she charged. "He calls, among other things, for AIDS estimates to be revised downward for all groups, not only heterosexuals." Fumento took quiet solace in the fact that just as his book came out—and several months before Treichler's review appeared—the CDC *had* revised downward its projections for all groups.

Fumento seemed to be getting attacked from all sides, *Forbes* editor Joe Queenan observed, for writing that AIDS would *not* be the bubonic plague of the twentieth century. "It doesn't pay to be the bearer of good news," he noted. It also didn't pay to write such things in *Forbes*. ACT-UP demonstrators assembled outside the *Forbes* building in New York City, protesting that "everyone is vulnerable to AIDS" and demanding an audience with publisher Malcolm S. Forbes, Sr. In his next column, Forbes retracted the Queenan article and denounced Fumento's views as "asinine." *Forbes* also published a statement by ACT-UP members condemning the article as being "highly speculative information provided by an unreliable source."

* * *

Meanwhile, Fumento says, AIDS activists had launched a nationwide, grassroots campaign to ban his book, going so far as to advise book distributors not to carry it. To an alarming extent, the tactic worked. The book was unavailable in Waldenbooks, Fumento says, until he pointed out the fact on national television. (A spokesperson for Waldenbooks says that initially the chain made "a small buy for selected stores.") Some stores sold out their initial supply and failed to reorder. Fumento got reports from all over the country that the book simply could not be found in stores. Just six months after publication, the Tattered Cover, one of the biggest bookstores in Fumento's hometown of Denver, no longer had a copy on its shelves, though it continued to stock scores of older, less-in-demand books. Ironically the store had a special display of books that had been banned. "Needless to say," Fumento notes, "mine was not among them." Even the co-founder of the Southern California Coalition for Intellectual Freedom joined the attack against the book, commenting, "If Fumento's book is sold in any store, it ought to be accompanied by a sign reading, THIS BOOK IS WRONG." Basic Books did no second printing, unusual when the first edition sells briskly. Nor did Basic Books exercise its right to bring out a paperback version.

Fumento's firing from the *Rocky Mountain News* drew no interest from news organizations, and the disappearance of his book from store and library shelves (it was apparently filched by activists) elicited no known response from the many groups claiming to be crusaders against book-banning, such as the American Library Association and People for the American Way. The book quietly vanished.

In an ironic postscript, two recent books by gay authors—William Rushing's *The AIDS Epidemic* and John Lauritsen's *AIDS War: Propaganda, Profiteering, and Genocide from the Medical Industrial Complex*—have praised Fumento's book, reflecting the realization that the anybody-can-get-it strategy had diluted the efforts to reduce the number of homo-sexuals who have died from AIDS. "Curiously," Rushing wrote, "*The Myth of Heterosexual AIDS* did not receive as much attention as it deserved."

During the battle over the Fumento book, another protagonist challenged the heterosexual-plague thesis. Irked at the uncritical way in which the news media failed to report the relative risks associated with AIDS, Dan Lynch, managing editor of the *Albany Times Union*, wrote a column on November 10, 1991, criticizing his fellow journalists. Specifically, he accused them of neglecting to point out that cancer kills more people in one month than AIDS does in a year, and of being too squeamish to say flat out that the primary mechanism for spreading AIDS was anal intercourse. "Instead of taking every opportunity to emphasize this key piece of information," Lynch wrote, "we used euphemisms such as 'exchange of bodily fluids' and 'intimate sexual contact,' which serve to educate no one." Lynch also criticized the barrage of stories about the spread of AIDS among heterosexuals spawned by basketball star Magic Johnson's intimation that he had become HIV-positive through heterosexual contacts. "Our stories have failed to communicate that male victims such as Magic Johnson, who say they could have contracted the disease only through heterosexual sex, are but 3 percent of the total number of persons with AIDS. . . . The reality, painful though it may be to people concerned about discrimination against gays and poverty-stricken minorities who make up the bulk of IV-drug users, is that AIDS in the United States remains overwhelmingly confined to members of those groups and their sexual partners."

The reaction in his own newsroom was explosive. The *Times Union* medical writer wrote a column attacking Lynch. Few colleagues confronted him directly —"People have learned not to get into an argument with me," he says —but anonymous notes referring to him as "Dan (Anal Intercourse) Lynch" appeared on bulletin boards. In letters to the editor, AIDS activists pilloried him for "poor taste" and "lacking compassion."

* * *

Lynch's column attracted attention elsewhere. The *Washington Journalism Review* (now the *American Journalism Review*) published an expanded version followed by a group of shorter articles mainly attacking it. *Cosmopolitan* and *Reader's Digest* also ran versions of Lynch's piece, and the conflagration spread. As Lynch later wrote, "I was swamped with hate mail from around the world."

But he thinks he made a difference. Elinor Burkett, he says, author of *The Gravest Show on Earth: America in the Age of AIDS* and formerly a reporter for *The Miami Herald,* told him that checking out the assertions in his column and discovering they were true had changed the way she covered AIDS. Lynch's piece also paved the way for other stories downplaying the heterosexual epidemic, notably Louis Kilzer's 1992 article, "The AIDS Mythology," in the Minneapolis *Star Tribune*, which also provoked a firestorm of protest.

In 1993, *The New York Times*'s Gina Kolata wrote a front-page story about how the entire AIDS epidemic had peaked and could be eradicated with proper prevention methods. Anticipating the thrust of the Bennett-Sharpe article three years later, Kolata stressed that a growing number of experts felt that the AIDS campaign needed to be targeted at specific risk groups rather than the general population. She cited clear and unambiguous reports—including one by a blue-ribbon panel assembled by the National Research Council—debunking the possibility of a heterosexual outbreak in the United States. In 1994, the results of the most comprehensive survey of American sexual behavior was released in two books—one for scientists and the other, *Sex in America* (co-written by the *Times*'s Kolata), for lay readers. Both books concluded that AIDS would not spread to the broader public.

Despite these corrective articles and reports, the message failed to get through to many journalists. "Heterosexual transmission of AIDS has tripled since 1981," Anne Rochell wrote in the February 22, 1995 *Atlanta Journal-Constitution*, "and the population most at risk is women." The article quoted a CDC official saying, "There's a huge myth out there that this is not a heterosexual epidemic." Numerous stories and editorials continue to recite verbatim the old CDC canards. As Kate Santich wrote in *The Orlando Sentinel* this past May 19 [1996] (the same month the Bennett-Sharpe article appeared), "The epidemic is now ... rising fastest among straights, especially straight women." The persistence of the belief that a heterosexual outbreak is imminent resembles something from a science fiction movie: The monster has escaped from the lab, and no one can get it under control.

Why did journalists exaggerate the threat of heterosexual AIDS? Some may have feared the storm of criticism if they bucked the trend. Others were simply ignorant. "Most editors don't know much about science or medicine," one reporter told me, but like to think they do. And some reporters, one journalist says, "will believe anything an academic tells them," never realizing that scholars may have just as much of a political agenda as, say, a Pentagon spokesperson or a politician. "You tend to think it's an academic's goal to go after truth in a dispassionate way," Kolata says, even when you may be aware that they have a stake in promoting their views and their field of study. As the *Tribune*'s Crewdson notes, "If you're Dr. X, or Professor Y, it doesn't matter if you're an adjunct professor of nothing in particular at some college no one has ever heard of—you're going in the story."

* * *

Another explanation, one editor confided, is that reporters found the AIDS activists pushing the heterosexual-epidemic thesis "ideologically congenial." As this editor explains, journalists tend to like victim groups, both because their own political views often match theirs, and because journalists instinctively love an underdog. And while no one interviewed for this story would admit to it, some journalists may have sympathized with the CDC's rationale that the ends (greater AIDS funding) justified the means (deception).

Crewdson believes that the wholesale support for the heterosexual-epidemic thesis can be explained by journalists simply doing what they get rewarded for. Their careers depend on their ability to get stories into the paper, he says, and "a writer is going to have trouble getting stories onto page one or on the cover of the magazine that just apply to gay men and IV-drug users. But if you can go to your editor and say the CDC has numbers providing evidence that AIDS is a threat to people like you and me, you've got a much better shot. Believe me. I do this for a living. I know."

Amanda Bennett has her own theory of why the news media kept the good news about heterosexual AIDS under wraps. This theory—the "template" theory—derives from her experiences in China as much as from her more recent work covering AIDS. "The 'template,'" she explains, "is what editors and other people who are not on the ground have decided is The Story." They use it to determine whether something is news or not. If it fits the template, it's news; if it doesn't, it's not.

"I was in China twice," Bennett recalls, "once when China was first opening up [in the mid-1980s], and then again right after Tiananmen Square [in 1989]. When I was first there, the reporters were complaining that their editors only wanted good stories about happy little children, beaming peasants, friendly people. They didn't want to hear about businessmen who were getting hassled or beaten up." The template, in other words, was that China was a great country emerging from a dark period in its history.

But when she returned to China during the Tiananmen Square uprising, the template had been reversed. "Now it was impossible to get a story in that said anything *good* about China. All anyone wanted to hear about was human rights abuses. And again the reporters who were actually there were complaining."

The AIDS template, she explains, was that the heterosexual plague is coming. Breaking that template was not easy, because it required considerable time and resources. And few publications these days are willing to let two reporters spend six months pursuing a story, particularly a story that contradicts The Story.

Gina Kolata of *The New York Times* is one reporter who came to see that The Story was wrong. Renowned for her willingness to challenge conventional wisdom and to resist special-interest pleading, Kolata says she can understand "the alarmist stuff" because at one point "I was part of it myself." Years ago, Kolata wrote articles indicating that AIDS was running amok among women and teenagers—articles she hopes no one will "ever find and read again. I can't believe I wasn't more skeptical."

And there were clues, she recalls. When she asked AIDS activists to help her find some teenagers with AIDS to interview, they could barely find any. "They came up with one gay kid who had been hanging around with older men," she remembers. "They said that the others couldn't deal with talking to the press." For a long time, Kolata gave the activists and public health officials promoting the heterosexual-epidemic thesis the benefit of the doubt, she says, but she ultimately found that on AIDS stories "you had to push a lot" to get the truth out of sources. "And on the reports about AIDS floating among women, you had to push hard. Are these women in risk groups? Is this anything different? Or is this the same old stuff?"

As she studied the data, Kolata became increasingly skeptical that a breakout was imminent. The National Research Council report in 1993 provided the clinching evidence that the HIV contagion was actually restricted to certain neighborhoods. As an alarmist, "that was the end for me," she says.

Did the Bennett-Sharpe exposé finally put a stake through the heart of the heterosexual-AIDS-epidemic thesis? Probably not. Reporters long familiar with the story say that too many people now have too much invested in keeping the myth alive. "Have you heard a high public official stand up and say it isn't true?" asks Fumento.

* * *

Similarly pessimistic, Kolata points to the recent experiences of her two teenage children. Her son's biology teacher at Princeton High School in New Jersey told his class this year that the heterosexual epidemic was on its way; when the lad pluckily attempted to protest, the teacher informed him he was wrong. And at a statewide convention of student leaders, Kolata's daughter heard the heterosexual-plague scenario with all its accoutrements. "She's given up arguing about it," says Kolata. "She just told us about it at the dinner table and we laughed."

There are signs that the underlying premise of the template—that good news about the spread of AIDS is not news—is mutating, much as HIV appears to do, and taking on new targets. For example, while prospects for treating AIDS with new drugs has received attention recently, reports issued this past April from the National Cancer Institute and the CDC itself indicating that the incidence of AIDS has diminished barely gained notice.

Indeed, both *The Washington Post* and *The New York Times* twisted the latest CDC release, making the good news masquerade as bad news. The *Post* ignored the CDC report in its news columns, but whined in an April 25, 1996 editorial that the report showed that the District of Columbia had a higher proportion of AIDS cases than all 50 states. It was unfair, the editorial stated, to compare a city to states. (This from an editorial board that for years has argued that Washington *should* be compared to other states, at least for determining its congressional representation.)

The *Times* metropolitan desk carefully combed the CDC report and did a short piece on its discovery that Jersey City had achieved the "grim distinction" of being second only to Washington, D.C., in its rate of AIDS cases. The article neatly skipped over the fact that even in Jersey City, the number of new AIDS cases was going down.

The *Times* science section, according to Kolata, skipped the CDC report on the grounds that the downturn was old news, something they had already written about many times. She concurred in that judgment. "How many times," she asks, "can we write the same thing?"

How many times, indeed. One answer might be: Perhaps until people start to notice.

Kolata herself felt a twinge of annoyance when she read in her own newspaper this past June [1996] an account of a speaker at the international AIDS conference in Vancouver who received applause when she started her presentation by saying, "I have AIDS and it doesn't matter how I got it."

Kolata shakes her head. "Here we are at a conference on how to stop the spread of AIDS and she's being cheered for saying that it doesn't matter how she got it? That may be the *only* thing that matters. I read that and I just said to myself, 'Here we go again.'"

POSTSCRIPT

Is AIDS a Major Threat to the Heterosexual, Non-Drug-Abusing Population?

AIDS was not officially diagnosed until the early 1980s. By that time, doctors had begun noticing rare cancers in young, male homosexuals. Other diseases, such as pneumonia and meningitis, had also begun to disproportionately affect male homosexuals and intravenous (IV) drug users. It wasn't until 1985, however, that President Ronald Reagan ever mentioned the word *AIDS*, even though the number of cases and AIDS-related deaths had risen to epidemic proportions. Finally, in 1986, Surgeon General C. Everett Koop issued a report on the AIDS virus and sent educational materials about AIDS to every household in the United States. Critics claimed, however, that had the government begun AIDS education and research sooner, many lives would have been saved. The late columnist Randy Shilts, in his book *And the Band Played On* (St. Martin's Press, 1987), agreed that the government knew about the AIDS epidemic years before anything was done about it.

Is there an epidemic-to-be among middle-class, non-drug-abusing heterosexuals that is currently being ignored? In 1991 Earvin "Magic" Johnson, the celebrated basketball superstar for the Los Angeles Lakers, disclosed that he was HIV positive. Johnson said that he contracted the disease through heterosexual contact. Is Johnson an early victim of an impending heterosexual AIDS epidemic? Suzanne Fields, a columnist for the *Washington Times*, would say no. In "Misrepresenting AIDS," *Washington Times* (August 17, 1986), Fields claims that AIDS is still primarily related to high-risk behavior practiced by specific population groups. Michael Fumento concurs. For more of Fumento's views on AIDS, see *The Myth of Heterosexual AIDS* (Basic Books, 1990); "'Teenaids': The Latest HIV Fib," *New Republic* (August 10, 1992); "Media, AIDS, and Truth," *National Review* (June 21, 1993); and "Heterosexual AIDS: Part VII," *The American Spectator* (July 1994).

AIDS has generated thousands of articles and books since the disease was first diagnosed. Two articles that discuss AIDS among minorities are "The Homecoming: Paranoia and Plague in Black America," *New Republic* (June 5, 1995) and "The White Cloud: Latino America's Stealth Virus," *New Republic* (June 5, 1995). The following articles offer several different viewpoints on the seriousness of the epidemic and the government's response to AIDS: "New Ways to Prevent and Treat AIDS," *FDA Consumer* (January 1997); "Update: Trends in AIDS Incidence, Deaths and Prevention," *Morbidity and Mortality Report* (February 28, 1997); "Signs of Life on the AIDS Front," *US News and*

World Report (March 10, 1997); "Fewer AIDS Victims," *Macleans* (March 10, 1997); "Health Hazard: AIDS Fight Is Skewed by Federal Campaign Exaggerated Risks; Most Heterosexuals Face Scant Peril but Receive Large Portion of Funds," *Wall Street Journal* (May 1, 1996); "US Heterosexuals Fail to Reduce Risk," *AIDS Weekly Plus* (May 13, 1996); "Has AIDS Won?" *New York Magazine*, February 20, 1995; "Reexamining AIDS Research Priorities," *Science* (February 1995); "AIDS: A Crisis Ignored," *U.S. News and World Report* (January 12, 1987); "AIDS and a Duty to Protect," *Hastings Center Report* (February 1987); "The AIDS Epidemic Has Hit Home," *Psychology Today* (April 1987); and "The Judgment Mentality," *Christianity Today* (March 20, 1987).

ISSUE 13

Can Abortion Be a Morally Acceptable Choice?

YES: Mary Gordon, from "A Moral Choice," *The Atlantic Monthly* (April 1990)

NO: Jason DeParle, from "Beyond the Legal Right: Why Liberals and Feminists Don't Like to Talk About the Morality of Abortion," *The Washington Monthly* (April 1989)

ISSUE SUMMARY

YES: Author Mary Gordon contends that abortion is an acceptable means to end an unwanted pregnancy and that women who have abortions are neither selfish nor immoral.

NO: Editor Jason DeParle argues that liberals and feminists refuse to acknowledge that the 3 out of 10 pregnancies that currently end in abortion raise many moral questions.

Few issues have created as much controversy and resulted in as much opposition as has the topic of abortion. Those involved in the abortion debate not only have firm beliefs, but each side has a self-designated label—pro-life and pro-choice—that clearly reflects what they believe to be the basic issues. The supporters of a woman's right to choose an abortion see individual choice as central to the debate. They believe that if a woman cannot choose to end an unwanted pregnancy, a condition that affects her body and possibly her whole life, then she has lost one of her most basic human rights. The pro-choice people feel that although the fetus is a potential human being, its life cannot be placed on the same level as that of a woman. On the other side, supporters of the pro-life movement argue that the fetus *is* a human being and that it has the same right to life as the mother. They believe that abortion is not only immoral; it is murder.

Although abortion appears to be a modern issue, it has a very long history. In the past, women in both urbanized and tribal societies have used a variety of dangerous methods to end unwanted pregnancies. Women sometimes consumed toxic chemicals, or various tools were inserted into the uterus in hopes of expelling its contents. Modern technology has simplified the procedure and has made it considerably safer. Before abortion was legalized in the United States, approximately 20 percent of all deaths from childbirth or pregnancy were caused by botched illegal abortions.

In 1973 the U.S. Supreme Court's decision of *Roe v. Wade* determined that an abortion in the first three months (trimester) of pregnancy is a decision between a woman and her physician and is protected by a right to privacy. The Court ruled that during the second trimester an abortion could be performed on the basis of health risks. During the final trimester, an abortion could be performed only to preserve the mother's life.

Since 1973 abortion has become one of the most controversial issues in America. The National Right to Life Committee, one of the major abortion foes, currently has over 11 million members, who have become increasingly militant. In the summer of 1991, a major battle between pro-life and pro-choice forces took place in Wichita, Kansas. A similar demonstration followed during the spring of 1992 in Buffalo, New York. Demonstrators have also become more aggressive and violent. In 1993 David Gunn, a physician who performed abortions in Pensacola, Florida, was gunned down by a pro-life fanatic. Dr. Gunn was replaced by Dr. John Britton who, along with his bodyguard, was killed in August 1994 by a regular protester at the abortion clinic. In Massachusetts later that year, several people, including a receptionist, were gunned down in two women's health clinics that performed abortions. In spring 1997 abortion protesters targeted high schools across the country with an educational message about pregnancy termination.

Despite opposition from the right-to-life groups, abortion remains safe and legal in the United States today. However, what continues to kindle the debate are these questions: Does an abortion involve killing what may be a human being? Is abortion moral? Does the fetus have a right to life, liberty, and the pursuit of happiness, as guaranteed by the U.S. Constitution? Or do women have a right to a safe means of terminating an unwanted pregnancy?

In the following selections, Mary Gordon writes that abortion is neither immoral nor selfish. Because abortions usually take place when the embryo is merely a clump of cells and not a developed fetus, Gordon argues, abortion is not immoral, and she maintains that a woman's life is more important than that of a *potential* human. Jason DeParle argues that there is nothing more vulnerable than the unborn child. DeParle cannot understand how liberalism can "hope to regain the glory of standing for morality and humanity while finding nothing inhumane or immoral in the extermination of so much life."

YES   Mary Gordon

A MORAL CHOICE

I am having lunch with six women. What is unusual is that four of them are in their seventies, two of them widowed, the other two living with husbands beside whom they've lived for decades. All of them have had children. Had they been men, they would have published books and hung their paintings on the walls of important galleries. But they are women of a certain generation, and their lives were shaped around their families and personal relations. They are women you go to for help and support. We begin talking about the latest legislative act that makes abortion more difficult for poor women to obtain. An extraordinary thing happens. Each of them talks about the illegal abortions she had during her young womanhood. Not one of them was spared the experience. Any of them could have died on the table of whatever person (not a doctor in any case) she was forced to approach, in secrecy and in terror, to end a pregnancy that she felt would blight her life.

I mention this incident for two reasons: first as a reminder that all kinds of women have always had abortions; second because it is essential that we remember that an abortion is performed on a living woman who has a life in which a terminated pregnancy is only a small part. Morally speaking, the decision to have an abortion doesn't take place in a vacuum. It is connected to other choices that a woman makes in the course of an adult life.

Anti-choice propagandists paint pictures of women who choose to have abortions as types of moral callousness, selfishness, or irresponsibility. The woman choosing to abort is the dressed-for-success yuppie who gets rid of her baby so that she won't miss her Caribbean vacation or her chance for promotion. Or she is the feckless, promiscuous ghetto teenager who couldn't bring herself to just say no to sex. A third, purportedly kinder, gentler picture has recently begun to be drawn. The woman in the abortion clinic is there because she is misinformed about the nature of the world. She is having an abortion because society does not provide for mothers and their children, and she mistakenly thinks that another mouth to feed will be the ruin of her family, not understanding that the temporary truth of family unhappiness doesn't stack up beside the eternal verity that abortion is murder. Or she is the dupe of her husband or boyfriend, who talks her into having an abortion because

From Mary Gordon, "A Moral Choice," *The Atlantic Monthly* (April 1990). Copyright © 1990 by Mary Gordon. Reprinted by permission of Sterling Lord Literistic, Inc.

a child will be a drag on his life-style. None of these pictures created by the anti-choice movement assumes that the decision to have an abortion is made responsibly, in the context of a morally lived life, by a free and responsible moral agent.

THE ONTOLOGY* OF THE FETUS

How would a woman who habitually makes choices in moral terms come to the decision to have an abortion? The moral discussion of abortion centers on the issue of whether or not abortion is an act of murder. At first glance it would seem that the answer should follow directly upon two questions: Is the fetus human? and Is it alive? It would be absurd to deny that a fetus is alive or that it is human. What would our other options be—to say that it is inanimate or belongs to another species? But we habitually use the terms "human" and "live" to refer to parts of our body—"human hair," for example, or "live red-blood cells"—and we are clear in our understanding that the nature of these objects does not rank equally with an entire personal existence. It then seems important to consider whether the fetus, this alive human thing, is a *person*, to whom the term "murder" could sensibly be applied. How would anyone come to a decision about something so impalpable as personhood? Philosophers have struggled with the issue of personhood, but in language that is so abstract that it is unhelpful to ordinary people making decisions in the course of their lives. It might be more productive to begin thinking about the status of the fetus by examining the language and customs that

*[*Ontology* refers to the nature of being or existing. —Ed.]

surround it. This approach will encourage us to focus on the choosing, acting woman, rather than the act of abortion— as if the act were performed by abstract forces without bodies, histories, attachments.

This focus on the acting woman is useful because a pregnant woman has an identifiable, consistent ontology, and a fetus takes on different ontological identities over time. But common sense, experience, and linguistic usage point clearly to the fact that we habitually consider, for example, a seven-week-old fetus to be different from a seven-month-old one. We can tell this by the way we respond to the involuntary loss of one as against the other. We have different language for the experience of the involuntary expulsion of the fetus from the womb depending upon the point of gestation at which the experience occurs. If it occurs early in the pregnancy, we call it a miscarriage; if late, we call it a stillbirth.

We would have an extreme reaction to the reversal of those terms. If a woman referred to a miscarriage at seven weeks as a stillbirth, we would be alarmed. It would shock our sense of propriety; it would make us uneasy; we would find it disturbing, misplaced—as we do when a bag lady sits down in a restaurant and starts shouting, or an octogenarian arrives at our door in a sailor suit. In short, we would suspect that the speaker was mad. Similarly, if a doctor or a nurse referred to the loss of a seven-month-old fetus as a miscarriage, we would be shocked by that person's insensitivity: could she or he not understand that a fetus that age is not what it was months before?

Our ritual and religious practices underscore the fact that we make distinctions among fetuses. If a woman took the bloody matter—indistinguishable from a heavy period—of an early miscarriage and insisted upon putting it in a tiny coffin and marking its grave, we would have serious concerns about her mental health. By the same token, we would feel squeamish about flushing a seven-month-old fetus down the toilet—something we would quite normally do with an early miscarriage. There are no prayers for the matter of a miscarriage, nor do we feel there should be. Even a Catholic priest would not baptize the issue of an early miscarriage.

The difficulties stem, of course, from the odd situation of a fetus's ontology: a complicated, differentiated, and nuanced response is required when we are dealing with an entity that changes over time. Yet we are in the habit of making distinctions like this. At one point we know that a child is no longer a child but an adult. That this question is vexed and problematic is clear from our difficulty in determining who is a juvenile offender and who is an adult criminal and at what age sexual intercourse ceases to be known as statutory rape. So at what point, if any, do we on the pro-choice side say that the developing fetus is a person, with rights equal to its mother's?

The anti-choice people have one advantage over us; their monolithic position gives them unity on this question. For myself, I am made uneasy by third-trimester abortions, which take place when the fetus could live outside the mother's body, but I also know that these are extremely rare and often performed on very young girls who have had difficulty comprehending the realities of pregnancy. It seems to me that the question of late abortions should be decided case by case, and that fixation on this issue is a deflection from what is most important: keeping early abortions, which are in the majority by far, safe and legal. I am also politically realistic enough to suspect that bills restricting late abortions are not good-faith attempts to make distinctions about the nature of fetal life. They are, rather, the cynical embodiments of the hope among anti-choice partisans that technology will be on their side and that medical science's ability to create situations in which younger fetuses are viable outside their mothers' bodies will increase dramatically in the next few years. Ironically, medical science will probably make the issue of abortion a minor one in the near future. The RU-486 pill, which can induce abortion early on, exists, and whether or not it is legally available (it is not on the market here, because of pressure from anti-choice groups), women will begin to obtain it. If abortion can occur through chemical rather than physical means, in the privacy of one's home, most people not directly involved will lose interest in it. As abortion is transformed from a public into a private issue, it will cease to be perceived as political; it will be called personal instead.

AN EQUIVOCAL GOOD

But because abortion will always deal with what it is to create and sustain life, it will always be a moral issue. And whether we like it or not, our moral thinking about abortion is rooted in the shifting soil of perception. In an age in which much of our perception is manipulated by media that specialize in the sound bite and the photo op, the anti-choice partisans have a twofold advantage over us on the pro-choice side. The pro-choice moral position is more complex, and the experience we defend is physically repellent to contemplate. None of us in the pro-choice movement would suggest that abortion is not a regrettable occurrence. Anti-choice proponents can offer pastel photographs of babies in buntings, their eyes peaceful in the camera's gaze. In answer, we can't offer the material of an early abortion, bloody, amorphous in a paper cup, to prove that what has just been removed from the woman's body is not a child, not in the same category of being as the adorable bundle in an adoptive mother's arms. It is not a pleasure to look at the physical evidence of abortion, and most of us don't get the opportunity to do so.

The theologian Daniel Maguire, uncomfortable with the fact that most theological arguments about the nature of abortion are made by men who have never been anywhere near an actual abortion, decided to visit a clinic and observe abortions being performed. He didn't find the experience easy, but he knew that before he could in good conscience make a moral judgment on abortion, he needed to experience through his senses what an aborted fetus is like: he needed to look at and touch the controversial entity. He held in his hand the bloody fetal stuff; the eight-week-old fetus fit in the palm of his hand, and it certainly bore no resemblance to either of his two children when he had held them moments after their birth. He knew at that point what women who have experienced early abortions and miscarriages know: that some event occurred, possibly even a dramatic one, but it was not the death of a child.

Because issues of pregnancy and birth are both physical and metaphorical, we must constantly step back and forth between ways of perceiving the world. When we speak of gestation, we are often talking in terms of potential, about events and objects to which we attach our hopes, fears, dreams, and ideals. A mother can speak to the fetus in her uterus and name it; she and her mate may decorate a nursery according to their vision of the good life; they may choose for an embryo a college, a profession, a dwelling. But those of us who are trying to think morally about pregnancy and birth must remember that these feelings are our own projections onto what is in reality an inappropriate object. However charmed we may be by an expectant father's buying a little football for something inside his wife's belly, we shouldn't make public policy based on such actions, nor should we force others to live their lives conforming to our fantasies.

As a society, we are making decisions that pit the complicated future of a complex adult against the fate of a mass of cells lacking cortical development. The moral pressure should be on distinguishing the true from the false, the real suffering of living persons from our individual and often idiosyncratic dreams and fears. We must make decisions on abortion based on an understanding of how people really do live. We must be able to say that poverty is worse than not being poor, that having dignified and meaningful work is better than working in conditions of degradation, that raising a child one loves and has desired is better than raising a child in resentment and rage, that it is better for a twelve-year-old not to endure the trauma of having a child when she is herself a child.

When we put these ideas against the ideas of "child" or "baby," we seem to be making a horrifying choice of life-style over life. But in fact we are telling the truth of what it means to bear a child, and what the experience of abortion really is.

This is extremely difficult, for the object of the discussion is hidden, changing, potential. We make our decisions on the basis of approximate and inadequate language, often on the basis of fantasies and fears. It will always be crucial to try to separate genuine moral concern from phobia, punitiveness, superstition, anxiety, a desperate search for certainty in an uncertain world.

One of the certainties that is removed if we accept the consequences of the pro-choice position is the belief that the birth of a child is an unequivocal good. In real life we act knowing that the birth of a child is not always a good thing: people are sometimes depressed, angry, rejecting, at the birth of a child. But this is a difficult truth to tell; we don't like to say it, and one of the fears preyed on by anti-choice proponents is that if we cannot look at the birth of a child as an unequivocal good, then there is nothing to look toward. The desire for security of the imagination, for typological fixity, particularly in the area of "the good," is an understandable desire. It must seem to some anti-choice people that we on the pro-choice side are not only murdering innocent children but also murdering hope. Those of us who have experienced the birth of a desired child and felt the joy of that moment can be tempted into believing that it was the physical experience of the birth itself that was the joy. But it is crucial to remember that the birth of a child itself is a neutral occurrence emotionally: the charge it takes on is invested in it by the people experiencing or observing it.

THE FEAR OF SEXUAL AUTONOMY

These uncertainties can lead to another set of fears, not only about abortion but about its implications. Many anti-choice people fear that to support abortion is to cast one's lot with the cold and techno-logical rather than with the warm and natural, to head down the slippery slope toward a brave new world where handicapped children are left on mountains to starve and the old are put out in the snow. But if we look at the history of abortion, we don't see the embodiment of what the anti-choice proponents fear. On the contrary, excepting the grotesque counterexample of the People's Republic of China (which practices forced abortion), there seems to be a real link between repressive anti-abortion stances and repressive governments. Abortion was banned in Fascist Italy and Nazi Germany; it is illegal in South Africa and in Chile. It is paid for by the governments of Denmark, England, and the Netherlands, which have national health and welfare systems that foster the health and well-being of mothers, children, the old, and the handicapped.

Advocates of outlawing abortion often refer to women seeking abortion as self-indulgent and materialistic. In fact these accusations mask a discomfort with female sexuality, sexual pleasure, and sexual autonomy. It is possible for a woman to have a sexual life unriddled by fear only if she can be confident that she need not pay for a failure of technology or judgment (and who among us has never once been swept away in the heat of a sexual moment?) by taking upon herself the crushing burden of unchosen motherhood.

It is no accident, therefore, that the increased appeal of measures to restrict maternal conduct during pregnancy—and a new focus on the physical autonomy of the pregnant woman—have come into public discourse at precisely the time when women are achieving unprecedented levels of economic and political autonomy. What has surprised me is that some of this new anti-autonomy talk comes to us from the left. An example of this new discourse is an article by Christopher Hitchens that appeared in *The Nation* last April, in which the author asserts his discomfort with abortion. Hitchens's tone is impeccably British: arch, light, we're men of the left.

> Anyone who has ever seen a sonogram or has spent even an hour with a textbook on embryology knows that the emotions are not the deciding factor. In order to terminate a pregnancy, you have to still a heartbeat, switch off a developing brain, and whatever the method, break some bones and rupture some organs. As to whether this involves pain on the "Silent Scream" scale, I have no idea. The "right to life" leadership, again, has cheapened everything it touches. ["Silent Scream" refers to Dr. Bernard Nathanson's widely debated antiabortion film *The Silent Scream,* in which an abortion on a 12-week-old fetus is shown from inside the uterus.—Ed.]

"It is a pity," Hitchens goes on to say, "that... the majority of feminists and their allies have stuck to the dead ground of 'Me Decade' possessive individualism, an ideology that has more in common than it admits with the prehistoric right, which it claims to oppose but has in fact encouraged." Hitchens proposes, as an alternative, a program of social reform that would make contraception free and support a national adoption service. In his opinion, it would seem, women have abortions for only two reasons: because they are selfish or because they are poor. If the state will take care of the economic problems and the bureaucratic messiness around adoption, it remains only for the possessive individualists to get their act together and walk with their babies into the communal utopia of the future. Hitchens would allow victims of rape or incest to have free abortions, on the grounds that since they didn't choose to have sex, the women should not be forced to have the babies. This would seem to put the issue of volition in a wrong and telling place. To Hitchens's mind, it would appear, if a woman chooses to have sex, she can't choose whether or not to have a baby. The implications of this are clear. If a woman is consciously and volitionally sexual, she should be prepared to take her medicine. And what medicine must the consciously sexual male take? Does Hitchens really believe, or want us to believe, that every male who has unintentionally impregnated a woman will be involved in the lifelong responsibility for the upbringing of the engendered child? Can he honestly say that he has observed this behavior—or, indeed, would want to see it observed—in the world in which he lives?

REAL CHOICES

It is essential for a moral decision about abortion to be made in an atmosphere of open, critical thinking. We on the pro-choice side must accept that there are indeed anti-choice activists who take their position in good faith. I believe, however, that they are people for whom childbirth is an emotionally overladen topic, people who are susceptible to unclear thinking because of their unrealistic hopes and fears. It is important for us in the pro-choice movement to be open in discussing those areas involving abortion which are nebulous and unclear. But we must not forget that there are some things that we know to be undeniably true.

There are some undeniable bad consequences of a woman's being forced to bear a child against her will. First is the trauma of going through a pregnancy and giving birth to a child who is not desired, a trauma more long-lasting than that experienced by some (only some) women who experience an early abortion. The grief of giving up a child at its birth—and at nine months it is a child whom one has felt move inside one's body—is underestimated both by anti-choice partisans and by those for whom access to adoptable children is important. This grief should not be forced on any woman—or, indeed, encouraged by public policy.

We must be realistic about the impact on society of millions of unwanted children in an overpopulated world. Most of the time, human beings have sex not because they want to make babies. Yet throughout history sex has resulted in unwanted pregnancies. And women have always aborted. One thing that is not hidden, mysterious, or debatable is that making abortion illegal will result in the deaths of women, as it has always done. Is our historical memory so short that none of us remember aunts, sisters, friends, or mothers who were killed or rendered sterile by septic abortions? Does no one in the anti-choice movement remember stories or actual experiences of midnight drives to filthy rooms from which aborted women were sent out, bleeding, to their fate? Can anyone genuinely say that it would be a moral good for us as a society to return to those conditions?

Thinking about abortion, then, forces us to take moral positions as adults who understand the complexities of the world and the realities of human suffering, to make decisions based on how people actually live and choose, and not on our fears, prejudices, and anxieties about sex and society, life and death.

NO

Jason DeParle

BEYOND THE LEGAL RIGHT: WHY LIBERALS AND FEMINISTS DON'T LIKE TO TALK ABOUT THE MORALITY OF ABORTION

It's hard to hold these two images—the dismembered body of the fetus and the enveloping body of the mother, each begging the allegiance of our conscience—in mind at the same time. One of the biggest problems with the abortion debate is how rarely we do it, at least in public discourse. While contentious issues naturally produce one-dimensional positions, the remarkable thing about abortion is that many otherwise sensitive, nuanced thinkers hold them. To one side, visions only of women in crisis, terrified and imperilled by an invasive growth; to the other, only legions of innocent children, chased by the steely needle.

The inhumanity that issues from baronies within the right-to-life movement is well known: the craziness of a crusade against birth control; the view of women as second-class citizens; even the descent into bomb-throwing madness. The insistence that an unborn child must always be saved, no matter the cost, isn't compassion but a compassionate mask, and it obscures a face of cruelty.

But what ought to be equally if not more disturbing to feminists, liberals, and others on the Left is the extent to which prominent prochoice intellectuals mirror that dishonesty and denial. One-and-a-half million abortions each year is not the moral equivalent of the Holocaust, precisely because of the way in which fetuses *are* distinguishable: growing inside women, they can wreck the lives of mothers and of others, including her children, who depend upon her. But the fact that three of 10 pregnancies end in abortion poses moral questions that much of the Left, especially abortion's most vocal defenders, refuses to acknowledge. This lowering of intellectual standards offers a useful way of looking at the reflexes of liberals in general, and also reveals much about the passions—many of them just—that underpin contemporary feminism.

WHAT THE SUCTION MACHINE SUCKS

The declaration of a legal right to an abortion doesn't end the discussion of what our attitude toward it should be, it merely begins it.... [M]any of the prochoice movement's writers and intellectuals would have us believe that the early fetus (and 90 percent of abortions take place in the first three months) is nothing more than a dewy piece of tissue, to be excised without regret. To speak of abortion as a moral dilemma, [Barbara Ehrenreich, prolific writer and contemporary feminist and socialist] has written, is to use "a mealy-mouthed vocabulary of evasion," to be compromised by a "strange and cabalistic question."

Yet everything we know—not just from science and religion but from experience, intuition, and compassion—suggests otherwise. A pregnant woman, even talking to her doctor, doesn't call the growth inside her an embryo or fetus. She calls it a *baby*. And she is admonished, by fellow feminists among others, to hold it in trust: Don't drink. Don't smoke. Eat well, counsels the feminist manual, *Our Bodies, Ourselves:* "think of it as eating for three—you, your baby, and the placenta...." Is it protoplasm that she's feeding? Or is it protoplasm only if she's feeding it to the forceps?

Grant for a moment that it is; agree that what the suction machine sucks is nothing more than tissue. Why then the feminist fuss over abortions for purposes of sex selection? If a couple wants a boy and nature hands them the makings of a girl, why not abort and start again? All that matters—no?—is "choice."

It wasn't sex selection but nuclear power that got a feminist named Juli Loesch rethinking her own contradictory views of fetuses. As an organizer attempting to stop the construction of Three Mile Island, she had schooled herself on what leaked radiation can do to prenatal development. At a meeting one day, she says, a group of women issued an unexpected challenge: "if you're so concerned about what Plutonium 239 might do to the child's arm bud you should go see what a suction machine does to his whole body."

In fact, we need neither *The Silent Scream* [Dr. Bernard Nathanson's antiabortion film, which was widely publicized and debated in the United States during the mid-1980s and which showed, from inside a uterus, an abortion being performed on a 12-week-old fetus] nor a degree in fetal physiology to tell us what we already know: that abortion is the eradication of human life and should be avoided whenever possible. Should it be legal? Yes, since the alternatives are worse. Is it moral? Perhaps, depending on what's at stake. Fetal life exists along a continuum; our obligations to it grow as it grows, but they must be weighed against other demands.

The number of liberals, feminists, and other defenders of abortion eager to simplify the moral questions is, at the very least, deeply ironic. One of the animating spirits of liberalism and other factions on the Left, and proudly so, is the concern for the most vulnerable. But what could be more vulnerable than the unborn? And how can liberalism hope to regain the glory of standing for humanity and morality while finding nothing inhumane or immoral in the extermination of so much life?

The problem with much prochoice thinking is suggested by the movement's chief slogan, "a woman's right to control her body," which fails to acknowledge that the great moral and biological conundrum is precisely that another body is involved. Slogans are slogans, not dissertations; but this one is revealing in that it mirrors so much of the prochoice tendency to ignore the conflict in an unwanted pregnancy between two competing interests, mother and embryo, and insist that only one is worthy of consideration. Daniel Callahan, a moral philosopher, has written of the need, upon securing the right to a legal abortion, to preserve the "moral tension" implicit in an unwanted pregnancy. This is something that too few members of the prochoice movement are willing to do.

One fine example of preserving the moral tension appeared several years ago in a *Harper's* piece by Sallie Tisdale, an abortion clinic nurse with a grudging acceptance of her work. First the mothers: "A twenty-one-year-old woman, unemployed, uneducated, without family, in the fifth month of her fifth pregnancy. A forty-two-year-old mother of teenagers, shocked by her condition, refusing to tell her husband. A twenty-three-year-old mother of two having her seventh abortion, and many women in their thirties having their first.... Oh, the ignorance.... Some swear they have not had sex, many do not know what a uterus is, how sperm and egg meet, how sex makes babies.... They come so young, snapping gum, sockless and sneakered, and their shakily applied eyeliner smears when they cry.... I cannot imagine them as mothers."

Then the fetus: "I am speaking in a matter-of-fact voice about 'the tissue' and 'the contents' when the woman suddenly catches my eye and asks, 'How big is the baby now?'.... I gauge, and sometimes lie a little, weaseling around its infantile features until its clinging power slackens. But when I look in the basin, among the curdlike blood clots, I see an elfin thorax, attenuated, its pencilline ribs all in parallel rows with tiny knobs of spine rounding upwards. A translucent arm and hand swim beside.... I have fetus dreams, we all do here: dreams of abortions one after the other; of buckets of blood splashed on the walls; trees full of crawling fetuses...."

It's not surprising that the defenders of abortion don't like pictures of fetuses; General Westmoreland didn't like the cameras in Vietnam either. Fetuses aren't babies, and the photos don't end the discussion. But they make it a more sober one, as it should be. Fetuses aren't just *their* image but our image too, anyone's image who is going to confront abortion.

If the prochoice movement doesn't like the way *The Silent Scream* depicts the fetus, turn to an early edition of *Our Bodies, Ourselves.* Describing an abortion at 16 weeks by means of saline injection, the feminist handbook explains: "Contractions will start some hours later. Generally they will be as strong as those of a full-term pregnancy.... The longest and most difficult part will be the labor. The breathing techniques taught in the childbirth section of this book might help make the contractions more bearable. After eight to fifteen hours of labor, the fetus is expelled in a bedpan in the patient's bed."

HEIL MARY

When Suzannah Lessard wrote about abortion in *The Washington Monthly* in 1972 ("Aborting a Fetus: the Legal Right, the Personal Choice"), a year before *Roe v. Wade,* she described what she called a "reaction formation along ideological lines... of the new feminist movement" as it related to abortion. This was a time when Gloria Steinem was insisting that a fetus was nothing more than "mass of dependent protoplasm" and aborting it the moral equivalent of a tonsillectomy. "I think a lot of women need to go fanatically ideological for a while because they can't in any other way overthrow the insidious sense of themselves as inferior," Lessard wrote, "nor otherwise live with the rage that comes to the surface when they realize how they have been psychically mauled." This is an observation about the psychology of oppression that could be applied to any number of righteous rebellions; the path to autonomy tends to pass, by necessity perhaps, through stages of angry defiance. "But I don't think that state of mind—hopefully temporary—is the strength of the movement," Lessard wrote. "It has very little to do with working out a new, undamaging way of living as women."

But to judge by much contemporary prochoice writing, the mere-protoplasm camp still thrives. Certainly, there are exceptions, Mario Cuomo's 1984 speech at Notre Dame perhaps being the most famous: "A fetus is different from an appendix or set of tonsils. At the very least... the full potential of human life is indisputably there. That—to my less subtle mind—by itself should demand respect, caution, indeed... reverence.... [But] I concluded that the approach of a constitutional amendment is not the best way for us to seek to deal with abortion." And others on the Left have gone even further: Nat Hentoff, who supports a legal ban, has written a number of attacks on abortion in the *Village Voice*; Mary Meehan, a former antiwar activist, published an article in *The Progressive* that

attacked the magazine's own editorial stance in favor of legal abortion.

But these are the exceptions. Pick up the past 10 years of *The Nation, Mother Jones,* or *Ms.* Read liberals and feminists on the op-ed pages of *The Washington Post* or *The New York Times*—you're likely to find more concern about the snail darter than the 1.6 million fetuses aborted each year....

LIBERAL PRECINCTS

... [T]he point is clear: questioning abortion—not only the legal right but also the moral choice—is often viewed, even by otherwise sensitive and thoughtful activists, as a betrayal of the highest order. (Except, at times, for Catholics, whose antiabortion views are usually dismissed as a quaint if unfortunate quirk of faith.)

A great irony about this public demonstration of zeal is that there may be more ambivalence on the Left than is usually acknowledged. When *The Progressive* published Mary Meehan's prolife piece in 1980, it drew more mail than any article save the famous guide to the workings of the H-bomb. About half were predictable: "your knees buckle at the mere thought of taking a forthright stand for women's rights," "prolife is only a code word representing the neo-fascist absolutist thinking." Etc, etc.

But the others: "I support most of the positions of the women's movement, but I part company with those who insist on abortion as a 'right of women to control their own bodies.' There's a lot more than just one body that is being controlled here." "I have no religious objection to abortion, but I do oppose it from a humanitarian point of view." "I was awfully glad to see a liberal publication printing an antiabortion article."

Why aren't there more voices like these heard in liberal precincts? The answers come in two general sets, one pertaining to liberal and progressive values generally and the other connected more specifically to the passions of contemporary feminism.

Right or wrong, abortion helps further values that liberals and progressives generally hold in esteem. Among them is public health. Even those with qualms about abortion tend to back the legal right, if for no other reason than to stem the mutilation that a return to back alleys would surely entail. There's also an equity-between-the-classes argument: if abortion is banned all women may experience trouble getting one, but the poor will have the most trouble of all. For others, there are always planes to Sweden.

Beyond questions of abortion's legality, the Left tends to hold values that encourage the acceptance of abortion's morality too. There's the civil liberties perspective, which argues that the state should "stay out of the bedroom." There's a population control argument; without abortion, wrote one *Progressive* reader, "there will be a more intense scramble for food and all the world's natural resources." There's a help-the-poor strand of thinking; what, liberals constantly ask, about the welfare mother who can't afford another child? And there's a fairness-in-the-marketplace argument, which maintains that without absolute control of their fertility, women cannot compete with men: if two Arnold & Porter associates conceive a child at a Christmas party tryst, bringing it into the world, whether she keeps it or not, will penalize her career much more than his.

These principles—a thirst for fairness between genders and classes, for civil liberties, for economic opportunity—are honorable ones. And they speak well of those who hold them as caring not only for life itself but also for its quality.

Careful, though. Quality-of-life arguments sometimes stop focusing on quality and start frowning on life. Concerns about population control have their place; but whether abortion is a fit means of seeking it raises questions that go well beyond environmental impact studies. One of the most troubling prochoice arguments is the what-kind-of-life-will-the-child-have line. Yes, poverty may appropriately enter the moral calculus if an additional child will truly tumble the family into chaos and despair, and those situations exist. (And there is little cruelty purer than child abuse, which afflicts unwanted children of all classes.) But liberal talk about the quality of life can quickly devolve into a form of cardboard compassion that assumes life for the poor doesn't mean much anyway. That sentiment says to an unborn child of poverty: life is tough, so you should die. Compassionate, that....

THE CHRISTMAS PARTY TRYST

While the values of the Left in general provide one set of explanations for the contours of the abortion debate, the specific passions and experiences of feminists provide another. These concerns don't, finally, answer the question of what our personal, as opposed to legal, obligations toward fetal life need to be. But they do underline the history of injustice that women have inherited.

In rough outline, one persuasive feminist argument for keeping abortion *legal* —an argument I accept—goes something like this: Without the option of abortion, women cannot be as free as men. Not just socially and economically but psychologically as well. And not just those with unwanted pregnancies. As Ellen Willis of the [*Village*] *Voice* has put it, "Criminalizing abortion doesn't just harm individual women with unwanted pregnancies, it affects all women's sense of themselves. Without control of our fertility we can never envision ourselves as free, for our biology makes us constantly vulnerable." Vulnerable to failed birth control. To rape or other coercive sex. Or simply to passion. Vulnerable in a way that men are not. And in a society that rightly prizes liberty as much as ours, it's unacceptable for one half of its members to be less free, at an essential level, than the other. Therefore the legal right.

Of course, having the legal right to do something doesn't tell us whether it's a desirable thing to do. Women have the legal right to smoke and drink heavily during pregnancy, but few of us would hesitate to dissuade them from doing so. Why don't more feminists take the same view toward abortion—defending the right, but urging women to incline against it whenever possible? The feminist defenders of abortion I spoke with reacted to that proposal with a litany of past and present injustices against women—economic, social, political, and cultural, all of them quite real. "You can sit around all day talking about what's the morally right thing to do—rights and sacrifices and the sanctity of life and all that—but I don't think it can be divorced from women's lives in this society," [poet and critic Katha] Pollitt said.

Leaving aside for a moment the wrenching emotional issues, one obvious burden is economics. Having a child—even one put up for adoption—costs not only trauma but time and money, and takes them from women, not men. The financial burden is one reason why poor women are more likely to have abortions than others.

But the same inequity is true among professional women. To return to the Arnold & Porter Christmas party tryst, what would happen if the female associate does the right thing by prolife standards and decides to have the child? At $65,000 a year, she can certainly afford to do it, and her insurance is probably blue chip. But in the eyes of some senior partners, the luster of her earlier promise begins to fade. They may be reluctant to keep her on certain accounts, for fear of offending the clients. What's more, even if the clients understand, she'll be missing at least six to eight weeks of work—just, as fate would have it, when she's needed in court on an important case. The long-term penalties may be overestimated—good employees are in short demand in most professions; it's the marginal who will suffer the most—but the fears are nonetheless real. What's more, the burden is unequally shared. Her trystee suffers no such repercussions. The clients love him, he shines in court, and his future seems assured. Unfair? Yes, extremely.

These inequities are one reason why the right-to-life movement has the obligation, often shirked, to support measures that would make it easier for women of all incomes to go through pregnancy—health care, maternity leave, parental leave, day care, protections against employment discrimination. But even if all these things were provided—as they should be—it's unlikely that the strength of feminist feeling on abortion would recede. Economic opportunity is an important facet of the abortion debate, but it's not, finally at its core. Of all the women I spoke with, the one I most expected to forward an economic argument was Barbara Ehrenreich—since she is co-chair of Democratic Socialists of America—but she never mentioned it. When I finally asked her about it she said that no amount of money or servants would change the essential moral equation, which centers, in her mind, on female autonomy. "The moral issue has to do with female personhood," she said.

CRUEL CHOICES

What surprised me in my talks with the female defenders of abortion, was how many of them seemed to view the abortion debate as some sort of referendum by which society judged women's deepest levels of self. Words like *guilt* and *sin, punishment* and *shame* kept issuing forth. They did so both about abortion and about sex in general. "The whole debate is more about the value of women's lives and the respect we have for women than it is about the act of abortion itself," said Kate Michelman, the head of the National Abortion Rights Action League.

A few days before my scheduled meeting with Michelman, I got a phone call from her press secretary. "We hear a nasty rumor," she said, "that you're writing something that says abortion is immoral." I mentioned the rumor when I sat down to speak with Michelman, who quickly told me about the very difficult circumstances surrounding her own abortion. Her first husband had walked out on her and her three small children when she was destitute, ill, and pregnant. She had to make a difficult moral judgment, she said, weighing her responsibilities to her family against

those to the fetus. Then, this being 1970, she couldn't even make the decision herself but had to obtain the consent of a panel of doctors and then, to further the pain, get her ex-husband's signature. Call me immoral, she seemed to say, in an I-dare-you way.

But it seemed to me that Michelman's decision, like those, certainly, of a great number of women, had involved a thoughtful handling of difficult questions —as she herself was underlining. "Sure the fetus has interests, absolutely," she said, as do other things, like a woman's commitments to her family and her health. It was only when I began asking why those leading the prochoice movement didn't discuss these moral tensions more often that her reasoning turned curious and defensive.

"The ethical questions are being raised," she said. "And if [a woman] makes a decision [to have an abortion] then she's made the right decision."

I asked her how she knew. With 1.6 million abortions a year, there seems to be a lot of room for error.

Merely asking the question, she said, implied that women had abortions for frivolous reasons. "To even raise the question of when it's immoral," she said, "is to say that women can't make moral decisions."

In considering the way a legacy of injustice fuels the adamance over abortion, it is helpful to consider three generations of women: those who preceded the feminist movement of the late sixties and early seventies; those who soldiered in it; and those who inherited its gains. Each has faced the tyranny of a man's world in a way that primes passions about abortion, but each has done so in a different way.

Women who became sexually active outside of marriage in the days of blanket abortion bans faced a world prepared to hand them the cruelest choice: the life-wrecking stigma of pregnancy out-of-wedlock or the back alley; a "ruined" life or a potentially lethal trip through a netherworld. Men, meanwhile, made the decisions that crafted that world while escaping the brunt of its cruelty. That *was* an unjust life, and the triumph over it is among feminism's proudest achievements....

ACCEPTING FEMALE SEXUALITY

... [W]hat's interesting about the observations of male irresponsibility [in casual sexual relationships], as it relates to abortion, is that both sides cite it. Prolife feminists, like Juli Loesch, argue that the acceptance of abortion actually *encourages* exploitation. The "hit and run" artist can pony up $200, send a woman off to a clinic, and imagine himself to have done the gallant thing. "The idea is that a man can use a woman, vacuum her out, and she's ready to be used again," Loesch says. "It's like a rent-a-car or something." (In such scenarios, Loesch argues, abortion has the same blame-the-victim effect that the Left is typically quick to condemn, with the victimized mother perpetrating the injustice through violence against the fetus.)

When I asked Katha Pollitt about this, she dismissed it with the argument that men will be just as irresponsible with or without abortion, and that the only difference will be the burden left to women. To some extent she's right: irresponsible sexual behavior—by men and women both—will no doubt continue under any imaginable scenario. Then again, it's not unreasonable to suspect that casual attitudes about abortion, particularly among men, could increase precisely the kind of "stallion" behavior that Pollitt rightly protests. And abortion can become a tool of male coercion in other ways as well. "He said that if I didn't have an abortion, the relationship would be over," a friend recently explained. Many women have experienced the same.

Of course, feminist emotion toward abortion isn't just a reaction to male sexuality but also an assertion that women's own sexual drive is equally legitimate. Feminists argue that antiabortion arguments reflect a larger cultural ambivalence, if not outright hostility, toward female sexuality. This is where words like *guilt* and *shame* and *punishment* continue to arise. I recently sat down with Katha Pollitt for a long conversation about abortion. She cited the many ways in which women (and the children antiabortionists want them to raise) are injured by society: poor health care, poor housing, economic discrimination, male abuse. We talked also about power, politics, religion, and the other forces that play into the abortion debate, like the unflagging responsibilities that come with parenthood. (She is a new, and proud, mother.) But when I asked her which, of the many justifications for abortion, she felt most deeply—what, in her mind, was the real core of the issue—her answer surprised me. "Deep down," she said, "what I believe is that children should not be a punishment for having sex."

Ellen Willis of the *Voice* advances a similar argument. Opposition to abortion, she's written, is cut of the same cloth as the more general "virginity fetishism, sexual guilt and panic and disgrace" foisted on women by a repressive society. The woman's fight for abortion without qualm, she says, is part of the fight for the "acceptance of the erotic impulse, and one's own erotic impulses, as fundamentally benign and necessary for human happiness."

Pollitt agreed. "The notion of female sexuality being expressed is something people have deeply contradictory feelings about," Pollitt said....

BIOLOGY AND DESTINY

What the argument for abortion-without-qualm comes down to is this: the fetus doesn't exist unless we want it to. But the whole crisis over abortion is that we know precisely the opposite to be true. It's there physically, feminists say, but not morally. But how could it be one without the other—there to nurture one day (remember, plenty of fresh vegetables, we're eating for three: you, baby, and placenta), but free to dismember the next? Qualm-less advocates argue that all that finally matters is whether the woman, for whatever reason, desires to bring it into the world. Yet the fetus is already there, no matter what we plan or desire. Forces may conspire against a woman and leave her *unable* to bring it into the world, or unable to do so without a great deal of harm to herself and others. That is, *other* moral obligations may overrule. But it is suspicious in the extreme to argue—as the qualmlessness position does—that our moral obligations are nothing more than what we want them to be, a wish-it-away view of the world. Inconveniently fetuses exist, quite outside our fluctuating emotions and desires.

Finally, Ellen Willis's argument that by giving fetuses any moral status at all we reduce women to vessels breaks down because women *are* vessels. They're not *just* vessels. They're much more than vessels. But the attempt to reconcile the just desire for full female autonomy with our moral obligations toward fetuses by insisting that we have none attempts to wish away a very real collision; it refuses to acknowledge a (so far) inalterable conflict buried in biology. Willis argues this is precisely the oppressive "biology equals destiny" argument that feminism has fought to overturn. Biology doesn't equal destiny; but it does affect destiny, and it leaves us with the extremely difficult fact that women, for any number of reasons, get burdened with unwanted pregnancies to which there are no easy moral solutions. Something important is lost—female autonomy or fetal life—in either event.

There are two highly imperfect ways of dealing with this conflict. The first is abstinence (since birth control fails). But not much chance of that. The second is adoption—another imperfect solution. The first argument against it is that there aren't enough parents to go around, particularly for minority and handicapped children. Ironically those quickest to point this out tend to be those for whom putting up a child for adoption really is a plausible option —white professionals. George Bush's "adoption not abortion" line brought quick ridicule by Pollitt in *The Nation* and Ehrenreich in *Mother Jones*. He's wrong to suggest it as a panacea— babies would quickly outstrip parents, as Pollitt insists—but right to encourage its wider use. The real challenge for liberals and progressives would be to turn the thought back toward Bush, and demand the governmental support, in health care and other ways, needed to get through pregnancy, and needed to raise a child.

The second argument against adoption focuses not on demand but supply: nine months of illness culminating in a "physiological crisis which is occasionally fatal and almost always excruciatingly painful," as Ehrenreich has written.... "It's almost unimaginable to me to think about giving up the baby," said Ehrenreich. "Talk about misery. Talk about 20 years of grief and ambivalence." The grief is real—particularly for people of conscience, like Ehrenreich. (And people of conscience are the targets of moral suasion in the first place.) But where does that argument lead? That in order to spare a child the risks of an adoptive life, we offer the kindness of a suction machine?

"A VERY SCARY TIME"

A few years ago, I was sharing an apartment with a friend who became pregnant just before breaking up with her fiance. Like many men... he just walked away, dealing with the dilemma through denial. My friend dealt with it with a lot of courage. I called her recently to see how the experience seemed in retrospect, and perhaps she should provide the coda, since her view complicates both Ehrenreich's position and my own. Though she said that putting her child up for adoption was "the right thing," she said she "would never, ever, pressure someone to go through the same thing."

It surprised me to hear her say that abortion "crossed my mind several thousand times," since that was the one option she had seemed to rule out from the start. When she realized she was pregnant, she said, she went riding her bicycle into potholes "trying to jar something loose. It was very, very easy for me to think of the sperm and the egg as having just joined. It was like a piece of mucous to me." She decided against abortion after about a week, "a very lonely, very scary time."

"At some point, I realized I was old enough, and mature enough, that I could do it [have the baby]," she said, but she emphasized that this calculus could have been altered easily by any number of factors—including less support from family and friends, a less understanding employer, or the lack of medical care. She spent months in counseling trying to decide whether to raise the child or put it up for adoption, and the decision to give the baby away "was the most difficult thing I've ever had to do." Since the baby was healthy and white the adoption market was on her side—"I could have dictated that I wanted two Finnish socialists," she said—and her certainty that the new parents would not only love the child but pass on certain shared values was an essential thing to know.

"When I think about her," she said, "just the miracle of being able to have brought her into this life, even if she's not here with me right now, she's with people who love her. It's a miracle."

"When she left to go to her adoptive parents, it was the most devastating and wonderful thing," she said. "I kept thinking this is my child, and I love her."

"It always kept coming back to that—I love her."

POSTSCRIPT

Can Abortion Be a Morally Acceptable Choice?

The abortion issue continues to be complex and polarizing. In 1983 and 1986 the Supreme Court reaffirmed its support of abortion rights. However, the Court has become more conservative and pro-life in recent years. With pressure and support from pro-life groups throughout the country, *Roe v. Wade* may continue to come before the Supreme Court for reconsideration.

The literature on abortion is often passionate and judgmental. Pro-life supporters often feel that in some cases, the ends justifies the means; see "The Right-to-Life Rampage," *The Progressive* (August 1993), by Operation Rescue founder, Randall Terry. Articles addressing the violence at clinics include "Abortion Case Verdict," *New York Times* (March 6, 1994) and "Bomb Squad," *Village Voice* (February 4, 1997).

Although there are literally thousands of articles and books addressing this issue, the following selections debate the moral concerns surrounding abortion: "Is There a Right To Die?" *Time Canada* (January 13, 1997); "A Dispatch from the Abortion Wars: Reflection on 'Common Ground,'" *America* (September 17, 1994); "Life Terms," *New Republic* (July 15, 1991); and "A Basic Human Right," *Ms* (August 1989).

Despite the increased violence at abortion clinics, the morality of abortion continues to be a central theme in many articles and books; see James Q. Wilson's "On Abortion," *Commentary* (January 1994). "Abortion and the Politics of Morality in the USA," *Parliamentary Affairs* (April 1994), discusses the role of abortion and the politics of morality in American life. "Killing Babies Isn't Always Wrong," *Spectator* (September 16, 1995), argues that in some circumstances, abortion is justified.

Whether or not legalized abortion has improved women's health is still the subject of controversy. Angela Bonavoglia claims that legal abortion saves women's lives in *The Choices We Made* (Random House, 1991). David C. Reardon, in *Aborted Women: Silent No More* (Loyola University Press, 1987), counters that the legalization of abortion has not improved the health of women.

Whether or not the opposing sides in the abortion issue will reach any common ground remains to be seen. Ernes van Der Haag in "Abortion: The Morality—Is There a Middle Ground?" *National Review* (December 22, 1989) and James R. Kelly in "A Dispatch from the Abortion Wars: Reflection on 'Common Ground,'" *America* (September 17, 1994), discuss this issue.

On the Internet . . .

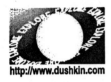

U.S. Environmental Protection Agency
The U.S. Environmental Protection Agency's home page is a useful site offering a comprehensive directory and a vast database. *http://www.epa.gov*

The Sierra Club
The Sierra Club's home page includes information on bird habitats, population growth, pesticides and the environment, and other related topics. *http://sierraclub.org*

Greenpeace International
Greenpeace offers multiple links to environmental issues, including global warming. The Antarctic warming link presents satellite photographs and maps of the northern Antarctic peninsula illustrate global warming effects. *http://www.greenpeace.org*

Council on Environmental Quality
Council on Environmental Quality offers databases and what's new on environmental issues. *http://ceq.eh.doe.gov/*

Nutrition Information Available on the World Wide Web
This is a great site for doing research on nutrition topics. It includes professional nutrition organizations, significant nutrition-related documents, journals, wellness newsletters, research resources, and even a link entitled "Desktop Resources," which offers the Merck Manual and the Periodic Table of the Elements. *http://weber.u.washington.edu/~kziemer/nutrlinks.html*

Food and Nutrition Information Center
The National Agricultural Library of the United States Department of Agriculture supplies publications and databases on topics such as foodborne illness, dietary guidelines for Americans, and a comprehensive index of food and nutrition information on the Internet. *http://www.nalusda.gov/fnic*

The American Society for Clinical Nutrition
The American Society for Clinical Nutrition page includes position papers and links to the National Institutes of Health. It also offers press releases. *http://www.faseb.org/ascn/*

PART 5

Environmental Issues

Many of today's environmental concerns are related to modern technology. Since World War II, thousands of new chemicals have been developed for the manufacturing and agricultural industries and for the military. But technological growth often has negative effects. Persian Gulf War veterans, for example, returned from the conflict claiming that environmental exposure to chemicals in the Persian Gulf have caused both minor and severe health problems in the soldiers. Energy needs have increased, resulting in the release of environmental pollutants, including the greenhouse gases. Also, as the world population continues to grow, how can food production keep pace without increased environmental degradation and exposure to toxic pesticides? This section discusses controversies related to environmental health issues.

■ Is the Gulf War Syndrome Real?

■ Is Pesticide Exposure Harmful to Human Health?

■ Public Policy and Health: Is Global Warming a Real Threat?

ISSUE 14

Is the Gulf War Syndrome Real?

YES: Dennis Bernstein and Thea Kelley, from "The Gulf War Comes Home: Sickness Spreads, But the Pentagon Denies All," *The Progressive* (March 1995)

NO: Michael Fumento, from "Gulf Lore Syndrome" *Reason* (March 1997)

ISSUE SUMMARY

YES: Journalists Dennis Bernstein and Thea Kelley claim that there are some four dozen disabling, sometimes life-threatening medical problems related to environmental and chemical exposure affecting thousands of soldiers who fought in the Persian Gulf War.

NO: Author Michael Fumento argues that Gulf War veterans are not suffering from illnesses at an extraordinary rate. They do not show evidence of more cancers, birth defects, and miscarriages than those who did not serve in the Persian Gulf.

Since Operation Desert Storm—the 1991 international effort to drive invading Iraqi forces out of Kuwait—more than 45,000 veterans out of the approximately 650,000 troops who served in the Persian Gulf War have complained of symptoms that have collectively become known as the Gulf War Syndrome. These symptoms include rashes, fatigue, headaches, vision problems, infections, joint and bone pain, birth defects in babies conceived after the war, and cancer.

The syndrome has been compared to the afflictions suffered by veterans of the Vietnam War. Unlike the health problems of the Vietnam veterans, however, the causes of the Gulf War veterans' varied symptoms are less clear. A number of entities are currently searching for an explanation. The American Legion claims that toxins from a long list of possible environmental origins —including fumes from burning oil wells and landfills, contact with hydrocarbons, pesticides sprayed over military vehicles, poor sanitary conditions, local parasites, inoculations, and insect bites—may be to blame. The U.S. government is exploring other causes, such as exposure to depleted uranium and the drug *pyridostigmine bromide*, an experimental pharmaceutical issued to soldiers to protect them against a possible nerve gas attack. The drug (as yet not approved for general use) was administered under a special waiver from the Food and Drug Administration, to be distributed with the informed consent of soldiers after the Department of Defense conducted its own research. Troops ordered to take the drug were reportedly never warned about its possible side effects. In addition, research on the drug was conducted only on men, so the drug's effects on women were unknown.

Another explanation being proposed is that veterans' health problems are the result of exposure to depleted uranium. Uranium was used to coat some artillery shells and tanks to protect them from enemy fire. On impact, however, depleted uranium releases radioactive particles of a related compound. The government claims that a relatively small number of personnel were exposed to this material and that none of them have shown any adverse symptoms. In Britain, allegations that the defence ministry is covering up evidence of Gulf War syndrome has created a political row. The Armed Forces minister in that country has admitted that troops were not properly advised of the dangers of radioactive contamination from depleted uranium shells. He has insisted, however, that there is no evidence of a link between serving in the Gulf War and veterans' subsequent health problems despite over 20 British war veterans who have been hospitalized with kidney and lung ailments typical of depleted uranium exposure.

There have been documented cases of illnesses among soldiers who served in the Gulf War, but less is known about the health of their families. One study conducted by outgoing Senator Donald Riegle found of 1,200 ill male veterans, 78 percent of their wives, 25 percent of children born to them before the war, and 65 percent born after suffered various illnesses and birth defects. Wives have reported bizarre symptoms concerning their husband's semen, which burns on contact. These women also complain of vaginal infections, cysts, bleeding sores, and blisters.

Despite widespread reports of health problems among Gulf War veterans, the Department of Veterans Affairs and the Pentagon insist that the symptoms are either psychological or due to chance. Major-General Ronald Blanck, commander of the Walter Reed Army Medical Center in Washington, D.C., in addressing Congress said, "Extensive evaluation and thorough epidemiological investigations have failed to show any commonality of exposure or unifying diagnosis to explain these symptoms." Many politicians, however, are fighting back and have vowed not to allow the Gulf War Syndrome to become another Vietnam-style denial by the government.

In the following selections, Dennis Bernstein and Thea Kelley argue that, although the Pentagon denies it, exposure to environmental and toxic substances in the Persian Gulf is responsible for illnesses experienced by thousands of veterans and their families. Michael Fumento counters that many illnesses suffered by Gulf War veterans have been attributed to the syndrome without sufficient evidence. He also claims there is no proof that any specific agent has caused physical sickness to soldiers or their families. Although Fumento admits that Gulf War veterans have more health complaints than the general population, he blames them on "current" traumatic stress disorders. He believes that the misinformation they are seeing in the media bombards them with the message that they *should* be sick.

YES

**Dennis Bernstein and
Thea Kelley**

THE GULF WAR COMES HOME:
SICKNESS SPREADS, BUT THE
PENTAGON DENIES ALL

The Persian Gulf War is not over. It drags on in the lives of tens of thousands of Gulf War veterans. Gulf War Syndrome, or Desert Fever as it is often called in Britain, is a set of some four dozen disabling, sometimes life-threatening medical conditions that afflict thousands of soldiers who fought in the war, as well as their offspring, their spouses, and medical professionals who treated them.

The symptoms suggest exposure to medical, chemical, or biological warfare agents, but the Pentagon denies such exposure occurred and claims it can't identify any common link among those who suffer from Gulf War Syndrome. Don Riegle, the recently retired Senator from Michigan who held hearings on the subject beginning in the fall of 1992, doesn't buy it. He believes the Pentagon may be engaged in a massive cover-up of this serious health problem.

The scale of the problem is enormous. More than 29,000 veterans in the United States with symptoms of Gulf War Syndrome have signed onto the Veterans Administration's Persian Gulf War Registry, 9,000 more have registered separately with the Pentagon, and the Pentagon's list is growing by 1,000 veterans a month.

"These are horrendous statistics that show the true scale of this problem," said Riegle last October when he released his final report on Gulf War Syndrome. Riegle condemned "the heartlessness and irresponsibility of a military bureaucracy that gives every sign of wanting to protect itself more than the health and well-being of our servicemen and women who actually go and fight our wars. To my mind, there is no more serious crime than an official military cover-up of facts that could prevent more effective diagnosis and treatment of sick U.S. veterans."

Birth defects are one of the most alarming problems associated with Gulf War Syndrome. One National Guard unit from Waynesboro, Mississippi, reported that of fifteen children conceived by veterans after the war, thirteen had birth defects. An informal survey of 600 afflicted veterans conducted by Senator Don Riegle's Banking, Housing, and Urban Affairs Committee last fall found that 65 percent of their babies were afflicted with dozens of medical problems, including severe birth defects.

Another disturbing phenomenon is the apparent transmission of the syndrome from soldiers to their family members. Riegle's study found that 77 percent of the wives of these veterans were also ill, as well as 25 percent of the children conceived before the war.

Riegle believes the Pentagon knows that U.S. veterans were exposed to chemical or biological weapons in the Gulf War. "The evidence available continues to mount that exposure to biological and chemical weapons is one cause of these illnesses," Riegle said. "I have evidence that despite repeated automatic denials by the Department of Defense, chemical weapons [were] found in the war." Riegle added that "laboratory findings from gas masks" showed the presence of biological warfare materials "that cause illnesses similar to Gulf War Syndrome."

The cover-up is not limited to the U.S. Government, however. Britain's Ministry of Defense is also being less than forthcoming. It has "a policy of denying Desert Fever for fear of big compensation claims," the British newspaper *Today* reported on October 10. A British Defense spokesperson told the paper, "We have no evidence that this illness exists." More than 1,000 out of the 43,000 British troops who served in the Persian Gulf have cited symptoms of Gulf War Syndrome.

＊ ＊ ＊

At 3 A.M. on January 19, 1991, Petty Officer Sterling Symms of the Naval Reserve Construction Battalion in Saudi Arabia awakened to a "real bad explosion" overhead. Alarms went off and everybody started running toward their bunkers, Symms said. A strong smell of ammonia pervaded the air. Symms said his eyes burned and his skin was stinging before he could don protective gear. Since that time, he has experienced fatigue, sore joints, running nose, a chronic severe rash, open sores, and strep infections. Symms and other soldiers described several such chemical attacks to Riegle's committee in May 1994.

One of the men interviewed by the committee who requested anonymity wrote home to his mother about the attack: "I can deal with getting shot at, because even if I got hit, I can be put back together—a missile, I can even accept that. But gas scares the hell out of me.... I know they detected a cloud of dusty mustard gas because I was there with them, but today everyone denies it. I was there when they radioed the other camps north of us and warned them of the cloud."

Front-line officers assured their troops that it was not a chemical attack, that what they heard was a sonic boom. "Members of Symms's unit were given orders not to discuss the incident," says Senator Riegle's report dated May 25, 1994.

Former U.S. Army Sergeant Randall L. Vallee served in the Persian Gulf as an advance scout. Vallee told Congress back in 1992 that he was convinced Iraqi Scud missiles were armed with chemical or biological warfare agents. "I was in numerous Scud missile attacks when I was in Dhahran," says Vallee. "It seemed like every time I was back there we'd come under fire."

Vallee has been afflicted by at least a half dozen serious medical conditions that started shortly after the Scud attacks. He had been in "perfect health" before his Gulf War service. Vallee supported what scores of veterans have already told Congress: that after every Scud attack, hundreds of alarms signaling chemical and biological attacks would sound, to the point where they were routinely shut off and reset as a matter of course.

Vallee and other members of his detail questioned their superiors about the alarms and about the presence of chemical-warfare agents in the Gulf. "After the whole ordeal was over, we asked about it and they said, 'No, the alarms are just acting that way because they're sensitive.' They gave us stories like, 'Oh, it's because of supersonic aircraft' or 'sand in the alarms.' There was always a story as to why the alarms sounded."

Last August, Vallee received a phone call from the Pentagon's Lieutenant Colonel Vicki Merriman, an aide to the Deputy Assistant Secretary of Defense for Chemical and Biological Matters.

"She asked me about my health and my family," says Vallee. But after some small talk, "the colonel's attitude turned from one of being concerned about my well-being to an interrogator trying to talk me out of my own experiences. She started using tactics of doubt regarding my statements. She said in regard to chemical and biological agents that there was absolutely no way that any soldiers in the Gulf were exposed to anything. Her exact words were, 'The only ones whining about problems are American troops, why aren't any of our allies?' And that was her exact word, 'whining.' "

* * *

British Gulf war vet Richard Turnball was surprised to hear Lieutenant Colonel Merriman's suggestion that only U.S. vets complained of Gulf War Syndrome. Turnball, who lives just outside Liverpool, served eighteen years in the British Royal Air Force. During the war against Iraq, Turnball built nuclear, biological, and chemical shelters, and instructed British troops in use of chemical monitoring and protective clothing. Turnball was based in Dhahran, Saudi Arabia.

Turnball is convinced there was widespread use of chemical-warfare agents. "People got sick in the chest and eyes, they got infections and skin rashes," he says. "One lad had his whole body covered with spots from head to toe" soon after a Scud attack that Turnball is convinced was chemical in nature.

"Within seconds of the warhead landing on January 20, every chemical-agent monitoring device in the area was blasting the alarm. We were put into the highest alert for twenty minutes," says Turnball, "and then we were told it was a false alarm caused by the fuel from aircraft taking off."

Corporal Turnball carried out two residual-vapor-detection tests for chemical and biological agents on January 20, shortly after the Scud hit "and both were positive," he says. Field supervisors dismissed the test results, claiming that jet fuel set off the indicators. Turnball was skeptical. "We tried on umpteen occasions, when aircraft were taking off in mass numbers," he says. "We stood on the side of the runway closer to the area where the aircraft were taking off, we carried out tests, and we got no readings."

At one point, Turnball says, he was warned to drop the case, and that if he kept it up he might be subject to secrecy laws under which he could be imprisoned. "I've had a very, very senior officer friend of mine ring me up and say, 'Richie, back off, you're kicking over a can of worms.'"

Before he went to war, Turnball said, he was in top condition, worked out every day, and was an avid scuba diver. Since his return, he has had twenty-four separate chest infections, and he has been forced to give up scuba diving because he "can't take the pressure below a few feet." Turnball can no longer run or swim or even take long walks. He said he has been put on steroids and uses two inhalers to help ease serious respiratory complications.

Turnball says the allies "used us as guinea pigs for new drugs" and chemical-weapons testing. He believes "probably both" chemical warfare agents and experimental drugs are responsible for his illness. "I feel we were subject to a chemical attack that affected us," he says. "As a serviceman, I can accept that, it's my job. But I believe more damage was done due to experimentation by our government. Many people got sick after taking some of the drugs. I came down with a high fever, I was sweating excessively. I actually stopped breathing a couple of times."

After three years of illness and fighting with the defense ministry, Turnball is still amazed by the denials that come out of the various bureaucracies. "We were always told that there was a 99.999 percent possibility of a chemical attack. We were expecting it. That was in our intelligence briefings. 'Inevitable' was the word used. And now they deny it."

* * *

Dr. Vivian Lane has never been to the Persian Gulf and is not a wife or mother of a Gulf War vet. The forty-three-year-old former squadron leader and former chief medical officer at the Royal Air Force base in Stafford, England, said she became seriously ill after treating a half dozen "very sick" British soldiers upon their return from the Persian Gulf. Dr. Lane says she was forced to move in with her elderly parents after she could no longer care for herself. Her parents, now in their eighties, are sick and suffering from lesions "very similar" to the ones she is suffering from, she says. "Nobody in this country can tell us why or what they are."

From December 1990 through June 1991 Dr. Lane treated at least six veterans who had the syndrome. Since that time, the aviation medical specialist, a former athlete, has been in great pain. She remembers waking up at four o'clock in the morning "with a terrific, excruciating, crushing type of chest pain and abdominal pain. When I got to the toilet, I didn't know whether to sit on it or stand over it. It just got worse from there. I managed somehow to get myself down to the medical center on base. All I remember was the excruciating chest pains. Next thing I know, I'm in intensive care. My parents had been brought to my bedside because everyone thought I was going to die. They didn't know what was wrong with me."

Dr. Lane offers a different angle on the hundreds of inoculations the soldiers were given before they left for the Persian Gulf. The protective shots were issued by the fistful, says Lane, and it's a wonder more people didn't have serious reactions. "With the amount we were banging into them, I'm surprised we didn't have more people falling over. We were attacking both arms, both buttocks, and their legs to get it all into them all at once. I think anybody with that amount of injections being shoved into them all within a couple of minutes of each other, would not feel terribly well."

Dr. Lane is one of several hundred former British soldiers suing the Ministry of Defense for medical redress. She says she is not holding her breath for results, though. "Frankly, I don't mean to be nasty, but I think they've bitten off more than they can chew."

Corporal Terry Walker was in the Persian Gulf from January to April 1991. Walker was a driver for the British Army's Fourth Armoured Brigade, First Armoured Division in Saudi Arabia. He has been sick ever since. He says his whole family suffers from Gulf War Syndrome.

In a recent interview, Walker described what he, too, believes was the Iraqi chemical Scud attack on January 20. "I was at the docks at Al-Jubayl about 2:30 in the morning," he said. "There was a couple of mighty bangs above our heads and suddenly all the chemical alarms went off and there were soldiers just running around in sheer panic, running around trying to get on their chemical suits." He says an "ammonia-like smell" filled the air after the sirens went off.

Walker, who had trouble getting his gas mask on, became ill soon after the Scuds hit. "I was feeling the burning sensation under the chin, around the back of the head as well. And ever since I've come back from the Gulf I've been ill." Walker suffers from chest infections, rashes, and headaches. Many of the people he served with were also sick after the attack, he says.

"As soon as the bangs happened, all these alarms went off and it was obvious that there was a chemical attack," says Walker, "but our superiors told us it was the jet fighters flying over with the sonic booms, and that it was also the fumes from the jets that set the alarms off."

"The thing is," says Walker, "they never went off before. The planes were flying day in and day out, and the alarms never went off at all, and on January 20, for about a ten-mile, fifteen-mile radius, these alarms went off."

Walker, who has since left the military, is furious with the military establishment in his country for "covering up what happened and the real risks" that would be faced by allied forces. "When they sent us out to fight the war, we expected them to look after us. Instead, when we came back they just tried to cover it up. They said there was nothing wrong at all because the general public would go against them if they found out about the exposures to chemical and biological warfare and how it gets into your whole family."

It is his family's illnesses that he objects to the most. "We knew there was a risk of being killed," he says, "but we didn't know that we would come back from the war so ill, and that our families would be getting sick, too. The wife has been ill since I've come back."

Walker's wife has had chronic abdominal pain and has been hospitalized at least seven times in the last three years. "She's been cut open twice but they couldn't find what was wrong," says Walker. The Walkers are extremely troubled about the health of their six-week-old child who has been plagued with a cold and respiratory problems "from day one."

* * *

Canadian legislator John O'Reilly recently raised the issue of Gulf War Syndrome in the House of Commons. O'Reilly asked the Defense Minister's Parliamentary Secretary, Fred Mifflin, what the government was doing to assist "deserving Canadians" who have been ill after serving in the Persian Gulf. Mifflin responded that the veterans had been cared for by Defense Department doctors and were experiencing "no difficulty whatsoever."

If Mifflin had spoken to Canadian Navy Lieutenant Louise Richard, he might have thought twice before painting such a rosy picture. Lieutenant Richard is an active-duty medical officer stationed at the National Defense Medical Center in Ottawa, the largest military hospital in Canada. Lieutenant Richard volunteered for service in the Persian Gulf as an operating-room nurse. She treated Americans, Britons, and Iraqi prisoners of war.

After eight years of commended service, Richard will be discharged from the Canadian Navy in September because of severe illness. She suffers from many of the same medical conditions afflicting some two dozen veterans interviewed for this article: severe respiratory problems, short-term memory loss, bronchitis, asthma, and pneumonia.

When Richard began to make a ruckus over her war-related illness and threatened to take it to the media, she ran into a stone wall of official denials and intimidation. "They've basically threatened me and said, 'It's all in your head, it's bullshit, don't go forward with it in the media.'" Richard says the threat from her medical superiors, whom she refuses to name for fear of further retribution, ran the gamut of intimidations. "It was the whole thing," says Richard, "your career, your pension—you know, the package."

She's frustrated at the lack of attention to the problem in Canada. "There doesn't seem to be anything happening since we're back," she says. "There's no research, no follow-up, there's nothing going on to help us." She said that she knows of many people in her position who have chosen to remain silent. "People fear to disclose anything because they don't want to ruin their pension or their career or whatever," she says. "I'm angry, because we were valued individuals when we were sent there, and now we're back, and we're not valued individuals at all. We're basically treated like mushrooms in a dark room."

* * *

Dr. Saleh Al-Harbi is an immunologist in Kuwait's Ministry of Public Health, and director of the immunogenetics unit of Kuwait University Medical Center. He says many people in Kuwait and Iran are suffering from what appear to be illnesses involving exposure to chemical and biological warfare agents.

"After the war we were getting diseases, respiratory diseases and unknown blood diseases such as leukemia, but not the typical kind, and for unknown reasons," he says. He is currently investigating with U.S. researchers the underlying causes of the medical conditions that have been plaguing Kuwaitis since the war. "Birth-related problems increased dramatically after liberation," he says, "and those kinds of cases have been reported to me."

He, too, is under pressure to keep a lid on his findings and concerns. "The authorities here are also standing with the Europeans' and Americans' point of view, but we believe that this is something political. I'm independent in mentioning this, and hopefully I will not get any threats from the superiors regarding this matter. They don't want the bad news and rumors to go around."

Dr. Al-Harbi characterizes the syndrome as a form of multiple chemical sensitivity, an explanation that is gaining favor in the United States as well.

Senator Riegle's report says that British and U.S. Army specialists, using sophisticated detection devices, made at least twenty tests that were positive for the presence of chemical-warfare agents. According to his report, "The Kuwaiti, U.S., and British governments all received reports on the discovery and recovery of bulk chemical agents."

Riegle's report also confirms than the alarms used in the war to warn troops of the presence of chemical warfare agents sounded thousands of times. In some cases, the report says, the alarms were sounding so frequently that they were simply turned off.

"The Defense Department told us at a hearing that they were all false alarms," says a former Riegle aide. "There were 14,000 of those chemical-alarm-monitoring units used during the war, and they're telling us that every time they went off, on all 14,000, they were false alarms. That's a little hard to believe."

According to a letter from Riegle to Veterans Affairs Secretary Jesse Brown, eighteen chemical, twelve biological, and four nuclear facilities in Iraq were bombed by the U.S.-led allied forces. Debris from the bombings was dispersed upwards into upper atmospheric currents, as shown by a U.S. satellite videotape obtained by Congress.

The Veterans Administration has only recently admitted that there is a problem with some "mystery illness" afflicting vets and their families. But the Pentagon denies there is any connection to chemical or biological warfare exposures.

In a May 25, 1994, "Memorandum for Persian Gulf Veterans," Defense Secretary William Perry and Joint Chiefs Chairman John Shalikashvili wrote:

"There have been reports in the press of the possibility that some of you were exposed to chemical or biological weapons agents. There is no information, classified or unclassified, that indicated that chemical or biological weapons were used in the Persian Gulf."

On June 23, 1994, the Defense Department's science board reported the results of an investigation into chemical and biological exposures in the Persian Gulf War. According to the report, "there is no evidence that either chemical or biological warfare was deployed at any level, or that there was any exposure of U.S. service members to chemical or biological warfare agents."

* * *

On December 13, 1994, the Pentagon released a report that says there was no single cause for Gulf War Syndrome. Veterans' groups were highly critical of this report. "It is more lies by the Pentagon to confuse and cover up the real causes of Gulf War Syndrome," says Major Richard Haines, president of Gulf Veterans International. In January, the Institute of Medicine of the National Academy of Sciences released a report critical of the Pentagon's research on Gulf War Syndrome.

Pentagon spokesman Dennis Boxx still maintains "we do not have any indication at this point that these things are transmittable to children or spouses."

Such declarations are consistent with the official British Ministry of Defense line. According to a July 14, 1994, letter from the Chemical and Biological Defense Establishment to the Pentagon's Lieutenant Colonel Vicki Merriman, "there was no evidence of any chemical warfare agent being present" in the Persian Gulf.

Ironically, when Senator Riegle first approached officials at the Department of Defense about veterans' possible exposures to chemical and biological warfare agents in the Persian Gulf, he was told by Walter Reed Army Medical Center commander Major General Ronald Blank that the issue was not even explored because "military intelligence maintained that such exposures never occurred."

While the Pentagon has refused to admit that chemical and biological warfare agents were present during the Gulf War, Senator Riegle stated on October 8, 1994, that "these Department of Defense explanations are inconsistent with the facts as related by the soldiers who were present, and with official government documents prepared by those who were present, and with experts who have examined the facts."

According to official Pentagon documents, at least eight members of the U.S. military who served in the Persian Gulf, in fact, received letters of commendation for locating and identifying chemical-warfare agents during the war. Army Captain Michael Johnson was awarded the Meritorious Service medal for overseeing the "positive identification of a suspected chemical agent." The certificate that accompanied Private First Class Allen Fisher's bronze star medal stated that his discoveries were the "first confirmed detection of chemical-agent contamination in the theater of operation."

In a memorandum dated January 4, 1994, to "Director, CATD," Captain Johnson of the Nuclear Biological and Chemical Branch of the Army wrote to his superiors: "Recent headlines have aroused considerable interest in the possible exposure of coalition forces to Iraqi chemical agents. Much of this interest is the result of health problems by Gulf War veterans that indicated exposure to chemical agents. Although no government officials have confirmed use, there is a high likelihood that some coalition forces experienced exposure to chemical agents."

Captain Johnson stated that he believed "coalition soldiers did experience exposure to Iraqi chemical agents." Johnson, who was commander of the 54th Chemical Troop, had cited in his report an example of a British soldier who was exposed. According to Johnson, "the soldier had an immediate reaction to the liquid contact. The soldier was in extreme pain and was going into shock." Captain Johnson first notified his superiors of his concerns in August 1991.

"This official dissembling and effort to obscure the facts are a continuation of Defense Department tactics," said Riegle in a written statement accompanying his October report. "The serious question remains as to why we were not provided with an official report dating from the time of the incident by the Department of Defense."

"If you look at the symptoms associated with biological and chemical contamination," says a former aide to Senator Riegle, "you'll see the same symptoms that are present in these veterans to varying degrees. The common denominator in all their illnesses is the breaking down of their immune system just as AIDS [acquired immunodeficiency syndrome] does, making them sicker and sicker as the days and years go by, and eventually incapacitating and killing some of them. And it's somehow being passed along to other people. We were getting hundreds of calls from people saying, 'He brought home this duffel bag, and we opened it up, and my eyes and hands started burning, and now I'm sick. What's wrong? What's happened?' "

NO

Michael Fumento

GULF LORE SYNDROME

"For Some, a Day of Betrayal," ran a headline in Denver's *Rocky Mountain News* the day before Veterans Day. A Persian Gulf vet said to be suffering the effects of the mysterious Gulf War Syndrome (GWS) was profiled, and the story by reporter Dick Foster contained a startling figure: "Cancers have developed in Gulf veterans at three to six times the rate among the general population." That news must have shot around Colorado faster than a Scud missile. Many vets probably spent their Veterans Day searching for lumps, bumps, sores, or anything else that might be a sign of cancer.

Three days later, a study appeared in *The New England Journal of Medicine.* Using the latest data available, it reported the cancer rate of Persian Gulf vets was slightly *below* that of comparable vets who didn't deploy to the Gulf, and far lower than that of the comparable civilian population.

Welcome to the world of Gulf Lore Syndrome. It is a world in which science is replaced by rumor, in which vets are presented as medical experts while real medical experts are ignored. It is a dimension in which authoritative review studies by eminent scientists are scorned and disdainfully labeled "Pentagon studies" because they reach the "wrong" conclusions—even if done by civilian organizations. Yet incredible accounts of such symptoms as skin-blistering semen and glowing vomit are taken as gospel. It is a "reality" constructed by crusading reporters, activists, demagogic congressmen, and, sadly, by Persian Gulf vets who have become convinced they are the victims of a conspiracy deeper and broader than anything on *The X-Files.* The sick vets live in this world of Gulf Lore Syndrome. Until reality is allowed to reach them, they will remain trapped in it.

I have been writing on GWS since 1993, and to the best of my knowledge I was the first writer to say that there is no Gulf War Syndrome in the accepted sense of the term. Since then, studies by some of the most prestigious scientists in the country have backed up that position. The early studies included two by the Department of Defense, one by the National Institutes of Health, and a preliminary report by the Institute of Medicine, an arm of the National Academy of Sciences. All said that the term *Gulf War Syndrome* was a misnomer. All said that the various theories of what might be making Persian

Gulf vets sick lacked any scientific basis. And every one of these studies' conclusions bounced off the reporters, the activists, and the sick vets like bullets off an M1 tank.

Some things *have* changed: When I began writing on the topic there were perhaps a hundred news reports about GWS; there are now over 4,000. Back then there were a few thousand Persian Gulf vets who claimed to have the illness; now, depending on who's counting, there are anywhere from 40,000 to more than 100,000. GWS studies continue to appear. The most recent include:

- The final report from the Institute of Medicine, which said in October that there is no "scientific evidence to date demonstrating adverse health consequences linked with [Gulf War] service other than [about 30] documented incidents of leishmaniasis [a parasitical disease caused, in this case, by sand fly bites], combat-related or injury-related mortality or morbidity, and increased risk of psychiatric [problems from] deployment."
- A draft copy of the final report of the Presidential Advisory Committee on Gulf War Veterans' Illnesses (commonly called the PAC), leaked in November to *The New York Times* and *The Washington Post*, which found "no support for the myriad theories proposed as causes of illnesses among Persian Gulf war veterans, or even evidence there is a 'Gulf War Syndrome,'" according to the *Post*.
- The article in the November 14 *New England Journal of Medicine*, which found that Persian Gulf vets had the same death rate from disease as non–Persian Gulf vets, and a much lower rate than the comparable civilian population. An accompanying article looked at hospitalizations, finding Persian Gulf vets and non-Persian Gulf vets hospitalized at the same rate.

Will these findings make any difference? Within days of the PAC draft report's release, President Clinton announced a doubling of the budget to investigate GWS. A few weeks later, he announced that the PAC final report would not be a final one after all, that he was going to keep the committee going albeit perhaps dumping some old members and assigning new ones. Rep. Chris Shays (R-Conn.) called two days of highly publicized hearings to denounce the government and parade one sick soldier after another to testify before his congressional panel, each claiming that his symptoms were beyond doubt the result of GWS. Apparently, science is still reaching the wrong conclusion.

MYTHS FIT TO PRINT

What pulled me back into the fray was the recent series of revelations concerning the demolition of bunkers at Khamisiyah, Iraq. The unit that blew up those bunkers was the 37th Engineer Battalion (Combat) (Airborne). In May, the Pentagon said U.N. inspectors had found that one of those bunkers and a nearby open pit contained Iraqi rockets marked to indicate a nerve gas called sarin. Thus, while the Pentagon could (and did) continue to say that there had been no offensive use of chemical weapons against U.S. troops, it was now clear that American soldiers had been close enough to exploding chemical weapons to be exposed to them. The 37th was my sister unit when I was in the 27th Engineers at Ft. Bragg, a decade earlier. I had lived in the same barracks and worn those same silver wings that mark the Army's proud elite, the paratrooper. I knew these soldiers in ways other reporters did not. What they would tell me in weeks of interviews taught me a great deal about GWS.

I interviewed eight of these men, beginning with former Pfc. Brian Martin. Martin is by far the most prominent 37th Engineer vet, having appeared on *60 Minutes* twice, on *Nightline, Geraldo, Montel Williams,* and *Tom Snyder,* and having been quoted by news wires, newspapers, and magazines, including the Associated Press, Gannett, *The Detroit News, Newsday, Playboy,* and one of a series of articles by *The New York Times*'s Philip Shenon. Martin, 33, is also co-president (with his wife) of International Advocacy for Gulf War Syndrome. Being a disabled vet is his life; indeed, his Web page lists his occupation as "disabled veteran," while his e-mail address is "dsveteran."

Martin is quick with a sound bite, such as, "I used to jump out of airplanes and now I can't even jump up and down." Sometimes he walks with a cane; other times he uses a wheelchair. We talked about our old brigade a bit. He explained to me the process of destroying the bunkers at Khamisiyah, and then I asked him to tell me about his symptoms. That was the first hint that something was seriously amiss about Pfc. Martin.

His long list of symptoms included such things as lupus—an autoimmune disease rarely found in men—and "early Alzheimer's." Sensationalist reporters just eat up things like this, but to a medical writer such symptoms were like flapping red flags.

Then *the* red flag unfurled. Martin told me what he would later tell a congressional panel headed by Shays on September 19, 1996. After returning from the Gulf, he told the panel, "during PT [physical training] I would vomit Chemlite-looking fluids every time I ran; an ambulance would pick me up, putting IVs in both arms, rushing me to Womack Community Hospital. This happened *every* morning after my return from the war." (Emphasis as noted in the official transcript.)

Chemlites are tubes that, when snapped, glow. In two conversations with me, Martin repeatedly referred to his vomit as being "fluorescent" and said these daily vomits lasted from "March 11 to December 31," 1991. Thus, we are dealing with a man who insists both that his vomit glows and that his NCOs and officers heartlessly insisted that he do physical training for 10 months, knowing that "every morning" he would end up in the hospital with IV tubes in his arms.

If Martin volunteered the vomiting story during both of my interviews with him, it's very likely he told it to every other reporter who interviewed him. Yet they all used Martin as a credible witness, omitting this peculiarity from their accounts.

There are two reporters that we know with certainty did this, because they attended the September 19 hearings and wrote about Martin's testimony. One was AP reporter Donna Abu-Nasr. I called her and asked why she didn't mention the glowing vomit remark. "I didn't notice it," she said. Did she think it impugned Martin's credibility? No, she said. "You have to remember he's been on talk shows, and they've written a lot about him." She then said, "Are you going to quote me?" I told her that was my job as a reporter, but I wouldn't if she insisted.

Not good enough. "I think that's very dishonest of you," she said, and hung up.

The other reporter who covered the hearing was John Hanchette at Gannett News Service, the chain that owns *USA Today.* Hanchette, a 1980 Pulitzer Prize winner, has probably written more articles on GWS—over 80—than any other single reporter, sometimes alone and sometimes with Norm Brewer. Given his reputation and sheer volume, he's certainly had a big impact on the perception of GWS. The titles of his stories show his slant: "Active-Duty Soldiers Tear into Pentagon Over Gulf Syndrome"; "Are Gulf Veterans Getting Needed Treatment?"; "Several Gulf Units Plagued by Unusually High Illness Rate"; "White House Panel: Pentagon Can't Be Trusted in Persian Gulf War Syndrome Probe"; "Persian Gulf Illnesses-the Lingering War"; "Gulf War Parents with Birth Defect Children: All They Want Are Answers."

In his coverage of Martin's testimony, Hanchette chopped Martin's symptom list down to nine, omitting the glowing vomit. Nor is that all he did.

Rather than merely attributing the laundry list of symptoms to Martin, Hanchette wrote that these symptoms were supported by "federal medical exams," making Martin's symptom list sound far more credible. But I had called Martin's doctors (with numbers Martin provided), and while Department of Veterans Affairs rules prohibit them from talking about any specific patient, I got around this by asking them if *any* of their patients had the various symptoms Martin claimed. Often, the answer was no. Some of the illnesses the doctors said they had not observed in any of their patients—such as lupus—were among those Hanchette listed as confirmed by

Martin's "federal medical exams." What exams could Hanchette possibly have been referring to?

I politely called Hanchette four times just to say I wanted to talk about his story. He didn't call back. I called twice more to say that I had reason to believe he had engaged in unethical conduct and that I wanted to give him a chance to respond. He still hasn't called back.

So I called Hanchette's editor, Jeffrey Stinson. In defending his reporter, Stinson noted twice that Hanchette was a Pulitzer winner, called my questions "a crock," and said he really couldn't comment further without seeing the relevant material. I faxed over Martin's testimony, Hanchette's write-up, and a list of questions. Stinson's response: "Our stuff is good; it's accurate. You're full of it, pal. Bye." Then he hung up....

SYNDROME OVER SCIENCE

To doctors, bizarre symptom claims like glowing vomit are a ready indicator that they are dealing with a patient suffering hysteria. "It's an old joke around ER; we ask if people's stools glow in the dark or if their hair hurts," Dr. Scott Kurtzman, assistant professor of surgery at the University of Connecticut School of Medicine, told me. But to the media, such symptoms are the makings of a great story. Kate McKenna's article, "The Curse of Desert Storm," in the March 1996 *Playboy*, didn't mention Brian Martin's vomit but said that he is "often confined to a wheelchair" because of "a *diarrhetic* condition that has damaged his spine." (Emphasis mine.) Perhaps the makers of Kaopectate should advertise that it may be effective in preventing spinal injury....

A key component of Gulf Lore Syndrome entails suspending the laws of science whenever necessary. Consider the first death widely attributed to GWS, that of Army Reservist Michael Adcock. Adcock died in 1992 at the age of 22 from what began as a lymphoma (cancer of the lymph glands) and then spread to the rest of his body. Without doubt he believed—as his mother Hester testified before Congress—that he had contracted the lymphoma from exposure to something in the Gulf. His last words, she said, were, "Mama, fight for me. Don't let this happen to another soldier." The congressmen listened solemnly, and the media faithfully reported the story. But Army Surgeon General spokeswoman Virginia Stephanakis told me that Adcock "had rectal bleeding [the first symptom of his lymphoma] six days after arriving, and the family blamed it on the Gulf." It is universally accepted by the medical community that lymphomas take years to develop, perhaps 10 or more years on average. Not months, not weeks, and certainly not days.

Likewise, former Navy Seabee (combat engineer) Reservist Nick Roberts claims to have contracted his lymphoma within weeks of what he claims was a nerve gas attack. Roberts is almost as popular with reporters as Brian Martin. The AP, *USA Today*, States News Service, *The Atlanta Journal and Constitution*, and *Esquire* in its cover story on GWS have all portrayed Roberts as a prototypical GWS victim, using such headlines as "Walking Wounded" and "Trail of Symptoms Suggests Chem-Arms." I've talked to Roberts, and I'm sure he's convinced of what he says. But his claim is a medical impossibility, and none of the stories about him bothered to make that clear.

Roberts appeared before Shays's committee on the same day as Martin, so I called Robert Newman, the Shays staffer who invited them both to testify. I asked Newman first about Martin's daily spewing of glowing vomit. "In the overall scheme of things," Newman told me, "that's got to be a minor point." Well, OK. What about Roberts's lymphoma? "Do you know how long it takes a lymphoma to develop?" I asked Newman. "It takes a long time to develop," Newman said. "So you're willing to concede that Roberts's lymphoma couldn't have had anything to do with exposure from something in the Gulf?" I asked. "I'm not going to concede anything," he said.

No, he certainly wasn't. It is part of the strategy of the lore spreaders that you never, ever admit that any vet's claims are incredible, or that even a single veteran anywhere might be suffering psychosomatic illness. Newman ended our conversation by saying, "You caught me at a bad time because I'm in another crisis. Call me tomorrow." I did, and several times after that. We never talked again.

It is bad enough that the media and Congress always treat Persian Gulf vets as experts in self-diagnosis, but they're even considered experts in diagnosing others. Roberts told a congressional panel in November 1993 that of the 33 members in his military reserve unit, 10 in addition to him have been diagnosed with lymphomas. Were that true it would probably be the most amazing cancer cluster in history. He also held up a list of what he said were 173 cancer-stricken Gulf veterans, and the media duly reported his comments. Yet five months later, an update of the Persian Gulf Registry showed only eight lymphomas out of all the Gulf vets in the country, with 38 cancers of all types.

There have been reports of mysterious illness clusters throughout the GWS scare. Vets or their spouses will call other vets, essentially doing their own epidemiological study. Often they conclude that they are suffering an abnormal amount of illness. They then contact the media, who publicize these "findings," gingerly referring to them as "unofficial investigations."

The Institute of Medicine looked at three such reports, including one involving Nick Roberts's reserve Seabee unit. In all three cases, the IOM found that, while the symptoms tended to be the same among the three groups, these were classic psychosomatic manifestations. The outbreak studies, said the IOM, "were not successful in demonstrating that these symptoms occurred at a higher rate among PGW [Persian Gulf War] veterans than among [other] PGW-era veterans, or that these symptoms could be linked to specific medical diagnoses or exposures."

The most famous of the self-diagnosed clusters occurred in Mississippi, involving alleged defects in the babies of vets. These reports added a whole new dimension to the disease. Among the heart-wrenching stories built around the "cluster" were "Gulf Syndrome Kills Babies," "A Town in Torment," and *Ladies Home Journal*'s "What's Wrong with Our Children?"

The basic story, as *Nightline*'s reporter told it, was, "In Waynesville, Mississippi, 13 of 15 babies born to returning members of a National Guard Unit were reported to have severe and often rare health problems." It didn't say the report was "prepared," as it were, by the parents themselves. The Mississippi Department of Health investigated the alleged cluster and found that of 54 births to returning Guardsmen in that state, both major and minor defects were well within the expected range. There were also no more premature or low-birth-weight children than would be expected.

Since then, several birth-defect and miscarriage studies have looked for exceptional rates among the offspring of Persian Gulf vets. They have found none. In addition, all live births to Persian Gulf vets are being tracked, with birth defect compared to those in the offspring of non-deployed soldiers. When last analyzed, the children of the Gulf War vets had the same percentage of birth defects as the children of the comparison soldiers.

But of all the media outlets that originally reported on the alleged Mississippi cluster, only CNN later told its audience of the state's report. So the "Town in Torment" remains a staple of Gulf Lore. Dr. Russell Tarver, who headed up the study, told me, "It's unconscionable to frighten people out of reproducing unless you have some good data to support that contention." He called it "a crime against those veterans." ...

POST GULF, ERGO PROPTER GULF

Much of what drives the GWS myth is the simplest of fallacies: that if something happens after a given event, it must have been caused by that event. The GWS fallacy works like this: The vets were obviously healthy when they went to the Gulf, or they wouldn't have been sent. Now they're sick. Therefore it must have been something in the Gulf that made them ill.

Appearing on *Nightline*, Sen. John D. (Jay) Rockefeller IV (D-W.Va.) invoked the fallacy repeatedly with such statements as: "They were totally healthy when they went over to the Persian Gulf. No problems whatsoever. They come back and all of the sudden their children are [born] defective, they can't have children, or they [the children] die."

So what happened to these vets? It depends not just on whom you ask, but what day you happened to ask them. Consider just the headlines from some of the stories authored or co-authored by Hanchette:

"Experimental Drugs on Gulf Troops Rapped by Panel"

"Key to Gulf War Syndrome May Be Flies"

"Doctor Says Gulf Illnesses Stem from Vaccines"

"CIA Document: Scud Fuel May Be Involved in Gulf War Illnesses"

"U.N. Intelligence Representatives Show Iraq Could Have Spread Deadly Aflatoxin"

Just can't make up our minds, can we? It's not uncommon for a vet or activist or reporter to insist that one thing is absolutely, definitely the cause of GWS, and later to insist that something else is absolutely, definitely the cause. Sometimes the media or activists will even use a sort of shotgun approach. *Nightline's* GWS show in October, which left no doubt that GWS was both real and spreading, first indicated the cause was nerve gas. That nerve gas symptoms couldn't possibly spread from person to person was apparently considered inconsequential. The *Nightline* reporter then proceeded to blame pyrodistigmine bromide (PB) pills the vets had taken. Then it was exposure to fumes from oil wells. Again, neither of these could possibly cause symptoms that are communicable, but that too seemed not to matter.

Vets and their families will often be influenced by these shifting fads, as in the case of Michael Adcock, the Persian Gulf vet who died of cancer. In May 1993, the fad cause of GWS was multiple chemical sensitivity, and that month Adcock's mother, Hester, told *The Washington Times*, "Beyond a shadow of a doubt, I believe Michael died of multiple chemical exposure" in the Gulf. She cited oil well fires, fresh paint on vehicles, and lead in the diesel fuel used in lanterns and heaters. Six months later the fad cause of GWS was nerve gas, and Mrs. Adcock testified before Congress, doubtless sincerely, that her son's disease was from nerve gas released by a Scud missile the day before his first symptom of lymphoma appeared.

Though the fads come and go, the main two so far have been PB and Iraqi chemical weapons. PB was given to many of the troops because of evidence from animal experimentation that it could provide some protection if they were hit by one type of nerve gas. A Nexis search shows no fewer than 175 stories implicating PB as a possible cause of GWS.

But the focus on PB has more to do with confusion over terms than with science. Time and again, the media have described PB using the fear-triggering word *experimental*. Hanchette and Brewer at Gannett did so in two different articles, calling it "unlicensed" in a third. The soldiers "had no idea they were taking an investigational drug," Ed Bradley told *60 Minutes* viewers, with a follow-up quote from a vet in combat fatigues saying, "We've been used as guinea pigs."

What virtually no one out there in media- and activist-land says is that PB was "experimental" or "investigational" only insofar as its ability to prevent illness from nerve agents went. The drug itself comes from a class of pharmaceuticals that has been in use since 1864. Far from being "unlicensed," it was licensed by the FDA in 1955 to treat a neuromuscular disease called myasthenia gravis. Moreover, the dose given to myasthenia gravis patients ranges from 360 to 6,000 milligrams daily. In contrast, U.S. soldiers in the Gulf were given a one-week supply of PB, with three 30-milligram pills to be taken daily.

This is why both the NIH and IOM panels rejected out of hand the notion that PB could be causing illness among Persian Gulf vets, with the NIH saying that even at the massive doses taken by the myasthenia gravis sufferers, PB has shown "no significant long-term effects." Yet one newspaper, in attributing the ills of Persian Gulf vet Carol Picou to the PB pills, went so far as to tell its readers that PB has never even been tested on women and was only the subject of a single test on men.

The second main culprit, nerve gas, has become a popular GWS suspect for reasons more psychological than scientific. "Chemical weapons are not useful as tactical weapons," FDA specialist Peter Procter told a wire service reporter during the 1990 Gulf buildup. Only 3 percent of Iranians gassed during the Iran-Iraq war died. It was hardly because Hitler was a humanitarian that he refrained from using sarin, the new nerve gas his scientists had invented, but rather because his experts convinced him that the old-fashioned high explosive shells and rockets were far more effective. But the received wisdom among American civilians, soldiers, reporters, and even government officials is that chemical weapons are incredibly efficient killing machines, so much so that they

are regularly lumped into the category "weapons of mass destruction," alongside hydrogen bombs.

Such weapons are mostly effective "as weapons of terrorism," the FDA's Proctor said six years ago. "The greatest fear among the soldiers on the line," wrote one reporter shortly before the Persian Gulf ground war began, "is the likelihood that the enemy artillery will be firing rounds of mustard gas and nerve gas. Thus, it's only natural that Gulf War vets seeking a cause for their symptoms would convince themselves that they must have been gassed.

But there are many problems with the gassing scenario. One is that, as the October IOM report stated, "there are no confirmed reports of clinical manifestations of acute nerve agent exposure." True, some vets are *now* claiming they remember being gassed, but not one of them reported to clinics then.

Chemical alarms went off constantly during the war, supposed evidence of gas attacks. But chemical alarms are made to be hypersensitive, for obvious reasons. Even a "confirmed" gas detection doesn't necessarily indicate the presence of gas; it's just a more specific test than the initial one....

That's it. Readers could conclude that GWS resulted from multiple chemical attacks, or a combination of such attacks and drugs. In fact, a [New York] Times reader could conclude anything or nothing about what the IOM had really said.

MEDICINE AND 'MIRACLES'

Journalists aren't the only ones feeding the vets good stories that don't quite add up. Dr. Howard Urnovitz is one doctor beloved by vets who believe they have

GWS. Last year he said his discovery of a mystery virus in Persian Gulf vets explains how, "Like rubella, it is being passed on as a virus and can, we believe, explain the birth defects in children of the veterans."

Urnovitz is not, however, a disinterested scientist. Although he may believe what he's saying, he also appears to be appealing to the vets' fears to raise money for his biotech company, Calypte Biomedical of Berkeley, California. After all, as Calypte's Web page (ChronicIllnet) informs readers, "ChronicIllnet feels that much of the current breakthroughs in understanding IMMUNE SYSTEM IMBALANCE SYNDROMES, such as cancer, will come from the MIRACLES occurring with the new treatments being explored in Persian Gulf War related illnesses." (Emphasis theirs.)

No responsible physician would use the term *miracle* to describe his treatments; that's huckster terminology. As it happens, *miracle* is a hypertext link. If you click on it, the link takes you to a story about a Gulf vet who claims that his GWS symptoms were cured by doxycycline. Somehow a general-purpose antibiotic developed in 1966 doesn't seem like the sort of thing that will lead to a cure for cancer.

But it's not just cancer that these "miracle" cures will finish off. "If we can find a cure for Gulf War Syndrome," Urnovitz said at a 1996 symposium in Denver, "we'll be able to cure cancer and AIDS and chronic fatigue syndrome and other immune system disorders. They're all linked together." Maybe that cure will start your car on a cold winter morning, too.

Another doctor who is revered by sick Persian Gulf vets and has testified before the Presidential Advisory Committee is Garth Nicolson. Nicolson is a highly regarded cancer researcher who says he and his wife Nancy, a molecular biophysicist, left the M. D. Anderson Cancer Center in Houston to pursue a cure for GWS after his stepdaughter, a Gulf War vet, fell ill.

Like Urnovitz, the Nicolsons claim great success with doxycycline. Unlike Urnovitz, the Nicolsons blame not a virus but a bacterium, specifically mycoplasma fermentans (MF). They claim that using a special form of the polymerase chain-reaction (PCR) test, they have detected MF in about half of the vets with GWS symptoms. With PCR you take some blood from a person and use a chemical procedure to enlarge parts of the DNA of an organism (such as MF) that you think might be in the blood. If you use the chemical that would enlarge the DNA of MF and it works, then you know the MF is there. If the chemical doesn't enlarge it, you don't have MF. So far, so good.

But the same sensitivity that makes PCR a useful tool in finding what's in blood also makes it liable to find what's not there. Improperly cleaned and sterilized equipment will have all sorts of DNA strands on it that didn't come from the blood of the specified patient. In the most famous case of PCR contamination, Dr. David Ho—recently named *Time*'s "Man of the Year" for his promising work on AIDS—published a study in the mid-'80s which, using PCR, detected the AIDS virus in numerous people who had tested negative in the standard blood test. It was a frightening result, but no one could duplicate his findings and Ho was forced to admit that his testing must have suffered contamination.

As with Ho's results, other doctors are finding they cannot duplicate Nicolson's PCR work on MF. This includes the man universally acknowledged as the leading expert on MF, Dr. Shyh-Ching Lo of the Armed Forces Institute of Pathology. "We've never found one" Persian Gulf vet with the bacterium, says Lo. "The Nicolsons claim their technique is different," allegedly using "a special form of PCR that's more sensitive," says Lo. Specifically, they claim their test can better find MF when it's hiding in the nucleus of the cell only. Lo says that's possible, "but we never truly get the detail of how [the Nicolsons] process PCR. They just give us the statements of their results." In late December [1996], Garth Nicolson announced that he will divulge his testing technique, but he had not done so at this writing.

I asked Nicolson if there were any scientists who had duplicated his work. He named only one, Aristo Vojdani, himself a GWS advocate and doctor who specializes in multiple chemical sensitivity. MCS is an alleged ailment that mainstream organizations, such as the American Medical Association, find questionable, if not outright nonsense. Vojdani is also now among the shrinking number of researchers claiming that silicone breast implants are harmful.

The other way of judging the merit of the Nicolsons' PCR work would be to see where it has been published. One National Institutes of Health MF expert, who asked not to be identified, conceded that Nicolson had indeed published in this area, but only in "garbage journals." Indeed, of the seven pieces Nicolson sent me, six were in journals that specialize in MCS or related fields. The seventh was in *The Journal of the American Medical Association*—but it was only an unrefereed letter to the editor.

None of which conclusively proves that the Nicolsons' research is invalid.

But even if their unique test does detect MF, it may have no connection to Gulf War Syndrome. For one, nobody knows how many perfectly healthy people carry around MF in their bodies, just as we carry around myriad types of benign and even helpful bacteria. More important, medical science so far has identified MF as a probable cause of just one health problem, rheumatoid arthritis. There is also some evidence it may be involved in acute respiratory problems. Sure, some Gulf vets have complained of aching joints and others of breathing troubles. But what of the 100-plus other problems they claim?

Further, the very idea of MF as a biological weapon, as the Nicolsons claim it was, is ludicrous. The purpose of biological weapons is to cripple, kill, and terrorize on the battlefield—not to cause aching joints in vets years later.

Nor does it help the Nicolsons' credibility that they suggest they are targets of a conspiracy because their work threatens the GWS coverup. Garth told the *Houston Press*, an alternative weekly, that while he and his wife were at M. D. Anderson, their faxes and letters were repeatedly intercepted, and their phone had been tapped so many times that "it was a record." Nancy also claims there have been six attempts on her life, but "assassins told her they saw her face and just couldn't pull the trigger." ...

THE MYSTERY SOLVED

Of the many reasons the media perpetuate Gulf Lore Syndrome, one is that reporters—and readers—love a mystery. Indeed, a Nexis search in November found 630 stories referring to the "mystery" of GWS. The allure of a mystery is often such that it refuses to die no matter how much light is shone on it. So it is with GWS. But there is no mystery.

Why are there so many sick Persian Gulf vets? First, because there are so many Persian Gulf vets, period. Take 697,000 vets, add their spouses and children, and you have a pool of well over a million people. In such a pool you're going to have every illness in the book. Because modern medicine is not an exact science, you're also going to have a certain number of illnesses for which no firm cause is identified.

"Among approximately 697,000 people over a period of several years, there will be poorly understood ailments and a number of obscure diseases," as the October IOM report put it. The question is, Are Gulf War vets having these illnesses at an extraordinary rate? The flat answer is: no—no more deaths (except vehicle accidents), no more cancers, no more birth defects, no more miscarriages. Persian Gulf vets have these problems because everybody has these problems. The difference is the media have convinced them that a neighbor's miscarriage is just a miscarriage, but *their* miscarriage is GWS.

Indeed, for all the talk of the "commonality" of symptoms of GWS, I have compiled a list of over 100, including hair loss, graying hair, weight gain, weight loss, irritability, heartburn, rashes, sore throat, kidney stones, sore gums, constipation, sneezing, leg cramps, insomnia, herpes, and "a foot fungus that will not go away." It is no exaggeration to say that every ailment any Persian Gulf vet has ever gotten —or that anybody has ever gotten—has been labeled a symptom of GWS.

According to Dr. Edward Young, former chief of staff at the Houston VA Medical Center, one of the three centers set up to investigate ailments among Gulf War vets, "We're talking about people who have multiple complaints. And if you go out on the street in any city in this country, you'll find people who have exactly the same things, and they've never been to the Gulf." In an interview with the *Birmingham Daily News*, he said, "It really rankles me when people stand up and call it 'Persian Gulf Syndrome.' To honor this thing with some name is ridiculous." Although Young later asked that the comments not be printed, the American Legion, the most powerful GWS lobbying group, got hold of them and complained to the VA. The VA unceremoniously yanked Young from his position, later citing his lack of compassion. As Shays staffer Robert Newman told me, "Nobody wants to go against vets; it's a very strong lobby." Amen.

Yet it's an oversimplification to say that vets are having exactly the same symptoms as anybody else. They appear to suffer more from illnesses commonly associated with stress—that is, psychosomatic ones.

Doctors have long understood that one can induce symptoms in many people by giving them reasons they *should* feel sick. David Murray, now with the Statistical Assessment Service in Washington, D.C., used to demonstrate this by telling his social anthropology students they might have suffered minor food poisoning at lunch and that, if so, they should go to the nurse's office. "Within five minutes there would be shifting of seats and belching and one or two people would walk out the door," says Murray. "Eventually a third of the class would have left or be complaining of illness."

Nothing enrages activists—or many sick vets—like suggesting that Gulf War vets are suffering psychosomatic illness. Responding to the Presidential Advisory Commission's conclusion, Denise Nichols told *The New York Times,* "I am appalled that after five years [the government] is still busy denying physical damage... this is not stress."

But "psychosomatic" does not refers to the symptom; it refers to its origin. You can get diarrhea because you're worried about tomorrow's final exam or because you ate a week-old taco. In the first case it is psychosomatic; in the second it is organic, meaning it came from some source other than stress. In either case, you're sick. Telling someone their symptoms are probably psychosomatic isn't an insult; it's just an explanation. Nor is there anything exotic about it; stress-induced symptoms—often more severe than organic ones—have been experienced by nearly everyone.

What is the source of this GWS stress? That has been muddled by the misapplication of the term, *post-traumatic stress disorder* (PTSD), coined to explain psychological (including psychosomatic) problems of Vietnam vets who had trouble adjusting to civilian life. *Nightline,* in October, said GWS couldn't possibly be PTSD because this wouldn't explain why vets' wives were sick.

Exactly right. What the vets and their wives are suffering is what I call *current traumatic stress disorder.* It isn't their experience in the Gulf that is haunting them, but rather what they're seeing on *Nightline* and other TV shows, what they're reading in the papers, what they're hearing from congressional demagogues and from activists, and finally what they hear from their fellow vets in conversations and Internet chatter. The Gulf War vets are sick for the same reason Murray's students became sick. They are bombarded with the message that they *ought* to be sick.

EPIDEMIC HYSTERIA

Medical historian Edward Shorter of the University of Toronto calls related cases of psychosomatic illness "epidemic hysteria." As a historian, he finds the GWS phenomenon tragic yet "fascinating." Says Shorter, "Just as cholera is spread by water droplets, epidemic hysteria is spread by the media."

In his 1992 book on epidemic hysteria, *From Paralysis to Fatigue,* Shorter recounts the similar history of a 19th-century syndrome called "spinal irritation," originally diagnosed by a handful of British doctors. Once informed they had this mysterious ailment, the patients, usually young women, would present an often bizarre array of symptoms, including temporary blindness, paralysis (of the sort Brian Martin appears to suffer), constant vomiting, dribbling saliva, and painful menstruation. Doctors used a wide array of treatments, including leeching, putting caustic agents on the skin, and applying magnets. "The more convincing and resolute the treatment," wrote Shorter, "the greater the success in cases of psychosomatic illness." "Spinal irritation" eventually spread to the United States, where it continued to afflict Americans for decades.

In November, the CDC announced that a study to be published in 1997 showed that Gulf vets from a Pennsylvania National Guard unit were three times more likely than comparable troops who didn't deploy to the Gulf to complain of such symptoms as chronic diarrhea, joint pain, skin rashes, fatigue, and memory loss. "This is absolutely a breakthrough study," said Matt Puglisi, an official with the American Legion. "For those who were more skeptical" than the Legion, he said, "and wanted scientific proof, now we've got it." *The New York Times*'s Shenon also played the story this way, in several articles with titles like, "The Numbers Support Gulf War Syndrome Claims." But this was far from the smoking gun GWS activists were hoping for and claimed to have found. All of these are classic psychosomatic symptoms. Combined with studies showing the Gulf vets have no higher rates of things not generally related to psychosomatic illness, such as cancer and death, the symptoms are actually further evidence that GWS reflects epidemic hysteria. Lost in the fuss over the CDC study was the statement from one of the authors to the Associated Press that "we have found there is nothing unique to the Persian Gulf, other than having gone there."

The GWS epidemic appears to have begun in mid-1992 as true PTSD among reservists who had such complaints as "hair loss, joint aches, severe bad breath, and fatigue." As reservists they were not as psychologically prepared to fight as were the active-duty soldiers; moreover, the reservists had to return to civilian jobs almost as if nothing had happened. At that point *USA Today*—the same newspaper that launched what proved to be the phony black church-burning epidemic of 1996—went into action, dubbing the symptoms "Gulf War Syndrome" and broadcasting them throughout the country.

A study of reservists found no extraordinary health problems, just illnesses attributed to stress. But Gulf Lore Syndrome was up and running. That's when the active-duty soldiers began to fall ill. By late 1993, CNN and others were seizing upon the alleged Mississippi birth defect cluster to say that GWS could be inherited. Gulf Lore Syndrome now included children.

By early 1994 some vets were linking their spouses' illnesses—including such things as irregular menstruation—to GWS. The media ran headlines like, "Gulf War Syndrome Spreading to Veterans' Families," and suddenly complaints about GWS symptoms began increasing among vets' wives. By late 1996 GWS had reached a point where people were contracting it from *objects* that had been in the Gulf. *Nightline* said Brian Martin's daughter got it from his military gear. CNN did a spot in November about a woman who contracted it from an Army surplus duffel bag.

For a year and a half, GWS remained strictly an American problem. By December 1993, however, *The Guardian* was reporting British cases. Eventually, GWS crossed to the continent. In a February 1996 article, Hanchette and Brewer began, "As recently as 15 months ago, asking the military about [GWS] often triggered this response: If there really is a sickness emanating from that war, why are our allies free of all symptoms?" To which the Gannett reporters responded: "Not any more. Well, here's a question for Hanchette and Brewer. Pick your favorite cause of GWS—chemical weapons, Scud fuel, sand flies, MCS—and explain why it would affect Americans three years before hitting soldiers in other countries.

"It's absolutely unmistakable" that "the symptoms are thoroughly psychosomatic," Shorter says. "The syndrome has no scientific status. It's entirely driven by political needs and the media's needs for sensationalism."

That's not entirely fair. Reporters like John Hanchette and Ed Bradley have probably convinced themselves they're doing vets a favor. They're not. Nor are the demagogic congressmen or the angry activists. You don't do people a favor by terrorizing them over their own health and that of their spouses and children. You don't do people a favor by replacing science with nonsense and reality with rumors.

It's been almost six years since the men and women who served us honorably in the Gulf War survived assault. They're still under assault, only now their enemy is more insidious, and, judging from the fear I saw in them, more successful.

POSTSCRIPT

Is the Gulf War Syndrome Real?

In *Hystories: Hysterical Epidemics and Modern Media* (Columbia University Press, 1997), author Elaine Showalter places the Gulf War Syndrome in the same category as tales of alien abduction and abuse by satanic cults; in other words, hysterias. She claims that stress is capable of causing genuine illnesses, but people feel shameful about sickness with an emotional or psychological cause. Instead, they search for another explanation such as the chemical weapons that produce anxiety attacks. Not everyone agrees with Showalter; see "Walking Wounded," *Esquire* (May 1994).

The U.S. government, however, has tried to deny ill veterans disability pay because it maintains that there is no proof that these illnesses are connected with service in the gulf. Articles that question the legitimacy of the syndrome include "Research Is Incomplete and Inadequate," *Chemistry and Industry* (January 16, 1995); "Pentagon Study Finds No Clinical Evidence for a Single Cause of Gulf War Syndrome," *Chemical and Engineering News* (December 19, 1994); and "Gulf War Syndrome: Is It a Real Disease?" *New York Times* (November 23, 1993). In "The Truth About Health Scares," *Health Confidential* (May 1993), Michael Fumento discusses several media-hyped environmental causes of death.

Many people feel that the government's denial of any relationship between environmental factors present in the Persian Gulf and subsequent health concerns among Gulf War veterans is similar to the government's original denial of the adverse effects of Agent Orange on Vietnam veterans. See "Congress Cites Agent Orange Coverup," *Science* (August 31, 1990).

Other articles calling for more and better research into the Gulf War Syndrome and Agent Orange include "Darkness at Noon," *Economist* (January 11, 1997); "The Gulf War Syndrome," *British Medical Journal* (vol. 310, 1995); "Institute of Medicine Calls for Coordinated Studies of Gulf War Veterans' Health Complaints," *Journal of the American Medical Association* (February 8, 1995); "The Persian Gulf Experience and Health," *Journal of the American Medical Association* (August 3, 1994); "Push for Gulf Syndrome Research," *Nature* (August 19, 1993); and "U.S. Congress Urged to Back Further Agent Orange Studies," *Nature* (July 29, 1993).

Readings that support the existence of the Gulf War Syndrome include "A Lingering Sickness," *The Nation* (January 23, 1995) and "Mal de Guerre," *The Nation* (March 7, 1994). Although the final word is not out on whether or not troops who served in the Persian Gulf War were exposed to environmental agents that triggered illnesses, many Americans are concerned that a Vietnam-style cover-up of the cause of these illnesses may exist.

ISSUE 15

Is Pesticide Exposure Harmful to Human Health?

YES: Martha Honey, from "Pesticides: Nowhere to Hide," *Ms.* (July/August 1995)

NO: Bruce Ames, from "Too Much Fuss About Pesticides," *Consumers' Research* (April 1990)

ISSUE SUMMARY

YES: Martha Honey, research fellow at the Institute for Policy Studies, claims that pesticides in the food chain are building up in animals and humans and are disrupting the immune system, causing cancers, and birth defects.

NO: Professor of biochemistry and molecular biology Bruce Ames argues that any risks from pesticides in foods are minimal and that fears are greatly exaggerated.

Throughout history, farmers and other food growers have fought with insect and weed pests that invade the food supply and cause disease and discomfort. Early attempts to reduce pest damage included purely physical attacks—burning and stepping on the pests—as well as saying prayers and performing ritual dances. A few more effective measures were discovered before modern times. These included sulfur compounds, plant extracts, wood ashes, and natural pest enemies.

For the past 50 years, the battle against pests has escalated, and some of the most lethal and sophisticated chemicals ever invented have been used against them. When modern pesticides, such as DDT, were first introduced in the late 1940s, scientists proclaimed total victory against crop destruction and diseases carried by insects. Many dispute this victory, but the evidence of these chemical weapons is present in streams, rivers, and soils—and in our bodies. Most of us carry traces of several chemical pesticides in our body tissues. Moreover, although pesticides are used specifically to kill insect pests, many of them are quite toxic to humans as well. Pesticides are responsible for an estimated 25 million human poisonings each year, mostly of children under 10.

To cause harm to humans, a pesticide must be taken internally through the mouth, skin, or respiratory system. Eating unwashed fruit or vegetables that were recently sprayed with pesticides or entering a field too soon after pesticide application are ways in which pesticides may enter the body. Symptoms of acute or one-time exposure include headache, fatigue, abdominal pain, coma, and death. Long-term exposure may cause cancer, mutations, or birth defects.

Pesticide poisoning from sprayed fruit and vegetables became a national issue when reports of the contamination of apple crops made headlines. Since 1968 some red varieties of apples have been sprayed with a chemical growth regulator that prevents the apples from dropping off trees before they ripen, improves color and firmness, and extends shelf life. The chemical, known as daminozide, is marketed under the trade name Alar. Alar penetrates the pulp of the apple and cannot be washed, cooked, or peeled off. In 1986 processors and stores in the United States, bowing to consumer pressure, vowed not to accept apples treated with the chemical. It was reported that a breakdown product of Alar, which is formed when treated apples are heated, is a low-level cancer-causing agent.

A report released in the spring of 1987 by the National Academy of Sciences claimed that pesticides may be responsible for as many as 20,000 cases of cancer a year. In their report, the academy identified 15 foods (tomatoes, beef, potatoes, oranges, lettuce, peaches, pork, wheat, soybeans, beans, carrots, chicken, corn, grapes, and apples) treated with a small group of pesticides that pose the greatest risk of cancer. Although these figures are certainly frightening, many scientists believe that too much fuss is being raised about pesticides. They point out that many foods contain natural cancer-causing agents, and they argue that people are still better off with a high intake of fruits and vegetables—ironically because they contain nutrients that may help prevent cancer.

In the following selections, Martha Honey contends that a lot of the food that is sold in supermarkets is not safe and that the government does not adequately test the fruit and vegetables that are sold to the public. Bruce Ames maintains that it is good for consumers to be concerned about what they eat, but the hysteria about pesticide residues may not be warranted by the actual risk they pose.

YES
Martha Honey

PESTICIDES: NOWHERE TO HIDE

Walk into almost any supermarket these days, any month of the year, and feast your eyes: towering pyramids of grapefruit, baskets of unblemished tomatoes and cucumbers, heaping bins of avocados and kiwifruit, stacks of ripened strawberries. Nowadays, the health-conscious U.S. consumer, transcending the inconveniences of the season, is serviced 12 months of the year by fruit and vegetable growers the world over. But if you're concerned that the produce section at your local market has come to resemble a wax museum, you have good reason. The abundance and variety of fresh, picture-perfect produce is brought to you and your family at a price—and not just at the cash register.

More than 30 years have passed since Rachel Carson called world attention to the health and environmental hazards of DDT and other pesticides in her landmark book, *Silent Spring*. "If we are going to live so intimately with these chemicals—eating and drinking them, taking them into the very marrow of our bones," Carson wrote, "we had better know something about their nature and their power." There is now ample proof that Carson's early warning was well founded: at least 136 active ingredients in pesticides have been found to cause cancer in humans or animals. But global pesticide use continues to escalate as farmers and food companies look for increasingly efficient methods to expand their markets. While Carson's book paved the way for the creation of the Environmental Protection Agency (EPA) in 1970, government efforts to protect the nation's food and water supply have moved at a snail's pace—of the 136 aforementioned carcinogenic chemicals, 79 are still being used on U.S. food crops. And the few, hard-won legislative gains that have been made by consumer, labor, and environmental advocates are currently being torpedoed in the Republican-controlled Congress.

The U.S. is one of the world's largest users of pesticides, and it's the top exporter. Sales in the U.S. total close to $8 billion. With annual overseas sales of $2.4 billion, or 44 billion pounds of chemicals, U.S. companies export more than 25 tons of pesticides *every hour*. In what has been dubbed the "circle of poison," at least one third of the pesticides exported have been banned or limited for use in this country—but they often return to consumers as residue on imported produce. While the U.S. imports only 9 percent of its vegetables, more than a quarter of the fruit sold here is imported; in winter, 40 to 60 percent of produce comes from abroad.

In the mid-1980s, the U.S. government made a major push to get many Latin American and Caribbean countries to grow new "designer" crops—strawberries, melons, and asparagus—all intended for the U.S. market and most, as they are not native to the region, heavily dependent on chemical fertilizers and pesticides. As a result, Latin America leads the Southern Hemisphere in pesticide use per acre and it supplies nearly 80 percent of U.S. fruit and vegetable imports. Not surprisingly, U.S. agricultural experts in Costa Rica, who conducted a survey of pesticide residues on strawberries in the late 1980s, refused to release their results. "But I can tell you one thing," confided one official involved in the study. "I won't eat the strawberries."

But while consumers are subject to long-term, low-level pesticide exposure from both domestic and imported produce, agricultural workers' concerns are more immediate. Each year 25 million people, primarily in the Southern Hemisphere, are poisoned through occupational exposure to pesticides; of those, 220,000 die, according to the World Health Organization (WHO). In the U.S., 300,000 farmworkers are poisoned each year.

Pesticides fall into three main categories—insecticides, herbicides, and fungicides—and they are designed to control or eliminate unwanted insects, weeds, and plant-killing fungi; each contains an "active ingredient," or the poison that kills the pest, and an "inert" carrying or spreading compound. When first developed after World War II, pesticides were hailed as miracle chemicals that would protect crops and homes, make food more plentiful and safe, and wipe out world hunger. Erika Rosenthal, Latin America Program Coordinator with the San Francisco-based Pesticides Action Network (PAN), has a late-1940s poster advertising DDT hanging in her office. The text at the bottom reads: "The great expectations held for DDT have been realized. During 1946, exhaustive scientific tests have shown that, when properly used, DDT kills a host of destructive insect pests and is a benefactor of all humanity."

But by the late 1950s, scientific evidence was already mounting that DDT was not only a potent carcinogen, but it also posed a serious threat to the environment—it is now cited as the cause of the near-extinction of the bald eagle, brown pelican, and condor. Despite its prominence in *Silent Spring* it wasn't until 1972 that DDT was finally banned in the U.S., and it is still manufactured in Mexico, India, and Indonesia and used in some developing countries. "DDT had the dubious fame of being one of the most widespread contaminants of the ecosystem," says PAN's Rosenthal. "Dangerously high concentrations have been found in the breast milk of mothers in Central America. It's also been found in the fat of Arctic polar bears. So it's covered the globe," she says. DDT remains in the food chain as a result of soil and water contamination. As recently as 1993, a study found higher levels of DDE (which is formed when DDT breaks down) in U.S. women who had developed breast cancer than in women who had not.

Pesticides are now everywhere—in our food, drinking water, homes, yards, and air. But it's difficult to rate the worst pesticides. "It's Russian roulette. Pick your poison: acutely toxic, chronically hazardous, cancer-causing, or effect unknown," says Sandra Marquardt, pesticide consultant at Consumers Union in Washington, D.C. Most often, we are exposed simultaneously to a variety of types, although the EPA sets safety levels by testing only one active ingredient at a time. And even when pesticides are banned, they are often used illegally by U.S. growers. Lax enforcement of EPA regulations by the Food and Drug Administration (FDA) makes it possible for many farmers to continue to use their pesticides of choice.

In addition to breast cancer, cancers of the reproductive system have been linked to pesticides. Infants and young children are especially vulnerable to pesticides. "Millions of children in the United States receive up to 35 percent of their entire lifetime dose of some cardnogenic pesticides by age five," reports a study by the Washington, D.C.-based Environmental Working Group (EWG). There is growing evidence that pesticides also cause a variety of birth defects and genetic mutations. And one of the newest and most worrisome findings is that some pesticides—known as "hormone imitating" chemicals or "endocrine disrupters" —are building up in animals and humans and disrupting reproduction, immunity, and metabolism. In a recent National Wildlife Federation study, "Fertility on the Brink," University of Florida zoologist Louis Guillette writes: "We've released endocrine disrupters throughout the world that are having fundamental effects on the immune system and the reproductive system. . . . Should we be upset? I think we should be screaming in the streets."

Neither the government nor the pesticide industry has responded with much urgency to the long-term health risks faced by consumers—or the daily risks faced by farmworkers. On the evening of November 14, 1989, a few miles outside Tampa, Florida, the insecticide mevinphos was sprayed on Goodson Farms' 16 acres of cauliflower. Early the next morning, farm managers sent migrant laborers into the dewy fields to tie up the plants. Within several hours, scores were complaining of headaches, dizziness, blurred vision, slurred speech, and breathing difficulties. They began vomiting, having convulsions, and staggering out of the field; several passed out. By late afternoon an estimated 112 farmworkers were treated at the scene or at area hospitals. Thirteen were admitted to hospitals. In the following months, dozens of the workers continued to suffer symptoms, and one pregnant woman miscarried.

Florida doctors called this one of the worst cases of pesticide poisonings they had ever seen. Goodson Farms managers were fined by state authorities for sending workers into the field too soon after spraying and not giving them proper protective gear. But Goodson's fine was later reduced from $12,600 to only $7,000. And the president of Amvac Chemical Corporation, which makes mevinphos under the brand name Phosdrin, continues to praise the product: Eric Wintemute describes it as "a neat compound" and "100 percent clean" because, he says, it leaves no permanent residue on crops; its "acute toxicity" simply means it must be applied with care.

"Even if this chemical is applied as directed it can still poison the workers," remarks Michael Hancock, executive director of the Washington, D.C.-based Farmworker Justice Fund. He calls mevinphos "the single most harmful pesticide to farmworkers." For years, labor advocates have urged the EPA to speed up its pesticide review process and ban chemicals like mevinphos, which is used on some 50 crops. Finally, in June 1994, the EPA made the unusual decision to issue an "emergency suspension order" that would have taken mevinphos off the market immediately.

But the day before the order was to be implemented, the EPA received a call from Amvac's lawyer, Steven Schatzow, saying the company had decided to "voluntarily" withdraw the pesticide from the U.S. market. Schatzow was no stranger to the EPA: he had been the agency's director of pesticide programs under Ronald Reagan. This was classic Washington revolving-door politics. Despite current EPA administrator Carol Browner's pledge to "break the gridlock on pesticide reform," Schatzow and the EPA struck a deal: Amvac agreed to stop producing mevinphos for use in the U.S., but the company was given until the end of 1994 to sell off its supply. And then after the Republicans' congressional sweep last November, the EPA agreed to give Amvac until the end of November 1995 "for sale, distribution, and use of existing stocks of mevinphos products."

Environmentalists are furious. "It's ridiculous. The EPA caved in," says Marquardt at Consumers Union. "It gave Amvac another year to dump this poison on the American people," adds Hancock, who sees the EPA's handling of mevinphos as a sign of the chilling effect the Republicans' Contract with America is having on the Clinton administration. "The EPA got the message not to do anything that would create headlines saying REGULATORY ACTION FORCES COMPANY OUT OF BUSINESS."

Amvac has continued to sell mevinphos overseas, in such countries as Thailand and South Africa. Under U.S. law,

the 43 active ingredients in pesticides that the EPA has deemed too dangerous for use in the U.S.—along with the hundreds of pesticide ingredients that haven't been registered by the EPA—can be exported. Dr. Robert McConnell, a World Health Organization pesticides expert, says he is most worried about unregistered pesticides exported to the Southern Hemisphere because "there is virtually no data on them." And the FDA doesn't monitor imported produce any better than domestic. Although FDA border inspectors are supposed to examine a "representative sample" of produce entering the country, few fruits and vegetables are screened. "Ninety-nine percent sail through untouched," says Marquardt. "There are so few inspectors out there, and they are more concerned with testing cosmetic appearance than pesticide residues." And about one third of the shipments detected with hazardous pesticide residues reach U.S. supermarkets anyway, due to halfhearted enforcement efforts and bureaucratic delays. "It is as if we were selling bombs around the world that come back and explode in our own backyards," Congressman Sam Gejdenson (D.-Conn.) testified at 1994 hearings on pesticide exports.

Ironically, as more humans are sickened or killed by pesticides, more strains of insects, mites, weeds, and rodents are developing immunity to these chemicals. In *Silent Spring*, Carson found that 137 species of insects and mites had already become pesticide-resistant; today it is more than 500. According to Cornell University Professor David Pimentel, the amount of crops lost to insects in the U.S. "has almost doubled during the last 40 years, despite a more than tenfold increase in the amount and toxicity of synthetic insecticides used."

Nevertheless, growers, both in the U.S. and abroad, are becoming increasingly reliant on pesticides. "My greatest concern is the expanded use of pesticides—the doubling [in the U.S.] over the last 30 years—and the effect it can have on our children, our water, air, and land," says the EPA's Browner. "And it's outrageous," she adds, "that a product banned here can be sold in other countries." But Browner, a longtime environmental activist, has not been able to "end the cycle of compromise" at the EPA, says Jay Feldman of the National Coalition Against the Misuse of Pesticides. She got points in early 1994 for proposing legislation that would create stricter safety standards for both domestic and imported produce, as well as stop the export of banned pesticides. But the administration's proposal never even made it out of the House agricultural committee last year, and this year it will not be reintroduced. It was "blocked by the pesticide lobby," which wields "tremendous power," says Browner, particularly in the current Republican-controlled Congress. "Now legislation is being written by the [pesticide industry] lobbyists." But labor advocates like Michael Hancock contend that the Clinton administration pressured the EPA to bow out too soon: "The agency seems to be in full retreat. They just surrender when they should stand and put up a fight over principle."

Behind the current antiregulatory fervor is the benign-sounding American Crop Protection Association, or ACPA (formerly the National Agricultural Chemical Association), the pesticide industry's main lobby. Comprised of 83 chemical companies, including such giants as DuPont, DOW, Monsanto, Velsicol, and American Cyanimid, this Washington, D.C.-based trade associa-

tion commands enormous political clout, in part through campaign contributions to key members of the House and Senate agricultural committees. ACPA member companies constitute a global pesticide supermarket, selling to virtually every country in both the Northern and Southern Hemispheres. And ACPA members have done little to ensure that workers-especially in the South—use their products safely. Scores of studies and press accounts show that workers often are given little or no training in handling the chemicals. Many cannot read labels, frequently mix pesticides with their bare hands, and carry home the poisons on their bodies and clothing. Hazardous chemicals spill or are dumped into fields, rivers, or ponds, and the poison-laced containers are reused for storing food, water, or seeds. "It's very difficult to have safe use under tropical conditions, by small farmers wearing backpacks. The packs leak and it's too hot and too expensive to wear protective clothing," says WHO's McConnell. Four years ago, DOW was sued by male Costa Rican banana workers who were showing up sterile after years of exposure to the highly toxic pesticide DBCP; women workers and family members who were also exposed were left out of the suit but are currently documenting their high rates of miscarriages, birth defects, and cancer in preparation for a suit of their own.

In 1991, ACPA opened its first "safe use" project to train growers in Guatemala, Thailand, and Kenya. "We recognized we had to roll up our sleeves and get involved," says John McCarthy of ACPA's international division. The association's commitment to "safe use" is minuscule: $400,000 a year and one staff person in each country. But it makes good PR—as ACPA President Jay Vroom told

Congress, these projects show industry's "advances" in "product stewardship and worker safety." "Three pilot projects four decades too late—how dare [they] make such claims?" says one health expert who has worked on pesticide safety programs in the Southern Hemisphere. "This 'safe use' is about buying companies another ten years" to export their goods, he says.

Little will change for either workers or consumers until farmers move away from an "agrochemical-intensive model of production," says PAN's Rosenthal. The right direction, say activists, is toward organic farming. The EPA's Browner agrees: "We know how to grow food with fewer chemicals, and that should be our goal." EWG's Richard Wiles, who directed a National Academy of Sciences' study of alternative farming methods, says, "It's possible to grow an affordable, abundant food supply using few or no synthetic chemicals. For all major field crops—corn, soybean, wheat, barley—the science is there. You can eliminate pesticides that pose serious health risks and maintain current levels of production." What's missing, Wiles explains, is the incentive. "American farmers have very minimal regulatory or market incentive to cut back on pesticides. They see the chemicals as legal, loosely regulated, and a low-cost form of insurance, and farmers don't pay any of the cost of the environmental consequences. So what the hell? Why change?"

Contract with America Republicans are hell-bent on pushing through more deregulation and corporate perks. But they may be misreading the mood of the country. A poll commissioned by the National Wildlife Federation just after the 1994 elections found that 41 percent of people in the U.S. believe that existing regulations "don't go far enough

in protecting the environment," that 46 percent agree that laws "do not require businesses to do enough to protect the environment," and that 64 percent say that government should pay subsidies to farmers for pesticide reduction.

The public's increasing health consciousness is reflected in organic food sales, which have skyrocketed over the past five years. And the emerging market is attracting a number of big food companies, a few of which have opened up organic divisions. Such rapid expansion—involving pesticide-happy companies—has prompted calls among some activists for federal regulation for the largely self-regulated organic food industry.

The growth of the organic market confirms what Betsy Lydon, of the New York City-based group Mothers and Others for a Livable Planet, has long maintained: "Change has to happen in the marketplace. Your food dollars *can* be very powerful." Her group, which has a mailing list of 25,000, is sponsoring a nationwide "shoppers' campaign" for healthier food choices. Members in Kentucky, Illinois, and New York are working with supermarket chains like D'Agostino's and Dominick's to encourage them to offer more organic food—which in many cases, Lydon says, is just slightly more expensive than nonorganic. When there is a real disparity, she says, "people need to talk to their retailer about price gouging. They should not be selling organic food as gourmet food." Lydon's group also spearheaded a project in Lexington, Kentucky, called a "buying club," involving 26 organic farmers and 100 families. The families give the farmers money in the early part of the season for seeds and supplies; come harvest, the farmers deliver their organic produce to the families at below-market rates.

Other groups, like the New York City-based Women's Environment and Development Organization (WEDO), are focusing on political action. WEDO is planning a series of nationwide "hearings" ... on the links between environmental factors, like pesticides, and breast cancer. WEDO is working in coalition with groups like One in Nine, a Long Island breast cancer awareness organization that is campaigning to get New York State to establish a pesticide registry that would be open to the public. "We found out that farmers have to register what they use and that information is supposed to go to the government. But they put the records into cartons and no one has access to them," says Geri Barish, head of One in Nine's Pesticide Project. "We want to know how much is used, where it's used, and what the studies say." A bill mandating such a registry made it through the state assembly [in 1994], but the farm lobby killed it in the senate. Barish is determined to get it reintroduced. Although "we're just volunteers and many of us are not well," says Barish, "we decided we're not going to go away."

Internationally, the pesticide industry is running into roadblocks—many countries in the south have banned importation of the most deadly chemicals. And there are other advances: a United Nations-sponsored rice farmer training program in Southeast Asia has cut pesticide use in the region by 90 percent; in Sweden, pesticide use was reduced by 50 percent between 1985 and 1990; in Colombia, sugar growers use beneficial insects instead of pesticides; and some Cuban farmers, forced to go organic because of trade sanctions, now say that they don't want to go back to chemicals. "The global movement against pesticide misuse has grown fantastically in the last 10 to 15 years," says PAN's Rosenthal. "Today we have thousands of organizations around the world pushing for sustainable and healthy agricultural techniques." But only the combined efforts of activists and consumers, working against official indifference to the public's health, can hope to one day repel the "chemical barrage that has been hurled against the fabric of life," in the words of Rachel Carson. Although life is "delicate and destructible," Carson wrote, it is also "tough and resilient, and capable of striking back in unexpected ways."

NO

Bruce Ames

TOO MUCH FUSS ABOUT PESTICIDES

In the wake of the Alar-in-apples scare last year [1989], consumers have become highly concerned about the threat posed to their health by the ingestion of trace amounts of man-made pesticides. While it is good for consumers to be concerned about what they eat, the hysteria about pesticide residues may not be warranted by the actual risk they pose. In helping consumers develop a fuller picture of the true risk of man-made pesticides (or other chemical additives to food), we present below an excerpt of a letter from Dr. Bruce Ames to *Consumer Reports* magazine. The letter was in response to an article run in that magazine (October 1989), which, according to Dr. Ames, "distorts my views and misstates facts." ...

—Ed. [of *Consumers' Research.*]

Consumer Reports' four-page attack on my scientific work both distorts my views and misstates the facts on which they are based. Good scientists are committed to challenging assumptions rigorously, and this is particularly important in the prevention of cancer, a murky, complex, multidisciplinary field to which I have devoted much of my scientific career. Sound public policy should be based on sound science, and new data or theory may require altering some prevailing assumptions.

In our efforts to prevent human cancer, it makes no sense to apply a double standard for human exposures to natural vs. synthetic chemicals. My colleagues and I have therefore attempted to provide an overview of possible carcinogenic hazards.

The following points clarify my views and their factual and theoretical basis:

1) Discovering the Causes of Cancer. Epidemiologists are continually coming up with clues about the causes of different types of human cancer, and these hypotheses are then refined by animal and metabolic studies. This approach will, in my view, lead to the understanding of the causal factors for the major human cancers during the next decade. Current epidemiologic data point to the major risk factors for human cancer as cigarette smoking (which is responsible for 30% of cancer), dietary imbalances, hormones, viruses, and lifestyle factors—not to such factors as water pollution or synthetic pesticide residues.

For example, epidemiologists in many countries have identified excessive salt as a risk factor for stomach cancer, one of the major types of cancer. Extensive experimental work in rodents on salt as a co-carcinogen supports the epidemiology. Yet *Consumer Reports* unfairly criticized Edith Efron for saying that salt is a carcinogen.

Consumer Reports criticized me for calling alcohol a carcinogen, yet alcoholic beverages, of numerous types, are carcinogenic in humans at a level of 5 drinks/day. Alcohol itself was positive in one rat test and also was co-carcinogenic in other tests. Acetaldehyde, the main metabolite of alcohol, is a carcinogen in rodents. Most of the leading scientists in the field believe that the active ingredient in alcoholic beverages is alcohol itself. I think that chronic high doses of alcohol are active by causing cell proliferation and inflammation and that, therefore, low doses are not of much interest.

2) Animal Cancer Tests. There are three fundamental problems with the use of animal cancer tests in trying to prevent human cancer from low-dose human exposures.

a) There are millions of chemicals in the world that we are exposed to in low or moderate doses, 99.9+% of which are natural. To identify significant risks, we need to identify the right chemicals to test in rodents.

b) About half of the chemicals tested in long-term bioassays in both rats and mice have been found to be carcinogens at the high doses administered, the maximum tolerated dose (MTD). Synthetic industrial chemicals account for almost all (82%) of the chemicals (427) tested in both species. However, despite the fact that humans eat vastly more natural than synthetic chemicals, only a small number (75) of *natural* chemicals have been tested in both rats and mice. For the 75 natural chemicals the proportion of positive results (47%) is similar, also about *half*. While some synthetic or natural chemicals were selected for testing precisely because of suspect structures, most chemicals were tested because they were natural or synthetic food additives, colors, high volume industrial compounds, pesticides, or natural or synthetic drugs. Thus, the high proportion of carcinogens among synthetic test agents in rodent studies is not simply due to selection of suspicious chemical structures, and the natural world of chemicals has never been looked at systematically. Recent research into the mechanism of carcinogenesis (see #4 below) supports the idea that when tested in rodents at the MTD, a high proportion of all chemicals we test in the future, whether natural or synthetic, will prove to be carcinogenic.

c) The problem of knowing whether there is any risk at all from the very low doses of human exposure to chemicals causing tumors in rodents at very high doses has been argued by toxicologists and regulators for years, precisely because one cannot measure effects at low doses. Regulators have opted for worst-case estimates, using assumptions that increasing scientific evidence suggests may be incorrect.

Because conventional risk assessment is focused mainly on man-made chemicals and is based on worst-case assumptions that we believe are proving to exaggerate hazard greatly, many leading scientists have argued that it is misleading to the public to try to present estimates of "worst-case risk" from animal studies in terms of expected numbers of human cancers. Our HERP [Human Exposure/Rodent Potency, Dr. Ames's index for estimating carcinogenic risk] uses essentially the same information as that in conventional risk assessment, but is explicitly intended as a relative scale. We have attempted to achieve some perspective on the plethora of possible hazards to humans from exposure to known rodent carcinogens by establishing a scale of the possible hazards for the amounts of various common carcinogens to which humans might be chronically exposed. We view the value of our calculations not as providing a basis for absolute human risk assessment, but as a guide for priority setting.

Carcinogens clearly do not all work in the same way, and as we learn more about the mechanisms, HERP comparisons can be refined, as can risk assessments.

Thus, if the public is told that the possible hazard of the UDMH residue [the breakdown product of Alar] in a daily glass of apple juice (about 30 parts per billion) is 1/18 that of aflatoxin (a mold carcinogen) in a daily peanut butter sandwich (the Food and Drug Administration [FDA] allows 10 times that residue level), 1/50 that of a daily mushroom, and 1/1,000 that of a daily beer, it puts these items in perspective. The possible relative hazard of a daily apple is at least 10× less than the apple juice. This is quite different from showing a witch's hand holding an apple [as was depicted on the May 1989 *Consumer Reports* cover on Alar—Ed].

3) Pesticides, 99.99% All Natural. All plants produce toxins to protect themselves against fungi, insects, and animal predators such as man. Tens of thousands of these natural pesticides have been discovered, and every species of plant contains its own set of different toxins, usually a few dozen. In addition, when plants are stressed or damaged, such as during a pest attack, they increase their natural pesticide levels many fold, occasionally to levels that are acutely toxic to humans. We estimate that Americans eat about 1,500 mg/day of natural pesticides, 10,000 times more than man-made pesticide residues, which FDA estimates at a total of 0.15 mg/day. Their concentration is usually measured in parts per thousand or million, rather than parts per billion (ppb), the usual concentration of synthetic pesticide residues and pollutants in water. We estimate that Americans are ingesting 5,000 to 10,000 different natural pesticides and their breakdown products, a subset of the tremendous number of natural chemicals we ingest. For example, there are 49 different natural pesticides (and breakdown products) ingested in eating cabbage.

Surprisingly few plant pesticides have been tested in animal cancer bioassays, but among those tested, again about *half* (25 out of 47) are carcinogenic. A search for the presence of just these 25 carcinogens in foods indicates that they occur naturally in the following (those at levels over 50,000 ppb are listed in parentheses); anise, apples (50,000+ ppb), bananas, basil (4 million ppb), broccoli, Brussels sprouts (500,000 ppb), cabbage (100,000 ppb), cantaloupe, carrots (50,000+ ppb), cauliflower, celery (50,000+ ppb), cinnamon, cloves, cocoa, coffee (brewed) (90,000 ppb), comfrey tea, fennel (3 million ppb), grapefruit juice, honeydew melon, horseradish (4 million ppb), kale, lettuce (300,000 ppb), mushrooms, mustard (black) (40 million ppb), nutmeg (5 million ppb), orange juice (30,000 ppb), parsley, parsnips (30,000 ppb), peaches, black pepper (100,000 ppb), pineapples, potatoes (50,000+ ppb), radishes, raspberries, strawberries, tarragon (1 million ppb), and turnips.

There is every reason to expect that we will continue to find mutagens and carcinogens among nature's pesticides if we ever test them systematically. In short-term tests for detecting mutagens, the proportion of natural pesticides that turn up positive is just as high as for synthetic industrial chemicals. In a compendium on the ability of 950 chemicals to break chromosomes in animal tests, there were 62 natural pesticides: half of them were positive. Thus, it seems highly probable that almost every plant product in the supermarket will contain natural carcinogens at much higher levels than those of man-made pesticides. We have suggested that many more natural pesticides (and chemicals from cooking of food) be tested in long-term bioassays.

Additionally, there is a fundamental trade-off between nature's pesticides and man-made pesticides. We can easily breed out many of nature's pesticides to protect our crops from being eaten by insects. In contrast, growers are currently breeding some plants for insect resistance and unwittingly raising the levels of natural pesticides. A new variety of insect-resistant celery that is being widely sold is almost 10× higher in carcinogens (6,200 ppb) than standard celery.

4) Mechanisms of Carcinogenesis. In the rapidly advancing field of mechanisms of carcinogenesis, there is now evidence to suggest that cell proliferation is extremely important. A large number of the major human carcinogens such as hormones, chronic viral infection, salt, asbestos, and alcohol are likely to be primarily active through causing cell proliferation. A cell is at considerably greater genetic risk during division, so chronic cell proliferation in itself is a mutagenic and carcinogenic stress. Cancers induced in animal cancer tests done at high doses seem to be primarily caused by cell proliferation, in part due to chronic cell killing, and inflammation that results from high toxic doses. This would be in agreement with the high proportion of all chemicals that are turning out to be carcinogens at high doses and the relation of toxicity to carcinogenic potency. The induction of cell proliferation is restricted to high doses, and this strongly suggests that low doses of carcinogens are of no risk, or are very much less hazardous than has been assumed.

In addition, humans, who live in a world of natural toxins, are well protected by many layers of inducible general defenses against low doses of toxins—defenses that do not distinguish between synthetic and natural toxins. Therefore, even the high levels of natural plant pesticides may not be of much concern in a balanced diet.

5) Trade-offs. Identifying and controlling the major causes of human cancer are not a matter of blame. We have tried in our scientific work to put into perspective the tiny exposures to pesticide residues by comparing them to the enormous background of natural substances. Minimizing pollution is a separate issue, and is clearly desirable, aside from any effect on public health, but it involves economic trade-offs. As a society, efforts to regulate pesticides or other synthetic rodent carcinogens down to the ppb level inevitably involve understanding these trade-offs. Synthetic pesticides (and chemicals such as Alar) have markedly lowered the cost of our food, a major advance in nutrition and, thus, health. Every complex mixture from gasoline to cooked food to orange juice contains rodent carcinogens. When people drive to work, put logs on a fire, or make a barbecue they are putting carcinogens into the air. There are costs and benefits to all of these. Exaggerating the risks from man-made substances, ignoring the natural world, and converting the issue to one of blaming U.S. industry does not advance our public health efforts. If we spend all our efforts on minimal, rather than important, hazards, we hurt public health. The Environmental Protection Agency (EPA) is trying to prevent hypothetical risks of 1 in a million at enormous economic cost. Yet the leading scientists trying to prevent cancer are working on numerous possible carcinogenic risks in the 1 in a 100 to 1 in 10 range: my lab is working on 4 that we think are in this range.

POSTSCRIPT

Is Pesticide Exposure Harmful to Human Health?

Increased consumer fear of pesticide residues on food has encouraged many activists to push for a ban on pesticide use. Although doing so might provide some health benefits, Ronald Knutson, director of the Agricultural and Food Policy Center at Texas A & M University, believes that such a ban would cause a significant rise in food prices. In "Pesticide-Free Equals Higher Food Prices," *Consumers' Research* (November 1990), Knutson and his colleagues argue that if there were a complete ban on the use of pesticides, food bills would rise at least 12 percent, crop yields would fall, and there would need to be a 10 percent increase in cultivated acreage, which would result in a corresponding rise in soil erosion.

An investigation by Constance Matthiessen challenges the opinions of Knutson and others. Matthiessen, writing in *Mother Jones* (March/April 1992), takes the position that despite the widespread use of pesticides, insects and weeds seem to be doing as much damage as ever. The reason: insects and weeds have the ability to adapt and evolve to become pesticide-resistant. As a result, the share of crop yields lost to pests has almost doubled over the last 40 years. Environmentalist Shirley A. Briggs agrees that pesticides have failed to decrease crop losses while causing widespread environmental damage. In "Silent Spring: The View from 1990," *The Ecologist* (March/April 1990), Briggs argues that we must find ways to reduce pesticide dependence. Other articles that support this viewpoint include "Organic: A Four-Letter Word," *Vegetarian Times* (March 1996) and "Breasticides," *Earth Island Journal* (Fall 1996), which discusses the relationship between pesticides and breast cancer.

Robert J. Scheuplein, a scientist with the Office of Toxicological Sciences at the Food and Drug Administration, shares the opinions of Ames. In "The Risk from Food," *Consumers' Research* (April 1990), Scheuplein argues that the public has an unrealistic view of pesticides and that other factors, particularly overall diet, contribute much more to the development of different cancers than pesticide-treated foods.

Most scientists agree that pesticide residues can affect human health to *some* degree. Many experts, however, maintain that current levels of residues are insignificant and that our food supply is safe. Articles such as: "Ban All Plants—They Pollute," *Forbes* (October 24 1993); "Proposed Food Safety Laws Are Starved for Scientific Merit," *Insight on the News* (November 1, 1993); "Are People Too Worried about Carcinogens for Their Own Good?" *Business Week* (October 19, 1992) and "Do Pesticides Cause Cancer?" *Consumers' Research*

(December 1991) argue that people are overly concerned about low levels of man-made chemicals in food when there are numerous natural carcinogens present. Dennis Avery, the director of global food issues at the Hudson Institute, believes that it is habitat loss, not chemicals that we should be most worried about. In his book *Biodiversity: Saving Species with Biotechnology* he claims that the "judicious use of modern pesticides can increase agricultural yields without creating any significant increase in the risk of developing cancer." Environmental journalist Ronald Bailey, writing in "Once and Future Farming," *Garbage: The Independent Environmental Quarterly* (Fall 1994), claims that pesticides and fertilizers are needed to feed the world population. An overall analysis of the pesticide risk/benefit relationship can be found in "EPA Begins Initial Approval," *Chemical Week* (February 12, 1997) and "Regulating Pesticides," *CQ Researcher* (January 28, 1994). Others argue that pesticides pose health risks, are environmentally unsound, and do not work in the long run, because many pests have become resistant to them. For an overview of the National Research Council of the National Academy of Science report on safety of current levels of pesticides in foods and the health of children see "Raising the Risk of Pesticides," *Environmental Science and Technology* (September 1993); "Pesticide Residues in Your Children's Food," *Consumers' Research* (August 1993); and "We've Been Down That Road Before," *Garbage: The Independent Environmental Quarterly* (Fall 1994). Researching alternatives to pesticides, as described in "Organics: Hot Debate," *Vegetarian Times* (August 1993) and "Could Marigolds Stop Killer Mosquitoes?" *New Scientist* (July 17, 1993), may be a safer, more ecologically sound, and ultimately more successful approach to limiting pest damage than is maintaining a total reliance on chemicals.

ISSUE 16

Public Policy and Health: Is Global Warming a Real Threat?

YES: **Ross Gelbspan,** from "The Heat Is On," *Harper's Magazine* (December 1995)

NO: **S. Fred Singer,** from "Dirty Climate," *National Review* (November 25, 1996)

ISSUE SUMMARY

YES: Journalist Ross Gelbspan contends that we need to act now to prevent future catastrophic climatic changes that may result from global warming.

NO: Atmospheric physicist S. Fred Singer argues that 18 years of weather-satellite data actually show a global cooling trend.

For the past several hundred million years, the relative concentrations of the four major gases in the atmosphere—nitrogen, oxygen, argon, and carbon dioxide (CO_2)—have remained constant. Within recent decades, however, scientists have been concerned that an increase in the amount of atmospheric CO_2 may be occurring due to the rapid rise in the burning of fossil fuels and the global slashing and burning of forests. When fossil fuels are burned, CO_2 is released. The natural processes that absorb excess CO_2 are currently being overwhelmed by the huge volume being released from industry, automobiles and other forms of transportation, and the burning of tropical forests. As a result, the concentration of CO_2 is rising at the rate of .05 percent per year, or a 12 percent increase since 1960.

Although CO_2 is not toxic to human beings, there is concern over its effect on global temperatures, a phenomenon known as the greenhouse effect. Carbon dioxide in the atmosphere appears to act as a blanket around the Earth, increasing the absorption of heat from the sun. This blanketing has already appeared to affect the Earth's average temperature. In 1988 a team of researchers from NASA found that the global mean temperature is now almost one degree Fahrenheit warmer than it was a century ago. A scientific panel made up of several hundred eminent researchers working under the sponsorship of the United Nations and the International Panel on Climate Change (IPCC) concluded that the reality of global warming cannot be ignored. In a 1990 report, the IPCC claimed that the projected increases in CO_2 would result in the average global temperature rising three to eight degrees within the next 100 years, making the Earth warmer than ever before in recorded history.

Although a warmer Earth may not seem to be a crisis, several health and environmental effects could be disastrous. The increasing frequency of excessive heat waves will have an impact on illness and death rates. Extreme heat will cause deaths due to heart attacks and stroke, and certain diseases spread by mosquitoes and other vectors, such as malaria, may spread from warmer to colder climates. Hotter weather could affect crop yields and the long-term survival of certain plants and animals. The most dramatic consequence of global warming will be a worldwide rise in sea level related to the melting of the Antarctic and Greenland ice caps. This could mean flooding of low-lying coastal areas and loss of coastal wetlands.

For the past 25 years, climatologists have been warning about the rise in global temperatures. They have urged policymakers to take action to prevent a doomsday scenario. Since 1980, the 10 hottest summers on record have added urgency to demands that the government launch efforts to reduce the emission of greenhouse gases. Although CO_2 is the primary greenhouse gas, several other gases (methane, nitrous oxide, and chlorofluorocarbons) are further enhancing the greenhouse effect by absorbing waves of heat. A call for action, however, is easier than actually implementing change. At the Earth Summit in Brazil in 1992, representatives from 12 countries agreed to stabilize concentrations of greenhouse gases at 1990 levels. In 1993, President Clinton vowed that the United States would comply. Unfortunately, even if all nations who signed the pact were to move immediately to cap emissions, global temperatures would continue to rise. Only if emissions were *slashed* would there be a genuine decline in atmospheric CO_2 levels. Because of the economic impact, no nation is currently contemplating this action.

Can anything be done to reduce the greenhouse gases? Several policy options, including improving energy efficiency, switching to alternative sources such as solar and wind energy, and replanting forests are possible. Green plants remove CO_2 from the air during photosynthesis. The worldwide cutting and burning of forests has removed this CO_2 consumer, contributing to a rise in atmospheric CO_2. Finally, as Vice President Gore has suggested, imposing a tax on fossil fuels might reduce their use.

Many eminent scientists believe that global warming will have a catastrophic effect on human health and the well-being of the planet. In the following selections, journalist Ross Gelbspan states that although the energy industry claims otherwise, the Earth's temperature continues to climb and this will have a catastrophic effect. S. Fred Singer, professor emeritus of environmental sciences at the University of Virginia, however, claims that there is little that would lead one to believe that global warming is actually happening now or that predictions for future warming will come true.

YES   Ross Gelbspan

THE HEAT IS ON

After my lawn had burned away to straw last summer, and the local papers announced that the season had been one of the driest in the recorded history of New England, I found myself wondering how long we can go on pretending that nothing is amiss with the world's weather. It wasn't just the fifty ducks near my house that had died when falling water levels in a creek exposed them to botulism-infested mud, or the five hundred people dead in the Midwest from an unexpected heat wave that followed the season's second "one-hundred-year flood" in three years. It was also the news from New Orleans (overrun by an extraordinary number of cockroaches and termites after a fifth consecutive winter without a killing frost), from Spain (suffering a fourth year of drought in a region that ordinarily enjoys a rainfall of 84 inches a year), and from London (Britain's meteorological office reporting the driest summer since 1727 and the hottest since 1659).

The reports of changes in the world's climate have been with us for fifteen or twenty years, most urgently since 1988, when Dr. James Hansen, director of NASA's Goddard Institute for Space Studies, declared that the era of global warming was at hand. As a newspaper correspondent who had reported on the United Nations Conferences on the environment in Stockholm in 1972 and in Rio in 1992, I understood something of the ill effects apt to result from the extravagant burning of oil and coal. New record-setting weather extremes seem to have become as commonplace as traffic accidents, and three simple facts have long been known: the distance from the surface of the earth to the far edge of the inner atmosphere is only twelve miles; the annual amount of carbon dioxide forced into that limited space is six billion tons; and the ten hottest years in recorded human history have all occurred since 1980. The facts beg a question that is as simple to ask as it is hard to answer. What do we do with what we know?

The question became more pointed in September, when the 2,500 climate scientists serving on the Intergovernmental Panel on Climate Change [IPCC] issued a new statement on the prospect of forthcoming catastrophe. Never before had the IPCC (called into existence in 1988) come to so unambiguous a conclusion. Always in years past there had been people saying that we didn't

From Ross Gelbspan, "The Heat Is On," *Harper's Magazine* (December 1995). Copyright © 1995 by *Harper's Magazine*. Reprinted by permission. All rights reserved. Some notes omitted.

yet know enough, or that the evidence was problematical, or our system of computer simulation was subject to too many uncertainties. Not this year. The panel flatly announced that the earth had entered a period of climatic instability likely to cause "widespread economic, social and environmental dislocation over the next century." The continuing emission of greenhouse gases would create protracted, crop-destroying droughts in continental interiors, a host of new and recurring diseases, hurricanes of extraordinary malevolence, and rising sea levels that could inundate island nations and low-lying coastal rims on the continents.

I came across the report in the *New York Times* during the same week that the island of St. Thomas was blasted to shambles by one of thirteen hurricanes that roiled the Caribbean this fall. Scientists speak the language of probability. They prefer to avoid making statements that cannot be further corrected, reinterpreted, modified, or proven wrong. If its September announcement was uncharacteristically bold, possibly it was because the IPCC scientists understood that they were addressing their remarks to people profoundly unwilling to hear what they had to say.

That resistance is understandable, given the immensity of the stakes. The energy industries now constitute the largest single enterprise known to mankind. Moreover, they are indivisible from automobile, farming, shipping, air freight, and banking interests, as well as from the governments dependent on oil revenues for their very existence. With annual sales in excess of one trillion dollars and daily sales of more than two billion dollars, the oil industry alone supports the economies of the Middle East and large segments of the economies of Russia, Mexico, Venezuela, Nigeria, Indonesia, Norway, and Great Britain. Begin to enforce restriction on the consumption of oil and coal, and the effects on the global economy—unemployment, depression, social breakdown, and war—might lay waste to what we have come to call civilization. It is no wonder that for the last five or six years many of the world's politicians and most of the world's news media have been promoting the perception that the worries about the weather are overwrought. Ever since the IPCC first set out to devise strategies whereby the nations of the world might reduce their carbon dioxide emissions, and thus ward off a rise in the average global temperature on the order of 4 or 5 degrees Celsius (roughly equal in magnitude to the difference between the last ice age and the current climatic period), the energy industry has been conducting, not unreasonably, a ferocious public relations campaign meant to sell the notion that science, any science, is always a matter of uncertainty. Yet on reading the news from the IPCC, I wondered how the oil company publicists would confront the most recent series of geophysical events and scientific findings. To wit:

• A 48-by-22 mile chunk of the Larsen Ice Shelf in the Antarctic broke off last March, exposing rocks that had been buried for 20,000 years and prompting Rodolfo del Valle of the Argentine Antarctic Institute to tell the Associated Press, "Last November we predicted the [ice shelf] would crack in ten years, but it has happened in barely two months."

• In April, researchers discovered a 70 percent decline in the population of zooplankton off the coast of southern California, raising questions about the survival of several species of fish that feed on it. Scientists have linked the change to a 1 to 2 degree C increase in the surface water temperature over the last four decades.

- A recent series of articles in *The Lancet*, a British medical journal, linked changes in climate patterns to the spread of infectious diseases around the world. The *Aedes aegypti* mosquito, which spreads dengue fever and yellow fever, has traditionally been unable to survive at altitudes higher than 1,000 meters above sea level. But these mosquitoes are now being reported at 1,150 meters in Costa Rica and at 2,200 meters in Colombia. Ocean warming has triggered algae blooms linked to outbreaks of cholera in India, Bangladesh, and the Pacific coast of South America, where, in 1991, the disease infected more than 400,000 people.

- In a paper published in *Science* in April, David J. Thomson, of the AT&T Bell Laboratories, concluded that the .6 degree C warming of the average global temperature over the past century correlates directly with the buildup of atmospheric carbon dioxide. Separate findings by a team of scientists at the National Oceanic and Atmospheric Administrations's National Climatic Data Center indicate that growing weather extremes in the United States are due, by a probability of 90 percent, to rising levels of greenhouse gases.

- Scientists previously believed that the transitions between ice ages and more moderate climatic periods occur gradually, over centuries. But researchers from the Woods Hole Oceanographic Institution, examining deep ocean sediment and ice core samples, found that these shifts, with their temperature changes of up to 7 degrees C, have occurred within three to four decades—a virtual nanosecond in geological time. Over the last 70,000 years, the earth's climate has snapped into radically different temperature regimes. "Our results suggest that the present climate system is very delicately poised," said researcher Scott Lehman. "Shifts could happen very rapidly if conditions are right, and we cannot predict when that will occur." His cautionary tone is underscored by findings that the end of the last ice age, some 8,000 years ago, was preceded by a series of extreme oscillations in which severe regional deep freezes alternated with warming spikes. As the North Atlantic warmed, Arctic snowmelts and increased rainfall diluted the salt content of the ocean, which, in turn, redirected the ocean's warming current from a northeasterly direction to one that ran nearly due east. Should such an episode occur today, say researchers, "the present climate of Britain and Norway would change suddenly to that of Greenland."

These items (and many like them) would seem to be alarming news—far more important than the candidacy of Colin Powell, or even whether Newt Gingrich believes the government should feed poor children—worthy of a national debate or the sustained attention of Congress. But the signs and portents have been largely ignored, relegated to the environmental press and the oddball margins of the mass media. More often than not, the news about the accelerating retreat of the world's glaciers or the heat- and insect-stressed Canadian forests comes qualified with the observation that the question of global warming never can be conclusively resolved. The confusion is intentional, expensively gift wrapped by the energy industries.

* * *

Capital keeps its nose to the wind. The people who run the world's oil and coal companies know that the march of science, and of political action, may be slowed by disinformation. In the last year and a half, one of the leading oil industry public relations outlets, the Global Climate Coalition, has spent more than a million dollars to downplay the threat of climate change. It expects to spend another $850,000 on the issue next year. Similarly, the National Coal Association spent more than $700,000 on the global climate issue in 1992 and 1993. In 1993 alone, the American Petroleum Institute, just one of fifty-four industry members of the GCC, paid $1.8 million to the public relations firm of Burson-Marsteller partly in an effort to defeat a proposed tax on fossil fuels. For perspective, this is only slightly less than the combined yearly expenditures on global warming of the five major environmental groups that focus on climate issues—about $2.1 million, according to officials of the Environmental Defense Fund, the Natural Resources Defense Council, the Sierra Club, the Union of Concerned Scientists, and the World Wildlife Fund.

For the most part the industry has relied on a small band of skeptics—Dr. Richard S. Lindzen, Dr. Pat Michaels, Dr. Robert Balling, Dr. Sherwood Idso, and Dr. S. Fred Singer, among others— who have proven extraordinarily adept at draining the issue of all sense of crisis. Through their frequent pronouncements in the press and on radio and television, they have helped to create the illusion that the question is hopelessly mired in unknowns. Most damaging has been their influence on decision makers; their contrarian views have allowed conservative Republicans such as Representative Dana Rohrabacher (R., Calif.) to dismiss legitimate research concerns as "liberal claptrap" and have provided the basis for the recent round of budget cuts to those government science programs designed to monitor the health of the planet.

Last May, Minnesota held hearings in St. Paul to determine the environmental cost of coal burning by state power plants. Three of the skeptics—Lindzen, Michaels, and Balling—were hired as expert witnesses to testify on behalf of Western Fuels Association, a $400 million consortium of coal suppliers and coal-fired utilities.[1]

An especially aggressive industry player, Western Fuels was quite candid about its strategy in two annual reports: "[T]here has been a close to universal impulse in the trade association community here in Washington to concede the scientific premise of global warming . . . while arguing over policy prescriptions that would be the least disruptive to our economy. . . . We have disagreed, and do disagree, with this strategy." "When [the climate change] controversy first erupted . . . scientists were found who are skeptical about much of what seemed generally accepted about the potential for climate change." Among them were Michaels, Balling, and S. Fred Singer.

Lindzen, a distinguished professor of meteorology at MIT, testified in St. Paul that the maximum probable warming of the atmosphere in the face of a doubling of carbon dioxide emissions over the next century would amount to no more than a negligible

.3 degrees C. Michaels, who teaches climatology at the University of Virginia, stated that he foresaw no increase in the rate of sea level rise—another feared precursor of global warming. Balling, who works on climate issues at Arizona State University, declared that the increase in emissions would boost the average global temperature by no more than one degree.

At first glance, these attacks appear defensible, given their focus on the black holes of uncertainty that mark our current knowledge of the planet's exquisitely interrelated climate system. The skeptics emphasize the inadequacy of a major climate research tool known as a General Circulation Model, and our ignorance of carbon dioxide exchange between the oceans and the atmosphere and of the various roles of clouds. They have repeatedly pointed out that although the world's output of carbon dioxide has exploded since 1940, there has been no corresponding increase in the global temperature. The larger scientific community, by contrast, holds that this is due to the masking effect of low-level sulfur particulates, which exert a temporary cooling effect on the earth, and to a time lag in the oceans' absorption and release of carbon dioxide.

But while the skeptics portray themselves as besieged truth-seekers fending off irresponsible environmental doom-sayers, their testimony in St. Paul and elsewhere revealed the source and scope of their funding for the first time. Michaels has received more than $115,000 over the last four years from coal and energy interests. *World Climate Review,* a quarterly he founded that routinely debunks climate concerns, was funded by Western Fuels. Over the last six years, either alone or with colleagues, Balling

has received more than $200,000 from coal and oil interests in Great Britain, Germany, and elsewhere. Balling (along with Sherwood Idso) has also taken money from Cyprus Minerals, a mining company that has been a major funder of People for the West—a militantly anti-environmental "Wise Use" group. Lindzen, for his part, charges oil and coal interests $2,500 a day for his consulting services; his 1991 trip to testify before a Senate committee was paid for by Western Fuels, and a speech he wrote, entitled "Global Warming: the Origin and Nature of Alleged Scientific Consensus," was underwritten by OPEC. Singer, who last winter proposed a $95,000 publicity project to "stem the tide towards ever more onerous controls on energy use," has received consulting fees from Exxon, Shell, Unocal, ARCO, and Sun Oil, and has warned them that they face the same threat as the chemical firms that produced chlorofluorocarbons (CFCs), a class of chemicals found to be depleting atmospheric ozone. "It took only five years to go from . . . a simple freeze of production [of CFCs]," Singer has written, " . . . to the 1992 decision of a complete production phase-out—all on the basis of quite insubstantial science."[2]

The skeptics assert flatly that their science is untainted by funding. Nevertheless, in this persistent and well-funded campaign of denial they have become interchangeable ornaments on the hood of a high-powered engine of disinformation. Their dissenting opinions are amplified beyond all proportion through the media while the concerns of the dominant majority of the world's scientific establishment are marginalized. By keeping the discussion focused on whether there is a problem in the first place, they have effectively silenced the debate over what to do about it.

Last spring's IPCC conference in Berlin is a good example. Delegations from 170 nations met to negotiate targets and timetables for reducing the world's carbon dioxide emissions. The efforts of the conference ultimately foundered on foot-dragging by the United States and Japan and active resistance from the OPEC nations. Leading the fight for the most dramatic reductions—to 60 percent of 1990 levels—was a coalition of small island nations from the Caribbean and the Pacific that fear being flooded out of existence. They were supported by most western European governments, but China and India, with their vast coal resources, argued that until the United States significantly cuts its own emissions, their obligation to develop their own economies outranked their obligation to the global environment. In the end, OPEC, supported by the United States, Japan, Australia, Canada, and New Zealand, rejected calls to limit emissions, declaring emission limits premature.

* * *

As the natural crisis escalates, so will the forces of institutional and societal denial. If, at the cost of corporate pocket change, industrial giants can control the publicly perceived reality of the condition of the planet and the state of our scientific knowledge, what would they do if their survival were truly put at risk? Billions would be spent on the creation of information and the control of politicians. Glad-handing oil company ads on the op-ed page of the *New York Times* (from a quarter-page pronouncement by Mobil last September 28: "There's a lot of good news out there") would give way to

a new stream of selective finding by privatized scientists. Long before the planet itself collapsed, democracy would break apart under the stress of "natural" disasters. It is not difficult to foresee that in an ecological state of emergency our political liberties would be the first casualties.

Thus, the question must be asked: can civilization change the way it operates? For 5,000 years, we have thought of ourselves as dependent children of the earth, flourishing or perishing according to the whims of nature. But with the explosion of the power of our technology and the size of our population, our activities have grown to the proportion of geological forces, affecting the major systems of the planet. Short of the Atlantic washing away half of Florida, the abstract notion that the old anomalies have become the new norm is difficult to grasp. Dr. James McCarthy of Harvard, who has supervised the work of climate scientists from sixty nations, puts it this way: "If the last 150 years had been marked by the kind of climate instability we are now seeing, the world would never have been able to support its present population of 5 billion people." We live in a world of man-size urgencies, measured in hours or days. What unfolds slowly is not, by our lights, urgent, and it will therefore take a collective act of imagination to understand the extremity of the situation we now confront. The lag time in our planet's ecological systems will undoubtedly delay these decisions, and even if the nations of the world were to agree tomorrow on a plan to phase out oil and coal and convert to renewable energies, an equivalent lag time in human affairs would delay its implementation for years. What too many people refuse to understand is that the global economy's existence depends upon the global environment, not the other way around. One cannot negotiate jobs, development, or rates of economic growth with nature.

What of the standard list of palliatives —carbon taxes, more energy-efficient buildings, a revival of public transportation? The ideas are attractive, but the thinking is too small. Even were the United States to halve its own carbon dioxide contribution, this cutback would soon be overwhelmed by the coming development of industry and housing and schools in China and India and Mexico for all their billions of citizens. No solution can work that does not provide ample energy resources for the development of all the world's nations.

So here is an informal proposal—at best a starting point for a conversation—from one man who is not an expert. What if we turned the deserts of the world into electricity farms? Let the Middle East countries keep their oil royalties as solar royalties. What if the world mobilized around a ten-year project to phase out all fossil fuels, to develop renewable energy technologies, to extend those technologies to every corner of the world? What if, to minimize the conflict of so massive a dislocation, the world's energy companies were put in charge of the transition—answering only to an international regulatory body and an enforceable timetable? Grant them the same profit margins for solar electricity and hydrogen fuel they now receive for petroleum and coal. Give them the licenses for all renewable energy technologies. Assure them the same relative position in the world's economy they now enjoy at the end of the project.

Are these ideas mere dream? Perhaps, but here are historical reasons to have hope. Four years ago a significant fraction of humanity overturned its Communist system in a historical blink of an eye. Eight years ago the world's governments joined together in Montreal to regulate CFCs. Technology is not the issue. The atomic bomb was developed in two and a half years. Putting a man on the moon took eleven. Surely, given the same sense of urgency, we can develop new energy systems in ten years. Most of the technology is already available to us or soon will be. We have the knowledge, the energy, and the hunger for jobs to get it done. And we are different in one unmeasurable way from previous generations: ours is the first to be educated about the larger world by the global reach of electronic information.

The leaders of the oil and coal industry, along with their skeptical scientists, relentlessly accuse environmentalists of overstating the climatic threat to destroy capitalism. Must a transformation that is merely technological dislodge the keystone of the economic order? I don't know. But I do know that technology changes the way we conceive of the world. To transform our economy would oblige us to understand the limits of the planet. That understanding alone might seed the culture with a more organic concept of ourselves and our connectedness to the earth. And corporations, it is useful to remember, are not only obstacles on the road to the future. They are also crucibles of technology and organizing engines of production, the modern expression of mankind's drive for creativity. The industrialist is no less human than the poet, and both the climate scientist and the oil company operator inhabit the same planet, suffer the same short life span, harbor the same hopes for their children.

NOTES

1. In 1991, Western Fuels spent an estimated $250,000 to produce and distribute a video entitled "The Greening of Planet Earth," which was shown frequently inside the Bush White House as well as within the governments of OPEC. In near-evangelical tones, the video promises that a new age of agricultural abundance will result from increasing concentrations of carbon dioxide. It portrays a world where vast areas of desert are reclaimed by the carbon dioxide-forced growth of new grasslands, where the earth's diminishing forests are replenished by a nurturing atmosphere. Unfortunately, it overlooks the bugs. Experts note that even a minor elevation in temperature would trigger an explosion in the planet's insect population, leading to potentially significant disruptions in food supplies from crop damage as well as to a surge in insect-borne diseases. It appears that Western Fuels' video fails to tell people what the termites in New Orleans may be trying to tell them now.

2. Contrary to his assertion, however, virtually all relevant researchers say the link between CFCs and ozone depletion is based on unassailably solid scientific evidence. As if to underscore the point, in May the research director of the European Union Commission estimated that last winter's ozone loss will result in about 80,000 additional cases of skin cancer in Europe. This fall, the three scientists who discovered the CFC-ozone link won the Nobel Prize for Chemistry.

NO

S. Fred Singer

DIRTY CLIMATE

When the 1992 UN Climate Treaty was signed in Rio de Janeiro, the U.S. Government refused to endorse a policy of mandating activities that would lead to reduced emissions of carbon dioxide (CO_2), the major anthropogenic greenhouse gas. Partly, this was because the goals of such activities were unclear: while the Treaty mentions stabilization of the quantity of greenhouse gases in the atmosphere at "non-dangerous levels" as a goal, what constitutes safe and dangerous levels is left unspecified. More importantly, there is a distinct lack of scientific consensus that global warming is in fact occurring.

However, at the July 1996 negotiations in Geneva, the State Department dramatically altered its position and called for *legally binding* targets and time-frames for reducing emissions of CO_2. A Department of Energy official, Dirk Forrister, insisted the Administration's policy switch does not call for any of the things rejected in 1992: new taxes, command-and-control regulations, fuel-economy targets for automobiles. The Senate Energy Committee held hearings this fall to learn just how, in that case, the Administration *did* plan to control energy consumption. It was unable to discover what schemes are afoot. But logically, since CO_2 comes mostly from the burning of fossil fuels, emission limits would have to restrict energy consumption—cutting the use of electric power, transportation, and heating, either by rationing or by taxes.

In the midst of the confusion over the Administration's policy switch, a surreptitious set of alterations of a key scientific document came to light. The changes and deletions gained wide attention with a June 12 essay in the *Wall Street Journal* by Dr. Frederick Seitz, former president of the U.S. National Academy of Sciences, president emeritus of the Rockefeller University, and recipient of the National Medal of Science. His claim that a "major corruption of the peer-review process" has taken place raised an international furor. Scientists on both sides of the controversy are spouting words like "scientific cleansing," "scurrilous" and "libelous."

Seitz's article revealed what had been known to only a few, namely that Chapter 8 of the scientific report on climate change issued by the UN-sponsored Intergovernmental Panel on Climate Change (IPCC) had been altered between its approval by government delegations in December 1995 and its printing in May 1996. Chapter 8 is crucial to the IPCC's major conclusion that "the balance of evidence suggests a discernible human influence on global climate."

Most scientists could probably swallow hard and accept this enigmatic phrase without compromising their reputations. Politicians, however, have understood this artful phrase to mean that a climate catastrophe is on its way: droughts and severe storms, continental flooding from rising sea levels, a spread of tropical diseases, and a tidal wave of environmental refugees from affected nations. Quite a frightening picture—and a perfect excuse for political action.

No one denies that alterations to Chapter 8, were made; its lead author, Dr. Benjamin Santer of the Lawrence Livermore National Laboratory in California, claims full responsibility. However, in a June 13 editorial, *Nature* disclosed the results of its own investigation; it contradicted Santer's story and reported hat the responsibility for the disputed changes lies with "IPCC officials."

In addition, we have now learned of the existence of a State Department letter, dated November 15, 1995, and addressed to Sir John Houghton, co-chairman of the IPCC. It says, *inter alia*, "it is essential that ... chapter authors be prevailed upon to modify their text in an appropriate manner."

The IPCC indignantly denies that "scientific cleansing" changed the sense of the report. But *Nature* concludes that "there is some evidence that the revision process did result in a subtle shift ... [that] tended to favor arguments that aligned with the report's broad conclusions." The *Nature* editorial further concedes that "phrases that might have been [mis]interpreted as undermining these conclusions ... have disappeared."

* * *

Particularly alarming to Dr. Seitz was the dropping of three passages from the report: "None of the studies cited above has shown clear evidence that we can attribute the observed [climate] changes to ... increases in greenhouse gases."

"No study to date has positively attributed all or part [of the climate change observed to date] to anthropogenic [man-made] causes."

"Any claims of positive detection of significant climate changes are likely to remain controversial until uncertainties in the total natural variability of the climate system are reduced."

Clearly, these statements cast serious doubt on the IPCC conclusion, which might explain why they were eliminated. But Dr. Santer has a more benign explanation, quoted by the journal *Science* (July 15): He made the changes because they "fine-tuned the wording to bring the report into line with the *scientific* consensus" (emphasis added) and because "reviewers requested them." Dr. Santer declines to specify who the reviewers were, which review comments were accepted, and which rejected—and on what basis.

IPCC officials quoted by *Nature* have an even more interesting story; they claim that the reason for the revisions to the report was "to ensure that it conformed to a policymakers' summary," a short document drafted by the IPCC leadership and hammered out as a *political* consensus of government delegations. This IPCC claim raises the obvious question: Shouldn't the Summary conform to the underlying scientific report rather than vice versa?

The real reason for the text changes may have been to back up the Summary's rather feeble conclusion about a possible human influence on climate. There is precious little in the Summary that would lead one to believe that global warming is happening now or that predictions of future warming can be trusted.

At that, the Summary is quite selective in the facts it presents. For example, it does not even mention the existence of 18 years of weather-satellite data that show a current global-cooling trend and contradict all theoretical models of climate warming. The IPCC blithely presents its conclusions as a "scientific consensus" of hundreds, if not thousands, of scientists. Those who disagree are marginalized as a "dwindling band of skeptics" or as a "tiny minority of dissidents" who view global warming (in Vice President Gore's words) as the "empirical equivalent of the Easter Bunny."

* * *

The tendency of promoters of the global-warming hypothesis to equate any criticism of the IPCC officials and of the report with an attack on science itself is beginning to create serious splints within the scientific community. In 1992 more than four thousand scientists signed the strongly worded Heidelberg Appeal to urge statesmen to go slow on climate-change policies that lack a proper scientific basis. More recently, nearly a hundred climate scientists have refuted the IPCC conclusions in the Leipzig Declaration, which grew out of a conference held in November 1995. The Declaration strongly challenges the notion that a "scientific consensus" predicts climate catastrophes, and condemns the 1992 Treaty as unrealistic and fraught with economic danger.

It is probably no coincidence that the signers include many well-established senior scientists who do not depend exclusively on federal funding. With billions of dollars of federal research money being spent on climate change, many scientists have developed a financial stake in adopting an alarmist attitude about global warming.

In spite of contrary evidence, the IPCC report's co-editor Sir John Houghton claims "serious impacts on human habitats and society" from a potential global warming and urges policy-makers to set fixed targets to reduce greenhouse-gas emissions. Not mentioned is the fact that stabilization at the present level of atmospheric carbon dioxide would require a reduction of emissions by 60 to 80 per cent, according to the IPCC's own studies. This translates into crippling reductions of energy use that could hardly be achieved simply through "aggressive efficiency measures," as Houghton claims.

Houghton's boss, British environmental minister John Gummer, goes even further, saying that "action by the international community is now urgent." He wants developed countries to reduce emissions by over 50 per cent, with 5 to 10 per cent reductions by the year 2010 "as a first step in the process." But even Gummer's unrealistic targets were not radical enough to satisfy some environmental activists. Friends of the Earth termed his attitude as "complacent in the extreme."

The global-warming zealots are leaving no stone unturned—they are even courting corporations. They are working hard on the insurance industry, arguing that rates need to be raised in view of impending disasters. (Ironically, one of the findings of the IPCC report is that the frequency of hurricanes has been decreasing over the past fifty years.) Of course, if insurance companies thought they could raise rates with impunity, they would presumably have done so long ago—with or without global warming.

But international organizations need to frighten the public in order to raise funds. The same holds true for UN bureaucrats who have built up sizable fiefdoms and are engaged in a continuous round of meetings, workshops, and other negotiations in resort locations around the world. The foreign-affairs departments of the approximately 150 nations adhering to the Treaty often see benefits from such negotiations, particularly if they lead to further treaties that establish international laws or controls, enhancing budgets and prestige.

It is not surprising, therefore, that as old predictions of catastrophe fail to materalize, these organizations keep coming up with new ones. Early on, it was rising sea levels, a scare the public largely ignored. Then it was announced that 1995 was the hottest year since temperature records were established (December and its blizzards were conveniently omitted from the temperature calculations). The current scare is about the spread of tropical diseases: global warming is supposed to increase the range of malaria-carrying mosquitoes.

The Clinton Administration's surprising about-face in Geneva is sure to raise hackles because it is likely to require the imposition of large energy taxes. The American public has already registered its opposition to energy taxes, whether a BTU tax or a carbon tax. Even a modest increase in the gasoline tax met with strong resistance from voters. An internationally mandated tax would fuel even greater resentment.

On July 10, a stern letter to President Clinton, signed by Frank Murkowski (Alaska) and seven other Senate Republicans, expressed dismay about the Climate Treaty negotiations. The senators surged Clinton to resist efforts to set "binding targets and time-frames" on energy use. They pointed out that the existing level of scientific certainty is not high enough to justify hasty actions that would damage the nation's economy. Independently, Bennett Johnston (La.) and five other Senate Democrats, in a July 17 letter to the White House, slammed proposals for mandatory emission reductions and warned Clinton that treaty amendments might not receive the consent of the Senate.

The senators are in tune with the growing number of scientists who view the IPCC findings with skepticism and the alteration of scientific documents with alarm. The Senate, however, can do much more; it can exercise the option under Treaty Article 25 and withdraw from the UN Climate Convention. In the absence of scientific evidence for a global-warming catastrophe, there is no reason to maintain a treaty which, if implemented rigorously, would lead to a world economic disaster.

POSTSCRIPT

Public Policy and Health: Is Global Warming a Real Threat?

Geochemist Wallace S. Broecker of Columbia University claimed in 1987 that "The inhabitants of Planet Earth are quietly conducting a gigantic environmental experiment. So vast and so sweeping will be the impacts of this experiment that, were it brought before any responsible council for approval, it would be firmly rejected as having potentially dangerous consequences. Yet, the experiment goes on with no significant interference from any jurisdiction or nation. The experiment in question is the release of carbon dioxide and other so-called greenhouse gases to the atmosphere." The vast majority of researchers agree with Broecker, but in 1991 the Science and Environmental Policy Project circulated a statement to over 300 atmospheric scientists in the United States. Approximately 50 have signed this statement, which states that policies to tax fossil fuels and environmental regulations are based on unsupported assumptions that catastrophic global warming is caused by the burning of fossil fuels. The scientists who signed the statement also claimed that the theoretical climate models used to predict a future warming trend are not valid.

There is obvious disagreement among scientists about the risks of global warming, or even if there is a problem, and some researchers believe that global warming will actually benefit the environment. They claim that longer growing seasons would be beneficial to crops and that humans would be able to live in greater numbers in arctic areas. They argue that the United States should not make major policy changes regarding fossil fuel emissions and taxation before all the data are available. Other scientists claim that if we wait until all available information is processed, it may be too late. Articles that support this viewpoint include the following: "Can We Stop Global Warming," *USA Today Magazine* (March 1997); "Stormy Weather," *Rolling Stone* (March 20, 1997); and "Global Warming—A Reality," *Natural Life* (November 1996). "Global Warming May Cause Epidemics," *Malaria Weekly* (January 6, 1997) supports the theory that as the Earth's temperature rises, vector-borne diseases such as dengue fever will move north.

Readings that deny problems associated with global warming include "It's Time to Reconsider Global Climate Change Policy," *USA Today Magazine* (March 1997); "Global Warming Chills Out," *National Review* (March 24, 1997); and "Warming Theories Need Warning Label," *Bulletin of the Atomic Scientists* (June 1992).

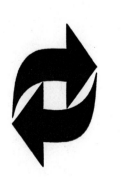

On the Internet . . .

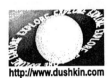

http://www.dushkin.com

Homeopathy Home Page

The homeopathy home page is a jumping-off point that provides links to available resources related to homeopathy. The site includes FAQs, discussion groups, and a reference library on homeopathy and alternative medicine.
http://www.dungeon.com/~cam/homeo.html

Babycare Corner

Family Internet: Babycare Corner presents a collection of information related to the care of babies and children. It contains special topics, including health risks, immunizations, and other issues related to the health of infants and children.
http://www.familyinternet.com/babycare/babycare.htm

Holistic Internet Resources

Holistic Internet Resources lists events, articles, and book reviews related to holistic health. It also identifies practitioners and schools of holistic health.
http://www.hir.com/

PART 6

Consumer Health and Nutrition Decisions

A shift is occurring in medical care toward informed self-care. People are starting to reclaim their autonomy, and the relationship between doctor and patient is changing. Many patients are asking more questions of their doctors, considering a wider range of medical options, and becoming more educated about what determines their health. Although most physicians support dietary changes and moderate exercise, critics claim that many people who follow diet and nutrition fads may actually develop nutritional deficiencies or a dieting mind-set and increase their risk of physical complications from dieting itself. Some individuals are rejecting traditional medicine altogether and seeking alternative health providers, while others are rejecting only some aspects of traditional medicine such as immunizations. This section debates some of the choices consumers may make regarding their health care.

■ Is Yo-Yo Dieting Dangerous?

■ Should All Children Be Immunized Against Childhood Diseases?

■ Are Homeopathic Remedies Legitimate?

ISSUE 17

Is Yo-Yo Dieting Dangerous?

YES: Frances M. Berg, from *Health Risks of Weight Loss*, 3rd ed. (*Healthy Weight Journal*, 1995)

NO: Editors of Harvard Heart Letter, from *Harvard Heart Letter* (February 1995)

ISSUE SUMMARY

YES: Nutritionist Frances M. Berg contends that yo-yo dieting, or weight cycling, is associated with an elevated risk of physical and mental health problems and that it increases the risk of regaining lost weight.

NO: The editors of the *Harvard Heart Letter* claim that there is no convincing evidence that weight cycling has any major effects on heart disease risk, the effectiveness of future diets, increased percentage of body fat, or metabolism.

Dieting has become a way of life for many people; close to 50 million Americans are currently dieting. But most will not lose as much weight as they want, and most will not keep off the weight they have lost. So why are so many Americans dieting?

Obesity has become widespread in the United States: 30 percent of the population is considered obese, up from 25 percent 10 years ago. Obesity has been linked with increased risks for certain diseases, including diabetes, heart disease, and some cancers. In addition, there are social and economic implications related to obesity. Many contend that overweight people are less likely to marry, earn less money, and are less likely to be accepted to elite colleges. As a result, more and more people are dieting.

It has been shown that most diets fail. Often, after lost weight is regained, dieters start over again and end up caught in a repeated lose/gain cycle known as "yo-yo dieting" or "weight cycling." Yo-yo dieting is considered by experts to be more dangerous than actually being overweight, and many urge overweight individuals to stop dieting and accept themselves as they are. Some theories as to why yo-yo dieting may be unsafe are that yo-yo dieting lowers metabolic rate, or the rate at which calories are burned; that yo-yo dieting increases the percentage of stored fat and reduces lean muscle tissue; that a lowered metabolic rate and an increase in fat stores can make subsequent dieting more difficult; and that yo-yo dieting may increase one's desire for fatty foods.

Frequent dieting has also been linked with psychological concerns. Some studies have reported a lower level of life satisfaction among weight cyclers.

There is also some evidence that frequent dieting may predispose an individual to disordered eating, including binge eating, or compulsive overeating. Research also indicates that among all dieters, both obese and of normal weight, anxiety, depression, and stress are associated with the up-and-down weight cycling that accompanies frequent dieting. These studies conclude that those who maintain a stable weight are better off psychologically, regardless of what they weigh.

Researchers have discerned a relationship between yo-yo dieting and an increased risk of heart disease based on findings from the Framingham Heart Study, a 30-year analysis of weight fluctuations in over 3,000 adults. They claim that weight cycling may be related to increased deaths from heart disease due to changes in cholesterol levels, distribution of body fat, and fat preference associated with yo-yo dieting. The study indicated that weight gain or loss in a short period of time increases the risk of a person's dying from heart disease.

Since evidence suggests that most diets fail and that many actually increase the risk of subsequent failure in dieting, is it safer to remain overweight than to try to lose weight? Recent research shows that it *is* more dangerous to remain overweight than to try to lose extra pounds. On the other hand, there is no evidence that *all* diets fail. Some people do lose and maintain weight, although the numbers and dieting methods are unclear. There are also important medical benefits associated with even modest weight loss, including improvements in blood pressure, blood fats (cholesterol), and blood sugar control.

In the following selections, Frances M. Berg asserts that dieting, especially yo-yo dieting, is more dangerous than being overweight. She maintains that people with a history of weight cycling have shown increased stress levels —even those who gained and lost as little as five pounds. The editors of the *Harvard Heart Letter* argue that among obese individuals, the benefits of even moderate weight loss are significantly greater than any risks associated with dieting.

YES

Frances M. Berg

WEIGHT CYCLING

The possible risks of repeated bouts of losing and regaining weight, called weight cycling or yo-yo dieting, have gained wide attention in the public press. And for good reason: if weight cycling is harmful and is the almost inevitable result of weight loss, then perhaps weight loss itself is harmful and weight loss an inappropriate goal even for large patients, placing more importance on prevention.

This possibility has major implications for the $30 to $50 billion weight loss industry and for the focus of health care in the United States.

Weight cycling has been under intense investigation at several institutions in the U.S. and other countries since 1986, following studies that suggested losing weight on a very low calorie diet and regaining that weight made subsequent weight loss more difficult.

However, research has shown inconsistent results on several issues. This has led some researchers to conclude weight cycling is not important. Others believe the variables have not yet been found which affect weight cycling changes—perhaps certain subgroups are more likely to be affected, or individuals are more vulnerable at times in their lives, such as during pregnancy.

The Diet and Health report of the National Academy of Sciences notes the possible detrimental effects of weight cycling. Similarly, the Surgeon General's Report on Nutrition and Health recommends that "the health consequences of repeated cycles of weight loss and gain" be given "special priority," and a poll of obesity experts lists weight cycling as one of the key causes of obesity.

There is little doubt that weight cycling is extremely prevalent in the U.S. Sixty to 80 million people are trying to lose weight, and most of those who lose weight apparently regain it fairly quickly.

In a review of weight cycling research, Kelly Brownell and Judith Rodin cite a six-year study which tracked the weight of 153 middle-aged adults and found the women lost an average of 27 pounds and gained 31 pounds during the six years. The men lost and gained an average of more than 22 pounds. For the women, this was a gain of 21 percent of their initial body weight, and a loss of 19 percent. For the men it was about 12 percent lost and gained.

Another study tracked 332 overweight persons and found the vast majority either lost or gained significant amounts of weight.

Weight cycling research focuses on two major issues:

1. Is weight cycling associated with increased risk to physical or mental health?
2. Does weight cycling make weight management more difficult by invoking survival mechanisms?

Major concerns have been raised that cycles of weight variability increase risk factors and the risk of mortality, especially cardiovascular deaths. Other concerns are that weight cycling may lower metabolic rate, decrease the ability to lose weight, increase the body's fat-to-lean ratio and waist-hip ratio, and increase the appetite for dietary fat.

CYCLING MAY THREATEN HEART

Research consistently shows an increase in mortality from all causes and from coronary heart disease with weight cycling.

Weight cycling is associated with greater risks for coronary heart disease and other severe health problems in a major study published recently in the *New England Journal of Medicine* by L. Lissner and colleagues.

The findings are based on a 32-year analysis of weight fluctuations in 3,130 men and women in the Framingham Heart Study.

Individuals with a high weight variability—many weight changes or large changes—were 25 to 100 percent more likely to be victims of heart disease and premature death than those whose weight remained stable. They had increased total mortality, and increased mortality and morbidity due to coronary heart disease.

The relative risk for a high degree of weight variability compared with 1.0 for a low degree of variability is as follows:

Men

Total mortality 1.30

Mortality due to CHD 1.48

Morbidity due to CHD 1.48

Morbidity due to cancer 1.04

Women

Total mortality 1.27

Mortality due to CHD 1.47

Morbidity due to CHD 1.42

Morbidity due to cancer 1.16

These results seemed to hold true regardless of the individual's initial weight, long-term weight trend and/or cardiovascular risk factors such as blood pressure, cholesterol level, glucose tolerance, smoking and physical activity.

Even though nearly 50 percent of women who diet are not overweight, the researchers note, the weight cycling risks are seen at all weight categories, whether thin or obese.

The degree of weight variability was evaluated in relation to total mortality, mortality from coronary heart disease, morbidity due to coronary heart disease and morbidity due to cancer. Risks were considerably increased for all except cancer, which did not differ significantly.

When age groups were considered separately, weight fluctuation was most strongly associated with adverse health outcomes in the youngest group (age 30 to 40). This is also the group seen as most likely to diet.

The researchers found that a person's weight at age 25 makes an important contribution to whether there will be great variability.

Both men and women gained weight at an average rate of .11 kg per square meter per year.

Researchers from Goteborg, Sweden, and Boston University are involved in the current study. They cite their research in Sweden which found large fluctuations in body weight, measured at three intervals, was associated with heart disease in men and total mortality in both men and women.

In an effort to control for weight changes that may have been caused by illness, diseases and deaths for the first four years were excluded. This study does not distinguish between several weight changes and a single large weight change.

The researchers say weight cycling may account for the observed increase in deaths in these ways:

1. Factors that influence coronary risk (such as cholesterol levels) may change with fluctuating weight and end up worse than before.

2. The amount and distribution of body fat as weight is lost and regained may change. During weight loss, a person loses both fat and lean body mass, but may regain mostly fat. This fat tends to settle in the abdomen, a location linked to increased heart disease risk.

3. People may increasingly prefer high-fat diets when they lose and re-gain weight. Studies have shown that weight-cycling laboratory animals tend to eat more fat.

In view of their findings, they suggest it may be important to look at public health implications of current weight loss practices. They note that about half of American women and one-fourth of men are dieting at any one time, with many of these efforts unsuccessful. Weight is commonly regained and the cycle repeated.

Kelly Brownell, PhD, a psychologist and weight specialist at Yale University involved in the study, says the harmful effects of weight cycling may be equal to the risks of remaining obese.

"The pressure in this society to be thin at all costs may be exacting a serious toll," Brownell says. The study's findings indicate that weight cycling is "potentially a very serious public health issue" because it affects such large numbers of people.

"It may be equally bad to lose the same five pounds 10 times as to lose 50 pounds and regain it once," he said.

The relative risk of increased risk with weight fluctuation is in the range of 1.25 to 2.00, which is similar to the risk attributed to obesity and to several of the cardiovascular risk factors, say Brownell and Rodin. Thus, determining weight cycling effects is an important question.

HARVARD ALUMS RISK DISEASE BY "ALWAYS" DIETING

Men risk heart disease, hypertension and diabetes by 'always' dieting, regardless of their weight, according to the Harvard Alumni studies reported by Steven N. Blair, an epidemiologist at the Cooper Institute for Aerobics Research in Dallas.

"One of the fundamental tenets of the weight loss industry is if you get people to eat less, they'll lose weight. And if they lose weight, they'll be better off. And there is no evidence to support either one," Blair said at the American Heart Association's annual epidemiology meeting in March 1994.

Earlier, Blair reported higher mortality with weight loss among the Harvard alumni. His latest report investigates non-fatal disease in 12,025 men, average age 67. The men who said they were always dieting had a heart disease rate of 23.2 percent, compared to 10.6 for those who "never" dieted. Their rates for hypertension were 38.3 percent, compared with 23.4 percent for the group who never dieted, and for diabetes 14.6 percent, compared with 3 percent.

Among men who dieted part of the time—"often," "sometimes," or "rarely" —the more they dieted, the higher their rates of disease. These findings held true even among the leanest group of men, and were basically unchanged by weight gain, physical activity, smoking or alcohol intake.

In addition to reporting dieting frequency, the men identified their shape variation at six points through life, total pounds lost, and the number of times they had lost 5, 10, 20 and 30 or more pounds.

In view of his findings, Blair advises people to keep a stable weight and avoid either weight gain or weight loss.

BONE LOSS WITH WEIGHT LOSS

Several studies of large population bases show higher mortality rates with weight loss, causing researchers to puzzle over the possible mechanisms whereby weight loss could cause long-term harm, even though it seems beneficial in reducing obesity-related risk factors in short-term studies.

One possible mechanism may be the bone mineral loss which accompanies weight loss. Weight cycling may increase this loss.

Mineral content in women's bones diminishes with weight loss, even when adequate nutrition and aerobic exercise are present. These findings from the USDA Human Research Center in Grand Forks, N.D., support clues which may explain recent findings in federal studies of potentially higher mortality with weight loss. The Grand Forks Center tested 14 women, age 21–38, in a five-month residential program using dual energy x-ray absorptiometry (DXA) to assess bone mineral status and soft tissue composition. The women lost 8.1 kg on a moderate nutrient-adequate diet with an aerobic exercise program. Both bone mineral content and bone mineral density decreased (36 g and .01 g/cm2 respectively).

Similar results were found at the Osteoporosis Research Centre in Copenhagen, Denmark. Using the DXA method, the study reports 51 obese patients averaged a 5.9 percent loss of total body bone mineral/TBBM during 15 weeks. One patient, who lost 45 kg, lost 754 g bone mineral in nine months. Greater mineral loss was reported in legs than arms. Postmenopausal women who did not get estrogen replacement tended to lose more bone mineral. Bone mineral loss correlated with body fat loss, not with fat-free mass loss, so that as more fat was lost, more mineral was lost as well.

When patients maintained their weight loss, they lost no more bone. If they regained, bone was regained as well. The Danish researchers concluded this level of bone loss was normal for weight loss in obese persons. They suggest an initiating factor in bone loss may be having less weight bearing on the bones.

WEIGHT CYCLING DROPS METABOLISM FOR WRESTLERS

Weight cycling is practiced with single-minded dedication by many high school and college athletes in the sport of wrestling.

Not only must the elite wrestler be talented, fit and superbly trained, but usually he is also actively engaged in weight reduction, even in the lower weight classes of 103 and 112 pounds.

The weight-cycling wrestler commonly loses 10 or more pounds in a few days to make weigh-ins for a match or tournament. He regains this weight quickly, and repeats the cycle many times throughout the wrestling season. Severe water deprivation and dehydration are often a part of his fasting episodes.

Long term effects of such strenuous weight loss efforts on the young wrestler are unknown.

Cold intolerance, weakness, and inability to concentrate are frequently reported. Other reported effects include changes in electrolyte balance, testosterone levels, nutritional status, renal function, thermal regulation, body composition and strength.

Growth and development may be delayed during one of the most active growth periods of a young man's life. The possibility of developing long-lasting eating disorders has been suggested.

FOOD EFFICIENCY

Metabolic effects of this severe weight cycling may cause an increase in food efficiency, and make losing more difficult.

Recent research with high school wrestlers on loss-and-gain cycles gives evidence of a lowered metabolism, as reported in the *Journal of the American Medical Association*.

The wrestlers were attending summer camp at the University of Iowa. It was several months after their last competitive match, and their weight had returned to normal.

The group of 27 wrestlers who cycled their weight were found to have significantly lower resting metabolic rate per unit of lean body mass than those defined as noncyclers.

Weight cyclers were defined as those who:

1. Cut weight 10 or more times during wrestling season.
2. Lost 4.5 kg or more weekly.
3. Reported they cut weight often or always.

(box continued on next page)

Noncyclers

1. Cut weight less than 5 times during the season.
2. Lost no more than 1.4 kg weekly.
3. Reported they cut weight sometimes, rarely or never.

Noncyclers were matched for age, weight, height, surface area, lean body mass, and percent body fat.

The cyclers competed farther below their natural off-season weight than did the noncyclers.

Results showed a significant difference in resting metabolic rate between the cyclers and noncyclers. The difference in resting energy expenditure was 14 percent. Oxygen consumption differed significantly. No differences were shown in respiratory quotient, oral temperature, pulse or blood pressure.

STUDIES NEEDED

The researchers suggest weight cycling was a likely cause of lower metabolic rates, although they grant it is possible that low metabolism came first and even made the severe cycling necessary, as wrestlers with low energy requirements could have had more difficulty controlling weight. They recommended longitudinal studies be conducted to assess any health changes resulting from weight restriction and fluctuation.

Although the body fat for both groups of wrestlers in this study is similar, an increase of fat over lean has been noted during fast weight regain, and a redistribution of fat is suggested as possible. Research is cited that shows increased preference for fat in the diet among weight cycling female rats.

The researchers speculate there may be psychological implications of repeated weight cycling, including frustration over the increasing difficulty in losing weight, which could lead to unhealthy methods of weight loss.

The high school or college wrestler differs from the typical weight cycler in the general population in that he is young, male, physically active, well-muscled, with low body fat. His diet and binge cycle is relatively short, usually lasting about three months a year for perhaps three to six years.

Psychologically, as a successful athlete, he is likely to have high self-esteem and strong social support.

Strong statements against excessive weight loss and the fluid and food deprivation practices often used by wrestlers have been issued by the American College of Sports Medicine and the American Medical Association.

Hank Lukaski, director of the Grand Forks Center, says people have the potential to regain some bone loss when they regain weight. But it is unknown whether bone mineral content and bone density are fully or only partially restored, or whether bone quality is as good as before, or how essential trace elements are affected. Further, the effect on bone quality of repeated bouts of weight loss and regain are unknown, Lukaski says.

WEIGHT CYCLING INCREASES STRESS

People with a history of weight cycling showed greater pathologic characteristics than those with stable weights, independent of weight, in recent research by John Foreyt, PhD, of Baylor College of Medicine, Houston, TX, and colleagues at Yale and the University of Nevada. The researchers suggest that weight cycling may be causal to the mental distress and pathology they found.

Men and women whose weight fluctuated up or down, as little as five pounds in a year, reported lower feelings of well-being, more out-of-control eating, and higher stress levels than people whose weight was stable in this study. And this was true regardless of their body weight.

The researchers say they did not expect such a large number of significant findings with the tight five-pound categories: "Psychologically, such small shifts in weight in both normal weight and obese individuals may be very important."

In obese women, weight maintenance was associated with fewer significant negative life stressors.

Weight fluctuation was strongly associated with negative psychological effects in both normal weight and obese individuals. Weight change and obesity were also associated with a poorer psychological score.

The researchers studied 497 adults, stratified into five age groups, 25 normal weight and 25 obese in each age and sex category.

The subjects were assessed twice with the Brownell Weight Cycling Questionnaire, which measures current dieting, weight satisfaction, abnormal eating patterns and body image. They reported on health, weight fluctuation, feelings of well-being and depression, stressful life events, and eating self-efficacy (ability to control urges to overeat in high-risk situations). Their weight was assessed over one year to classify them, through a weight change of 5 pounds or more, as maintainers, gainers or losers.

The researchers suggest that attempts at weight loss may be stressful for various reasons, including the self-denial required, the disruption of routine, and a concern about failure. Repeated failures to control weight may reduce one's feeling of self-efficacy, and add to feelings of depression.

"Once inappropriate dieting is initiated, regardless of body weight, fluctuations and increasing obesity may follow," says their report. They cite research that shows that among obese individuals, more than half fluctuate up or down 12 pounds over intervals of 1 to 5 years.

While the researchers suggest that weight change likely causes these adverse effects, they grant the reverse is possible—psychological distress may cause weight change. They recommend further research on assessing and treating weight fluctuation for individuals of all weights.

Weight cycling appears consistently linked to increased psychopathology, lower life satisfaction, more disturbed eating in general, and perhaps increased risk for binge eating in the research, Brownell and Rodin report.

They cite research by Everson and Matthews that found lower levels of life satisfaction related to increased weight cycling in women, but not men. A study of a large sample of runners found weight cycling associated with higher levels of disturbed eating practices. Other studies show repeated or chronic dieting may predispose an individual to disordered eating, including binge eating. One study showed restrained eating (dieting) to be a stronger predictor of weight fluctuation than body weight itself.

FINDINGS STIR CONTROVERSY

The recent findings are likely to be controversial and to further fuel the weight cycling debate among scientists, says Claude Bouchard, PhD, of Laval University, Quebec, in an editorial in the same issue of the *New England Journal of Medicine* as the Lissner study.

Bouchard notes that a recent review of 18 studies of weight cycling in rodents, by Hill and Reed, found no clear evidence that weight cycling makes future weight loss harder and weight gain easier.

They found no evidence that weight cycling increases total body fat or central adiposity, increases subsequent caloric intake, increases food efficiency, decreases energy expenditure, or increases blood pressure, insulin resistance, or cholesterol levels. However, Bouchard suggests there may be a preference for dietary fat in refeeding and that the observed risks could result from higher fat intake.

Rat studies may not provide the weight cycling information needed for humans and, given that human studies are difficult to design, this may be why weight cycling studies give such confusing and conflicting results, says Carolyn Berdanier, PhD, a researcher at the University of Georgia.

Berdanier says rats and mice differ from humans in several important ways. Most critically to weight cycling research, they continue to grow in length throughout their lives. This growth is expensive in calories, and affects the degree of body fat storage, keeping them leaner.

NO   Editors of *Harvard Heart Letter*

YO-YO DIETING REVISITED

Obesity is a well-established risk factor for several illnesses, including heart disease, stroke, diabetes, arthritis, and some cancers. To decrease their risk for these conditions—and to look and feel better—many Americans lose weight by dieting, exercise, and even by using medications. The problem is that after the weight-loss program is over, they often regain the lost weight.

The tendency to diet repeatedly, losing and regaining the same pounds over and over again, is often called "weight cycling" or "yo-yo dieting." Some medical researchers have been concerned that weight cycling might increase the risk of heart disease and other problems. These experts have raised the question of whether it is safer to remain overweight than to embark on repetitive cycles of weight loss if the weight is likely to be regained. Of course, neither of these options is as desirable as losing excess pounds and maintaining ideal weight.

No single study has settled this issue. However, a federally sponsored panel of experts, the National Task Force on the Prevention and Treatment of Obesity, recently did the next best thing. They carefully reviewed the available data and made reasonable recommendations. After examining 43 studies that had evaluated the effects of yo-yo dieting on humans and animals, the task force found no definitive evidence that weight cycling has long-term adverse effects on health.

EVIDENCE FOR AND AGAINST

The task force was strongly influenced by concern that fears about weight cycling might cause some overweight people to give up on weight loss without even trying. The experts did not dismiss studies that raised concerns about yo-yo dieting, but they emphasized the serious risks to health and life posed by obesity and concluded that the evidence linking variation in body weight with increased death and illness "is not sufficiently compelling to override the potential benefits of moderate weight loss in significantly obese patients."

Four of the studies reviewed by the task force had made a strong case against yo-yo dieting. These large population-based studies had found an association between marked changes in body weight and an increase in risk of death—both from all causes and from cardiovascular disease:

- The Gothenburg Prospective Study, with more than 6,000 participants, reported in 1989 that weight change was a risk factor for coronary heart disease in men and for total mortality in both men and women.
- The Western Electric Study, involving 1,877 men, indicated in 1989 that those individuals who experienced a large weight change were about twice as likely to die from heart disease as those whose weights were stable.
- The MRFIT (Multiple Risk Factor Intervention Trial) Cohort Study, in which researchers examined the records of 10,000 men, reported in 1993 that individuals whose weight varied by more than 5% had a 55% increased risk of death from coronary artery disease and an increase of about 50% in overall mortality.
- The Framingham Heart Study, a long-term study of 3,000 men and women, reported in 1991 that men who lost and regained 20–30 pounds over a two-year period faced as much as twice the risk of dying from heart disease as those whose weight remained reasonably constant; women had about one-and-a-half times the risk of heart disease and heart-related death if they lost and regained 15–20 pounds.

However, more recent analyses of data from the Framingham Study and other investigations indicate that only lean people who lose weight seem to be endangering their health. In addition, two smaller studies showed no relationship between weight cycling and the risk of death.

There are other reasons to question whether the worrisome findings from the larger investigations are relevant to the overweight person contemplating a diet. Most of these studies did not distinguish intentional from unintentional weight loss, and the one study that examined voluntary dieting did not find harmful effects. Therefore, experts strongly suspect that much or all of the increased mortality associated with weight change in these studies was due to medical problems that contributed both to weight loss and to premature death.

The task force suggested that if weight cycling is, in fact, deleterious to health, the negative effects may be limited to people who are not obese. The panel noted that most of the people in the population-based observational studies were either non-obese or only mildly obese and that, in two of the studies, increased mortality associated with body-weight variability occurred among the participants with the lowest weights.

WHEN IS A CYCLE A CYCLE?

Some of the confusion about the health effects of weight variations can be traced to uncertainty about the definition of weight cycling. The task force emphasized that future researchers should agree on several criteria: the number of cycles that constitute an official case of weight cycling; the duration and frequency of each cycle; the magnitude of weight change in each cycle; and the distinction between a loss followed by a gain, and a gain followed by a loss.

Other questions that require clarification: What are the psychological effects of repeated cycles of weight loss and gain? Do any detrimental effects of weight cycling on health occur immediately or years later? Is the effect of a cycle caused by intentional weight change the same as a cycle that occurs unintentionally? In which populations (if any) does cycling exert its deleterious effects—in women or men, normal-weight or obese individuals, or particular ethnic groups?

New research may someday permit a more sophisticated assessment of the effects of yo-yo dieting. However, given current knowledge, the Harvard Heart Letter editorial board agrees with the central point of the panel's report: Obese individuals should not allow concerns about the hazards of weight cycling to deter them from efforts to control their body weight.

Furthermore, individuals who have no excess body fat and no risk factors for obesity-related illness should not undertake weight-loss efforts. Instead, they should focus on the prevention of weight gain by engaging in regular physical activity, such as brisk walking, biking, jogging or swimming, and by consuming a healthful diet.

Such a diet should include no more than 10% of calories from saturated fat and trans-fatty acids, as well as plenty of fruits, vegetables, legumes, and grains. Finally, and most importantly, obese individuals who undertake weight-loss efforts must make a lifelong commitment to changing their behavior, diet, and physical activity.

POSTSCRIPT

Is Yo-Yo Dieting Dangerous?

The issue of dieting involves the public, health providers, the media, and the diet and food industry. Repeated (or yo-yo) dieting has been linked to several physical and mental health concerns. These include heart disease, premature death, increased fat stores, lowered metabolism, increased risk of subsequent diet failure, psychological stress, and a reduced sense of well-being. Yo-yo dieting has also been related to an increased risk of disordered eating, including binge eating. Obesity, however, is also linked to heart disease, a decreased sense of well-being, as well as many other physical and mental problems.

Many articles discuss the potential harm related to yo-yo dieting. In "Change in Body Weight and Longevity," *Journal of the American Medical Association* (October 21, 1992), researchers I-Min Lee and Ralph S. Paffenbarger Jr. report that individuals who cycle between being overweight and normal weight during their lifetime may die sooner than they would if they maintained a steady weight. Other articles concluding that it is more dangerous to diet than to remain overweight include "The Great Diet Deception," *USA Today Magazine* (January 1995); "Theories on Yo-Yo Dieting," *Tufts University Diet and Nutrition Letter* (December 1994).

Articles arguing that yo-yo dieting is not as harmful as previously thought and that it is better to keep trying to lose weight include "Coasting Downhill," *Prevention* (March 1995); "Yo-Yo Diets Aren't Risky After All," *Health* (January/February 1995); "Don't Let Fears of Yo-Yoing Stop Before You Start," *Environmental Nutrition* (December 1994); "Yo-Yo Diets May Beat No Diets at All," *U.S. News and World Report* (October 31, 1994); and "Weight Cycling Reviewed," *Obesity and Health* (January/February 1993).

For an overview of weight cycling, see "Medical, Metabolic, and Psychological Effects of Weight Cycling," *Archives of Internal Medicine* (June 27, 1994); "Weight Cycling: The Public Concern and the Scientific Data," *Obesity Research* (September 1993); and "Weight Cycling in Humans: A Review of the Literature," *Annals of Behavioral Medicine* (vol. 14, 1992).

While the experts are not in agreement over which is more harmful, yo-yo dieting or remaining overweight, there is further conflict regarding whether or not it is even possible—or advisable—to lose weight. For further information on dieting in general, see "Dying to Lose Weight," *Vogue* (May 1997); "Obesity: No Miracle Cure Yet," *Priorities* (vol. 8, 1996); "Gaining on Fat," *Scientific American* (August 1996); "New Study Questions Weight Guidelines," *Healthy Weight Journal* (March/April 1996); and "Dieting and Health: Is Dieting the Best Way to Lose Weight?" *CQ Researcher* (April 14, 1995).

ISSUE 18

Should All Children Be Immunized Against Childhood Diseases?

YES: Gary L. Freed, Samuel L. Katz and Sarah J. Clark, from "Safety of Vaccinations: Miss America, the Media, and Public Health," *The Journal of the American Medical Association* (December 18, 1996)

NO: Richard Leviton, from "Who Calls the Shots?" *East West: The Journal of Natural Health and Living* (November 1988)

ISSUE SUMMARY

YES: Physicians Gary L. Freed and Samuel L. Katz and epidemiologist Sarah J. Clark maintain that the benefits of vaccination substantially outweigh the risks and that childhood vaccination has significantly reduced the incidence of many common childhood infections.

NO: Health journalist Richard Leviton maintains that many vaccines are neither safe nor effective and that parents should have a say in whether or not their children receive them.

A number of infectious diseases are almost completely preventable through routine childhood immunizations. These diseases include diphtheria, meningitis, pertussis (whooping cough), tetanus, polio, measles, mumps, and rubella (German measles). Largely as a result of widespread vaccination, these once-common diseases have become relatively rare. Before the introduction of the polio vaccine in 1955, epidemics of the paralyzing disease occurred each year. In 1952 a record 20,000 cases were diagnosed, as compared to the last outbreak in 1979, when only 10 paralytic cases were identified.

The incidence of measles, which can cause serious complications and death, has also declined considerably since the measles vaccine became available. In 1962 there were close to 500,000 cases in the United States, as compared to under 4,000 cases in late 1980. Measles still kills some children and causes permanent damage to others who have not been immunized. In some parts of the country, particularly in urban areas, measles epidemics rage among nonimmunized children of all ages, who pass the disease along to each other.

Unfortunately, measles is not the only disease making a comeback. In 1983 an outbreak of whooping cough in Oklahoma affected over 300 people. By 1988 nearly 3,000 cases nationwide had been diagnosed. Whooping cough is a serious and sometimes fatal disease, especially among young infants. Although the risks of whooping cough and other childhood diseases are serious, many children remain unimmunized. Currently between 37 percent and 56 percent of preschool children in the United States have not received the immunizations they need because their parents either cannot afford vaccination, are unaware of the dangers of childhood diseases, or believe that the risks of vaccination outweigh the benefits—the last of these reasons is the basis for this debate.

The whooping cough vaccine has been the subject of more concern than any other immunization. Although almost all of the 18 million doses administered each year cause little or no reaction, about 50 to 75 children who receive the vaccine suffer serious neurological injury, a few of which lead to death. Some consider this risk to be too high, but before the vaccine was available, nearly 8,000 children died annually from whooping cough. Still, many parents who are concerned about the dangers of the vaccine have chosen not to protect their children against the disease. In 1994 when the first deaf Miss America was chosen, the media erroneously reported that Heather Whitestone's deafness was caused by an adverse reaction to the DPT vaccine she had received as a child. Her pediatrician set the record straight, stating that the vaccination was not linked to her hearing loss.

In the following articles, Gary L. Freed, Samuel L. Katz, and Sarah J. Clark determine that there is a much greater risk to children if they are not immunized. They also claim that serious adverse reactions are very rare.

Richard Leviton asserts that many vaccines, particularly whooping cough, are not safe or effective and that parents must have a say in whether or not their children receive them.

YES
Gary L. Freed, Samuel L. Katz and Sarah J. Clark

SAFETY OF VACCINATIONS: MISS AMERICA, THE MEDIA, AND PUBLIC HEALTH

On September 17, 1994, Heather Whitestone was chosen as Miss America, the first ever with a disability. Her deafness has been the subject of much media attention. On September 16, 1994, the *Atlanta Constitution* ran a story in its front section about Whitestone stating, "At age 18 months, [she] almost died from an adverse reaction to a routine DPT (diphtheria, pertussis, tetanus) vaccination. It wiped out all but a tiny sliver of her hearing.[1] On September 18, the *New York Times* ran an Associated Press story in its first section stating "Miss Whitestone... lost her hearing at 18 months because of a reaction to a diphtheria-tetanus shot."[2] On September 19 the *New York Times* ran another story ascribing her deafness to a vaccination.[3] Not until September 26 did the *New York Times* publish a story stating that Whitestone's deafness was not due to a vaccination but actually resulted from *Haemophilus influenzae* type b meningitis, a disease now preventable by vaccination.[4] Unlike the previous news stories, this report, entitled "Revisiting Miss America's Story," appeared in the paper's second section.

Significant public concern regarding the safety of vaccines clearly exists.[5] Some of that concern arises from erroneous news reporting of adverse events allegedly due to immunization, as was the case with Heather Whitestone. Additional concern has been manifest by efforts from some parents, attorneys, and health care professionals to link childhood immunization to a number of neurologic conditions that first become evident in the early months of life. Although serious and permanent reactions to vaccines do occur, recent studies and rigorous review of previous research indicate the rarity of these events.[6]

Modern clinical reports concerning the safety of childhood vaccines date back almost 50 years, corresponding with the advent of the first large-scale immunization programs in the United States. A 1948 article in *Pediatrics*[7] described an encephalopathy following a pertussis vaccine. Because the per-

From Gary L. Freed, Samuel L. Katz and Sarah J. Clark, "Safety of Vaccinations: Miss America, the Media, and Public Health," *The Journal of the American Medical Association*, vol. 276, no. 23 (December 18, 1996), pp. 1869–1872. Copyright © 1996 by the American Medical Association. Reprinted by permission.

tussis vaccine is associated with mild or moderate fever (between 38° C and 40.5 ° C) in up to 50% of immunizations and less frequently with a high-pitched cry (1%) or seizures (<0.1%),[8] a seemingly natural connection was made with a broad range of neurologic conditions by those seeking answers to the etiology of previously unexplained neurologic disorders. Thus, the pertussis vaccine began to be identified with many neurologic conditions of childhood. Over time, numerous case reports and case series were published in the medical and lay literature, all struggling to answer the ultimate question posed by any rare event: how does a temporal association differ from a causal reaction?

Why did so many neurologic and other problems become anecdotally linked to vaccination? Why is there so much difficulty in separating causal from temporal relationships with regard to vaccine reactions? Like most complex questions, the answers are many and varied. Children receive the first doses of the primary immunization series at ages 2, 4, and 6 months. Therefore, at any time during the first 8 months of life, infants are within 2 months of having received a vaccine. By unfortunate coincidence, this is also the same time that many neurologic diseases (eg., white matter degenerative diseases, seizure disorders) show their first symptoms. These conditions all existed in the prevaccine era and, for the most part, were inexplicable. Although genetic predisposition explained an occasional condition, most cases seemed to occur at random. Parents naturally long for an explanation as to why their child, and not another, experiences a disease or disability. Often, the clinician has no definitive answer, leaving parents to grasp at any

action or event that may have been the cause.

Another understandable reason for a predisposition of fear regarding vaccines is that minor reactions to vaccines are common. Many children experience pain and swelling at the site of a diphtheria and tetanus toxoids and pertussis (DTP) injection; a significant number also have an elevation in temperature.[6,8,9] As such, parents may already be fearful of their child's potential reaction to a vaccine or may be more willing to assume that unrelated symptoms are an extension of the discomfort or fever noted earlier.

THE DATA ON ADVERSE REACTIONS

Just how dangerous is DTP vaccine? How do we know if the concerns are justified? From 1976 to 1989, more than 10 population-based studies were published. These studies were conducted to establish the incidence and actual risk of adverse neurologic outcomes following vaccination. A separate systematic review of the literature, published by Golden[10] in 1990, found that research did not support the existence of pertussis encephalopathy syndrome and suggests "that the neurological events after immunization are chance temporal associations of neurologic conditions that occur in the target age group, even in the absence of immunization." Golden concluded that the population-based studies did not prove a causal relationship between DTP vaccine and acute encephalopathy, and although there was clearly an increased risk of febrile convulsion after DTP immunization, there was no evidence that this produced brain injury or was the forerunner of epilepsy.[10]

Baraff and colleagues[11] conducted a long-term, follow-up study of 18 children who experienced convulsions or hypotonic-hyporesponsive episodes following DTP vaccination. After psychometric and neurologic evaluation these children were determined to be without significant neurologic deficit.

In 1991 the Institute of Medicine (IOM) published a comprehensive review of the existing scientific data on 22 adverse events anecdotally associated with DTP and measles-mumps-rubella (MMR) vaccines.[9] The IOM review found evidence consistent with a causal relationship with vaccination for only 3 of the 22 adverse events examined (acute encephalopathy and shock following DTP vaccination; chronic arthritis following rubella vaccination) and evidence indicating a causal relationship in 3 others (anaphylaxis and inconsolable crying following DTP vaccination; acute arthritis following rubella vaccination). Specifically, the report found insufficient evidence to indicate a causal relationship between DTP vaccine and chronic neurologic damage. A commentary by the authors of the IOM report states, "this finding should offer reassurance to health professionals, parents, and other persons concerned with the safety of the pertussis and rubella vaccines."[12]

A second IOM report, released in September 1994,[6] reviewed all available medical and scientific data, including published and unpublished individual case reports and controlled clinical trials of several childhood vaccines (excluding pertussis and rubella vaccines, the focus of the 1991 report). The IOM report reviewed and rejected a causal relationship for most conditions alleged to be a result of immunization. However, causal relationships were found for some reactions, including an increased risk of Guillain-Barré syndrome following oral polio vaccine[6,13,14] and brachial neuritis following tetanus toxoid vaccine.[15] Estimating the true risk of these reactions, though, was difficult due to the lack of controlled epidemiologic data. Overall, the risks were extraordinarily small, as the incidence of adverse reactions was very low despite the large number of children immunized during the last 40 years. For example, excess risk for brachial neuritis associated with tetanus toxoid vaccine was determined to range from 0.5 to 1.0 case per 100,000 vaccine recipients.[6]

The news media have assumed the task of warning the public about potential health risks. In light of the available scientific evidence on vaccines, the question for the media is how to report rare adverse events without distorting the public's perception of the true risk of adverse reaction on an individual basis. Otherwise, fear and misinformation will guide parents' decisions about immunizations for their children.

THE IMPACT OF LITIGATION

Claims of reactions to childhood immunization became a legal and economic issue in the mid 1970s with the emergence of malpractice and product liability lawsuits for presumed injury from DTP vaccine.[16] Damages were assessed and awards were granted through the legal system despite a lack of true epidemiologic, pathologic, or physiologic evidence linking specific vaccines to specific adverse outcomes. Temporal relationships presuming cause and effect were often considered sufficiently convincing in court to warrant large monetary awards. As was demonstrated in later studies, these temporal relationships lacked cause-and-effect evidence and were often subject to methodological flaws (eg, confounding and selection bias). Regardless, damage awards became accepted for a host of neurologic conditions. The proof of actual causality became irrelevant to the legal process.[17]

Vaccine injury litigation became a growth industry in the late 1970s and early 1980s as attorneys rushed to enter the market. In 1978 only 2 suits related to DTP vaccine were filed; by 1986 more than 250 suits were being brought annually.[18] The average amount sought per claim also increased, from $10 million in 1978 to $46 million in 1984.[18] By 1985, the total amount sought through litigation was $3.162 billion, an amount more than 30 times greater than the market value of all DTP vaccine sold in the private sector that year.[19] Juries awarded more than $3.7 million in only 2 cases, and several more were settled out of court for undisclosed amounts.[20] Direct advertisements from lawyers to parents of neurologically impaired children began to appear on television, billboards, classified telephone directories, newspapers, magazines, and other venues. Left behind in this assault on the vaccines, on the health professionals who administered them, and on the manufacturers who produced them was the quest to determine the presence of an actual causal relationship between many of the alleged damages and the vaccines themselves.[20]

The litigious climate and the prospect of a never-ending stream of lawsuits drove 2 of the last 3 manufacturers of DTP vaccine from the market during the late 1970s and early 1980s.[20,21] Shortages of DTP vaccine followed as the remaining manufacturer did not have sufficient inventory to meet demand when a production problem occurred. Although

Newsweek covered the shortage, it was done without the alarm and level of concern devoted to adverse reactions.[22] One article appearing in the *National Law Journal* included plaintiff attorneys' assertions that the "alleged DTP shortage is a ploy by drug manufacturers to avoid paying damages for a product that the companies knew was less safe than they led the public to believe."[20]

In response to this growing problem, Congress established the National Vaccine Injury Compensation Program in 1986.[23] The program was designed to serve as a no-fault insurance fund to compensate for actual vaccine-related injuries.[24]

The National Vaccine Injury Compensation Program developed a specific vaccine injury table that lists conditions allowable for compensation. Unfortunately, the original vaccine injury table helped to perpetuate certain myths and misperceptions regarding vaccine reactions. For example, even though there were no accepted scientific data to indicate a causal relationship between DTP vaccine and chronic neurologic damage, the vaccine injury table included the clause "may result in permanent impairment"[25] as part of the definition of encephalopathy, a condition for which compensation is provided. Therefore, in a legal sense, the vaccine injury table legitimized a condition not grounded in accepted scientific data.[24] The 1991 IOM report does not support this definition of encephalopathy. In 1995, changes were made in the vaccine injury table to correct this problem.[26]

INVOLVEMENT OF THE NEWS MEDIA

For many years, questions about vaccine reactions were limited to medical journals. However, case reports, damage awards, and attorney advertisements received increasing publicity in the major news media throughout the 1970s. The first significant investigative effort by the news media was a 1982 television special, "DTP: Vaccine Roulette."[27] This program aired 3 times on a local Washington, DC, station and was excerpted on NBC's "Today Show." It featured statements by a former US Food and Drug Administration employee and a British neurologist, both of whom alleged that vaccines caused serious neurologic disorders. The program's host reporter then queried employees of the Centers for Disease Control (CDC) and other officials from the Food and Drug Administration on whether information about the dangers of vaccines was being withheld from the public. Interspersed throughout the program were interviews of families who claimed their children suffered serious neurologic injury as a result of pertussis vaccine. The cases were retrospective reviews, some with damages allegedly occurring more than 15 years previously. Even though no sound epidemiologic evidence for most of these claims existed at the time, the emotional effect of showing impaired children was dramatic.

"DTP: Vaccine Roulette" received an Emmy award but was quickly denounced by national medical experts as "imbalanced" and "inaccurate."[28] This controversy was reported in the *Washington Post*.[28,29] The American Academy of Pediatrics protested to NBC officials that the program was "unfortunate and dangerous... [its] distortion and total lack of balance of scientific fact... [has caused] extraordinary anguish and perhaps irreparable harm to the health and welfare of the nation's children."[29] A wire service story reported the concerns of Sen Dale Bumpers (D, Ark) over the program.[30] Bumpers cited a particular example of this lack of balance involving the program's statement that "serious reactions from the whooping cough vaccine are common, as low as 1 in 700 children." By focusing only on brain damage, rather than on the more common reactions to pertussis vaccine (fever and high-pitched crying), the show conveyed an erroneous impression that 1 in 700 children who receive pertussis vaccine will suffer brain damage.[30]

In addition to its impact on parents, "DTP: Vaccine Roulette" also may have had an effect on other media, both the popular press and the professional medical literature. Following the program, reports in the medical literature on the controversy and the perceived accuracy of both television and print media coverage of vaccine injury grew more common.[19,31,32] As the case of Heather Whitestone still illustrates, news reporters published unsubstantiated, often erroneous, descriptions of vaccine reactions. In the case of Whitestone, her pediatrician had to come forward and hold a press conference to correct the public misinformation promulgated by the news media.[33] The correction was covered by the print media but not with the page 1 placement of the original story.[4,34,35]

A SOCIAL CONTRACT

Although some journalists disagree,[36] we believe that the news media have an obligation to report and publicize adverse reactions to immunization but that such information must be presented in a manner that accurately portrays the preponderance of evidence documenting the safety of childhood vaccines. There is a fine line between public perception and misperception of risk. For immunizations, the distinctions are often blurred by simplistic notions. Indeed, the incidence of vaccine-preventable diseases in this country is extraordinarily low precisely because so many of our children are being immunized.[37] For example, in 1934 the incidence of pertussis in the United States was 265,269 cases.[38] Establishment of routine immunization in children led to the sharp decline in reported cases to less than 2,000 by 1976.[38] Therefore the majority of parents, and often the media, accurately perceive the risk of contracting vaccine-preventable diseases to be small. Because of the success of vaccines, today's parents have rarely witnessed children with vaccine-preventable diseases, which creates an artificial perception regarding risk of disease. Unfortunately, although the risk of a debilitating adverse reaction to vaccines is far lower than the risk of contracting the disease itself, it is the rare adverse reactions (truly related or not) that often receive attention through television, radio, and wire service news reports,[31] contributing to a skewed sense of risk among many parents.

In our society, children who do not receive immunizations are protected by the immunity of those who do. In essence, a de facto social contract exists among parents who immunize their children. They provide individual protection to their children as well as contribute to the overall protection of other children for whom the vaccine is ineffective or those who cannot receive vaccines due to true medical contraindications or religious exemptions. Because of the skewed perceptions of risk, parents of healthy children who do not have their children immunized violate this social contract. They act on the assumption that since other parents have their children immunized, they do not have to immunize their children. Their children share none of the perceived or actual risk of adverse reaction yet benefit from the population immunity.

Obviously, when this scenario plays out to a certain epidemiologic juncture, epidemics occur, as is illustrated by the pertussis epidemic that occurred in the United Kingdom during the 1970s. Increasing numbers of parents began to perceive the risk of the vaccine to be greater than its potential benefit and immunization rates in the United Kingdom fell by over 50% (from 80% to 40%) from 1973 to 1977.[39] This decline in immunization was followed by a pertussis epidemic during 1971 through 1979 involving more than 100,000 cases and 36 deaths[40]

THE ROLE OF HEALTH CARE PROFESSIONALS

The way in which US health care professionals disseminate vaccine information has varied significantly. Until recently, a standardized manner to inform parents of the safety and efficacy of vaccines did not exist. However, as mandated by the National Vaccine Injury Compensation Program,[41] beginning in April 1992 federal law required that clinicians providing pediatric vaccines give parents a standardized information brochure before immunization and obtain written consent for each vaccine administered. Separate brochures were developed for the DTP vaccine, the oral polio vaccine, and the MMR vaccine; each took approximately 15 minutes to read.[42] On review, several officials from the American Academy of Pediatrics found the brochures to be too long, too complex, and too frightening to parents to be practical and effective.[43] In effect, the informational brochures gave mixed messages regarding the safety of this necessary preventive service.[42] These brochures subsequently were revised to place the context of risk and benefit more succinctly and in clearer, more balanced terms for parents.

Physicians have a special responsibility to provide accurate information, based on rigorous research, regarding vaccine safety. Unfortunately, some physicians continue to report and publish methodologically flawed studies alleging linkage of immunizations to rare diseases. Fortunately, a journal's readership often catches the errors missed in the peer-review process. A recent medical journal article suggesting an association of measles vaccination to inflammatory bowel disease[44] was followed by the publication of 6 letters to the editor highlighting the methodological flaws of the study.[45-50] However, the initial publication of the research created an illusion of controversy within the medical profession regarding the safety of vaccines, which the news media reported. In what we believe was an attempt at balanced reporting, a Reuters Information Service news article stated that "doctors at London's Royal Free Hospital said... they could not confirm that measles vaccination causes inflammatory bowel disease, a gut disorder for which there is no cure."[51] Although there was additional news coverage of the original article,[52] we found no media coverage of the letters to the editor explaining the flaws of the study.

LEGITIMATE CONCERN VS SENSATIONALISM

We do not take issue with the reporting of factual information to parents regarding vaccines; all parents should make informed choices for their children. At issue is the manner in which information about vaccines is presented and the perceptions of risk that are conferred.

It is fair to question how many children have not received vaccines because their parents were frightened by erroneous media reports. How many children contracted measles, pertussis, or other vaccine-preventable illnesses as a result? How many children might not have received DTP vaccine if Heather Whitestone's pediatrician had not taken it on himself to set the record straight?

With all the controversy surrounding vaccines, it is easy for parents to forget that childhood immunization has made a major contribution to child survival in this century. From the widespread DTP immunization programs that began in the 1940s, to the marked reduction of *H influenzae* type b invasive disease in the 1990s, vaccines have become a widely accepted, beneficial, safe, and effective clinical preventive measure. Further, the incidence of all vaccine-preventable diseases has been reduced by more than 90% compared with prevaccination era rates.[53] These positive aspects of childhood immunization have also been covered by the news media.[54,55]

Parents, health care professionals, and the public at large are responsible for the public health of our children. We believe the news media are included in this social contract. Although parents almost always seek to act in the best interests of their children, their decisions are influenced greatly by the information they receive from many sources. We should all help parents understand the risks and benefits of any medical intervention, including continued vigilance, follow-up, and assessment of reported adverse events. Providing parents with an accurate and balanced perspective will help them make the best choices for their children's future.

REFERENCES

1. Patureau A. Around the South: in step with the 'real world': Alabamian overcomes deafness to compete with a select few in Miss America pageant. *Atlanta Constitution.* September 16, 1994:A3.

2. Associated Press. Miss America is chosen. *New York Times.* September 18, 1994:A38.

3. Associated Press. First deaf Miss America. *New York Times.* September 19, 1994:A12.

4. Associated Press. Revising Miss America's story. *New York Times.* September 26, 1994:B9.

5. Keane V, Stanton B, Horton L, Aronson R, Galbraith J, Hughart N. Perceptions of vaccine efficacy, illness, and health among inner-city parents. *Clin Pediatr.* January 1993:2–7.

6. Institute of Medicine. *Adverse Events Associated With Childhood Vaccines: Evidence Bearing on Causality.* Washington, DC: National Academy Press; 1994.

7. Byers RK, Moll FC. Encephalopathies following prophylactic pertussis vaccine. *Pediatrics.* 1948; 1:437–457.

8. Centers for Disease Control. Diphtheria, tetanus, and pertussis: guidelines for vaccine prophylaxis and other preventive measures. *MMWR Morb Mortal Wkly Rep.* 1985;34:411.

9. Howson CP, Howe CJ, Fineberg HV. *Adverse Effects of Pertussis and Rubella Vaccines: Report From the Institute of Medicine.* Washington, DC: National Academy Press; 1991.

10. Golden GS. Pertussis vaccine and injury to the brain. *J Pediatr.* 1990;116: 854–861.

11. Baraff LJ, Shields WD, Beckwith L, et al. Infants and children with convulsions and hypotonic-hyporesponsive episode following DTP immunization: follow-up evaluation. *Pediatrics.* 1988;8 1:789–794.

12. Howson CP, Fineberg HV. The ricochet of magic bullets: summary of the Institute of Medicine report, 'Adverse Effects of Pertussis and Rubella Vaccines.' *Pediatrics.* 1992;89:318–324.

13. Kinnunen E, Ferkkila M, Houi T, Juntunen J, Weckstrom P. Incidence of Guillain-Barré syndrome during a nationwide oral polio vaccine campaign. *Neurology.* 1989;39:1034–1036.

14. Uhari M, Rantala H, Niemela M. Cluster of childhood Guillain-Barré cases after oral polio vaccine campaign. *Lancet.* 1989;2:440–441.

15. Tsairis P, Dyck PJ, Mulder DW. Natural history of brachial plexus neuropathy: report on 99 patients. *Arch Neurol.* 1972;27:109–117.

16. Kitch EW, Mortimer EA. American law, preventive vaccine programs, and the National Vaccine Injury Compensation Program. In: Plotkin SA, Mortimer EA, eds. *Vaccines.* 2nd ed. Philadelphia, Pa: WB Saunders Co; 1994:933–957.

17. Clayton EW, Hickson GB. Compensation under the National Childhood Vaccine Injury Act. *J Pediatr.* 1990;116:508–513.

18. Washington Business and Trade Report. *Vaccine Bulletin.* May 1993;3:6.

19. Hinman AR. DTP vaccine litigation. *Am J Dis Child.* 1986;140:528–530.

20. Tarr A. DTP vaccine injuries: who should pay? *National Law J.* April 1, 1985:1.

21. Manley H. The shot parents worry most about. *Good Housekeeping.* June 1985:220.

22. A shortage of vaccine. *Newsweek.* December 24, 1984; 104:24.

23. Pub L No. 99-660 §311, 100 Stat 3755; 42 USC §300aa-1 (1989).

24. Freed GL, Bordley WC, DeFriese GH. Child immunization programs: an analysis of policy issues. *Milbank Q.* 1993;71:65–96.

25. Fulginiti VA. How safe are pertussis and rubella vaccines? a commentary on the Institute of Medicine report. *Pediatrics.* 1992;89:334–336.

26. US Dept of Health and Human Services. Vaccination compensation criteria revised. *Pub Health Rep.* 1995;110:373–374.

27. Thompson L, Nuell D. DTP: *Vaccine Roulette* [videorecording]. Washington, DC: WRC-TV (NBC); 1982.

28. Walsh E. State defends vaccine. *Washington Post.* June 30,1982; Maryland Weekly:6.

29. Hilts D. TV report on vaccine stirs bitter controversy. *Washington Post.* April 28, 1982; District Weekly:1.

30. United Press International. Washington, DC: *United Press International.* May 12,1982; Regional News (AM cycle).

31. Hinman AR. The pertussis vaccine controversy. *Public Health Rep.* 1984; 99:255–259.

32. Gonzalez ER. TV report on DTP galvanizes US pediatricians. *JAMA.* 1982;248:12–22.

33. American Academy of Pediatrics. Miss America and immunizations. *AAP News.* November 1994; 10:33.

34. Miss America's doctors: deafness not due to vaccine: they say bacterial infection was cause. *Atlanta Constitution.* September 24, 1994:E5.

35. Evans S. Miss America's hearing loss story disputed: deafness not linked to shot, doctor says. *Washington Post.* September 23, 1994:A3.
36. Bishop J. A journalist's view of responsibility. In: Ethiel N, ed. *Medicine and the Media: A Changing Relationship.* Chicago, Ill: Robert R McCormick Tribune Foundation; 1995:23–27.
37. American Academy of Pediatrics. Active and passive immunization. In: Peter G, ed. *1994 Red Book: Report of the Committee on Infectious Diseases.* 23rd ed. Elk Grove Village, Ill: American Academy of Pediatrics; 1994:7.
38. Rabinovich R, Robbins A. Pertussis vaccines: a progress report. *JAMA.* 1994;271:68.
39. Stuart-Harris C. Benefits and risks of immunization against pertussis. *Dev Biol Stand.* 1979;43:75–83.
40. Joint Committee on Vaccination and Immunization. The whooping cough epidemic, 1977–79. In: *Whooping Cough: Reports From the Committee on Safety of Medicine and the Joint Committee on Vaccination and Immunization.* London, England: Her Majesty's Stationery Office; 1981:170.
41. The National Childhood Vaccine Injury Act of 1986, 42 USC §300aa.
42. Goldsmith M. Vaccine information pamphlets here, but some physicians react strongly. *JAMA.* 1992;267:2005–2007.
43. Lieu TA, Glauber JH, Fuentes-Afflick E, Lo B. Effects of vaccine informational pamphlet on parents' attitude. *Arch Pediatr Adolesc Med.* 1994;148: 921–925.
44. Thompson NP, Montgomery SM, Pounder RE, Wakefield AJ. Is measles vaccination a risk factor for inflammatory bowel disease? *Lancet.* 1995;345:1071–1074.
45. Miller D, Renton A. Measles vaccination as a risk factor for inflammatory bowel disease. *Lancet.* 1995;345:1363.
46. Baxter T, Radford J. Measles vaccination as a risk factor for inflammatory bowel disease. *Lancet.* 1995;345:1363–1364.
47. MacDonald TT. Measles vaccination as a risk factor for inflammatory bowel disease. *Lancet.* 1995;345:1363.
48. Minor PD. Measles vaccination as a risk factor for inflammatory bowel disease. *Lancet.* 1995;345:1362–1363.
49. Farringten P, Miller E. Measles vaccination as a risk factor for inflammatory bowel disease. *Lancet.* 1995;345: 1362.
50. Calman KC. Measles vaccination as a risk factor for inflammatory bowel disease. *Lancet.* 1995;345:1362.
51. Reuters Information Services. British doctors link measles vaccine, gut disease. *Reuter Newswire, United Kingdom, Reuters Economic News.* April 28, 1995.
52. Mihill C. Illness linked to measles vaccine. *Guardian.* April 28, 1995;1:8.
53. Cutts FT, Zell ER, Mason D, Bernier RH, Dini EF, Orenstein WA. Monitoring progress toward US preschool immunization goals. *JAMA.* 1992;267: 1952–1955.
54. Blanchard F. Rejection of vaccine could cause whooping cough epidemics. *Associated Press.* December 2, 1982 (AM cycle).
55. Cheevers J. Preventable diseases reach 10-year low; cases of measles and other illnesses have plummeted due to immunization efforts in LA County. *Los Angeles Times.* November 19, 1995:B16.

NO

Richard Leviton

WHO CALLS THE SHOTS?

One day in 1980 Barbara Fisher held down her two-and-a-half-year-old son, Christian, so the doctor could give him his fourth DPT (diphtheria-pertussis-tetanus) shot. Neither Fisher nor the doctor knew that Christian, with respect to DPT vaccine, was a high-risk child. He had experienced a violent "local reaction" to his third injection, an experience a physician would diagnose, had one noticed it, as a contraindication against further vaccination.

Within hours of his fourth shot, Christian suffered what his mother now realizes was a classic collapse/shock reaction to pertussis. "I didn't report it to my doctor," says Fisher today. "I had not been informed of what a severe reaction was, and I didn't know I was witnessing one." She thought Christian might be undergoing a relapse of the flu. Fisher didn't want her doctor to regard her as "one of those hysterical mothers who calls up every time the child sneezes."

In the ensuing months it became obvious to Fisher that something had gone wrong with the DPT vaccination. Christian forgot his alphabet. He became hyperactive and emotionally fragile. He had staring spells, lost weight, and developed chronic diarrhea, upper respiratory infections, and allergies. Fisher still trusted her physician, who assured her that Christian was "just going through a stage." "But," says Fisher, "my whole family knew something drastic had happened to Christian, that he had become a totally different child overnight."

Today Barbara Fisher is a much wiser and infinitely better-informed mother. She knows that after his fourth DPT shot her "once precocious" Christian suffered a mild encephalopathy that left him with minimal brain damage, multiple learning disabilities, and an impaired immune system. Fisher, like many mothers, was left raging with many unanswered medical questions.

"Why was I so willing to suspend my common sense and deny reality in order to believe in the infallibility of medicine and my doctor? I believed vaccines were completely safe and effective because that is what I was led to believe by all I had read or heard in the media, by what I had been told by my pediatrician, and because I came from a family full of doctors and nurses and

From Richard Leviton, "Who Calls the Shots?" *East West: The Journal of Natural Health and Living* (November 1988). Copyright © 1988 by Richard Leviton. Reprinted by permission.

other health professionals who had dedicated their lives to medicine. I had absolutely no idea that a vaccination could result in brain damage or death."

Young Christian Fisher, however, was one of the lucky ones. He is not dead or mentally retarded or suffering from convulsions. There are 67,000 infants vaccinated with DPT every week in America but nobody—not medical professionals, the government, or mothers—has accurate casualty statistics. But that there have been significant vaccine-associated damages is meticulously documented in Fisher's provocative book, coauthored by Harris Coulter, *DPT: A Shot in the Dark* (Warner Books, 1985).

For Barbara Fisher, educating the public about the dangers of adverse reactions to DPT has become a paramount social responsibility. Christian's experience instantly politicized her. And she cites the familiar equation: Knowledge equals power.

"It is time we as parents begin to take back the right and responsibility for our children's health instead of taking the easy way out and leaving the decisions up to our doctors." Thus in 1982 Fisher founded Dissatisfied Parents Together (DPT) in Washington, D.C., to spearhead the drive for greater public awareness and to initiate legislative change. Fisher's DPT coalition, with chapters in many states, has a huge natural constituency. Each year another 3 1/2 million babies are born in America, who will be legally required to have some ten vaccinations by the age of six.

Barbara Fisher has become a major figure in the controversy over mandatory vaccination policies. On the other side of the controversy are some of the leading policymakers in American medicine —the American Academy of Pediatrics, the federal Centers for Disease Control, and the American Medical Association. They unilaterally endorse vaccination programs. "There is an ineluctable conflict between public health and individual rights and this is a regrettable fact," observes Stanley Plotkin, M.D., chairman of A.A.P.'s Committee on Infectious Diseases and director, Division of Infectious Diseases at Children's Hospital of Philadelphia.

"Public health makes the assumption that the health of a group of people is more important," he says. "When you're dealing with contagious diseases the action of a single individual may impact on others. We do not recognize the right of parents to put their children at risk of developing an infectious disease. We feel that a policy that protects children is superior."

Navigating the waters across which such volleys are fired requires today's parents to be both wary and well-informed.

AN ARSENAL OF VACCINES

The concept behind vaccination is to artificially produce immunity to an infectious disease by introducing a small amount of the disease virus or bacteria into the body. The immune system wages a mini-campaign against the foreign materials and develops antibodies tailored for that disease organism, for future reference, in case the child contacts the pathogens in the environment.

This is called active immunization and theoretically provides lasting, effective protection against specific diseases. "The goal is to mimic the natural infection by evoking an immunologic response which presents little or no risk to the recipient," informs the 1986 *Red Book,* the pediatrician's standard reference work on vaccinations, published by the A.A.P.

...Today's vaccines use either live or killed infectious agents, usually a virus or bacteria. They are typically injected; a type of polio vaccine is taken orally. The oral polio vaccine is cultured from the kidney cells of the African green monkey.

In addition to the active immunizing antigen, vaccines contain a suspending fluid (sterile water), trace amounts of preservatives (including formaldehyde and mercury-derivatives), stabilizers, antibiotics, and adjuvants (aluminum phosphate).

While there are no national vaccination laws, the fifty states are fairly uniform in their requirements for mandatory vaccinations as a prerequisite for school admission. Children must be vaccinated against the five traditional childhood diseases of mumps, measles, rubella, diphtheria, and pertussis, plus tetanus and polio.

Mumps is a routine, relatively innocuous viral disease that lasts one to two weeks and requires no medical treatment. Two-thirds of infected children develop a self-limiting illness with swollen salivary glands, fever, headache, and appetite loss, but afterwards they have lifetime immunity. A single vaccination of live virus is given at age fifteen months, usually as part of a triple injection called MMR (measles-mumps-rubella). The mumps component, however, is not required in sixteen states.

Measles is a contagious viral disease that lasts two weeks. Characteristic symptoms are a high fever and a rash of pink spots, but more serious complications include eye and ear inflammations, pneumonia, or, in rare instances, encephalitis. The live virus vaccine was introduced in America in 1963 although the measles mortality rate had already dropped radically from 13.3/100,000 cases to 0.3/ 100,000 by 1955.

Rubella (German measles) is often a benign disease with symptoms so mild they often escape detection. There is a three-day rash, fever, a slight cold, and sore throat. The principal danger is congenital rubella syndrome (CRS), whereby a pregnant woman can expose her fetus to injury if she contracts rubella in her first trimester. A children's mass immunization program for rubella began in 1969 after a CRS epidemic among 20,000 babies in 1964.

Diphtheria has nearly disappeared from America, where it was once greatly feared as a highly contagious bacterial disease with a mortality rate at 3–10 percent. Medical treatment with penicillin or erythromycin is usually indicated. Although mortality rates from diphtheria had dropped by 50 percent before a vaccine was developed, today three to five doses are required in all fifty states.

Pertussis, or whooping cough, is probably the most virulent of the traditional childhood diseases and it can be life-threatening. The infectious agent, *Bordetella pertussis*, was first isolated in France in 1906. Pertussis vaccination, using whole-cell killed virus, began in 1936 and became widespread by 1957. Pertussis symptoms, including a paroxysmal cough, usually afflict infants younger than two years. Today thirty-nine states require three to five injections, beginning at age two months.

Tetanus, technically not a childhood disease, is a potentially dangerous, sometimes fatal, random bacterial infection. Tetanus infection can produce severe neurologic symptoms and muscular spasms (the spasms in the jaw gave the disease the name of "lockjaw"), and worldwide it has a 30–50 percent mortality rate. It is especially prevalent in tropical countries. A regimen of one to five tetanus inoculations are required by forty-seven states, beginning at age two months.

Poliomyelitis infection actually produces no symptoms in 90 percent of its recipients and only 1–2 percent of children infected develop its classic, virally produced symptoms. Polio vaccine, required at three to four doses nationwide, comes in two forms: Salk killed-virus injection and Sabin live-virus oral vaccine.

BRAVE NEW VACCINES

... The A.A.P. is categorically opposed to any kind of optional vaccination approach, states G. Scott Giebink, M.D., professor of pediatrics at the University of Minnesota Medical School and a member of the A.A.P. infectious diseases committee. "This is because the virtual eradication of many of the vaccine-preventable diseases has been based on universal rather than optional, or partial, immunization. All of the programs have been incredibly effective—but not because only a few people had the vaccines."

Childhood diseases are still a significant public health threat, requiring prevention, Giebink stresses. "That's the primary reason for continuing a strong and universal immunization program as these diseases are rampant in the world. I'd place the public health benefits first."

Alan Nelson, M.D., president of the A.M.A., agrees. "The data that support the advantages of vaccinations in terms of neurologic injury or mortality to those unprotected are so clear-cut that our public policy still has to support mass immunization. There are few things in medicine that are totally risk-free. That's why we have to measure the benefits against the risks, but with vaccinations the benefits clearly outweigh the risks."

Nelson cites the example of Britain. "There the choice of parents was expressed and DPT vaccination rates have dropped, but the experience has been bad in terms of epidemics and outbreaks of pertussis ever since."

The primary issue at stake is the communicability of infectious diseases, says Walter Orenstein, M.D., director of the Division of Immunization at the CDC in Atlanta. "It's a community decision. When we have children vaccinated, we not only protect the children, we protect the community at large. Parents who decide not to have their children vaccinated not only are not protecting their children, but potentially their actions are leading to danger for other children in that community. If this happened on a large scale, that would put an entire community at risk." ...

CONTRAINDICATIONS

Not everyone shares this rosy prognosis for preventive vaccination for nearly all diseases. In the mid-1980s a combination of television documentaries, major newspaper stories, and several books—most prominently, Fisher and Coulter's *DPT* —raised public awareness to a shocked appreciation of problems with the mass vaccination approach. Major fissures in the otherwise solid medical edifice were suddenly revealed. The issues are complex and myriad, and often emotionally tinged.

The DPT shot, among all vaccinations in use, produces the most serious adverse reactions. Before 1985 parents were never adequately advised (if at all) of the potentially harmful side-effects of DPT, state Fisher and Coulter. Even today pediatricians still usually downplay the risks. Adverse reactions, which are medical contraindications against further injections, run the gamut from localized skin reactions to seizure, brain inflammation, and death. In 1988, more than forty years after the DPT vaccine was introduced, no accepted parameters have been developed for prescreening hypersensitive children who might be at major risk from DPT.

Prior to 1988 there was not a nationally mandated reporting system either, one which required physicians or health departments to file reports on adverse reactions. Thus accurate data on the prevalence of adverse reactions is lacking and estimates vary widely. Often pediatricians fail (or refuse) to make the connection between a DPT injection and adverse reactions, even when they occur within hours of each other. Coulter and Fisher did their own calculations, based on the best available published data, and came up with some staggering damage estimates.

They calculated that, based on an infant population of 3.3 million per year eligible for DPT shots, 4,248 children have either post-injection convulsions or collapse, 10,377 have high-pitched screaming within forty-eight hours, and 18,873 infants have some form of significant neurological reaction within two days. Possibly as many as 943 deaths and 11,666 cases of long-term damage are attributable to DPT.

There is also considerable disagreement over the level of efficacy of the DPT vaccine, state Fisher and Coulter. Estimates range from 63 to 94 percent. DPT was never adequately tested for safety, its artificially induced immunity lasts only two to five years, and it is regarded as "one of the crudest vaccines on the market." American medical authorities are inexplicably reluctant to adopt the newer and apparently safer Japanese acellular pertussis vaccine.

Given these conditions, Fisher's DPT coalition is understandably strongly in favor of making vaccinations a voluntary act. Fisher would like the DPT vaccine to function freely in the marketplace, like other consumer goods. "Then you will have the good, safe, effective vaccines used, and the poor ones will be dropped. That will give an incentive to the drug companies and government to come up with the most effective and the safest vaccines possible."

Most European nations now allow optional vaccinations for DPT. Voluntary programs are actually generating "control group" data for natural infection rates in countries without mass vaccination. Communist countries such as the Soviet Union, Poland, and East Germany still require vaccinations.

The examples of Britain, West Germany, and Sweden are often cited on both sides of the DPT debate. In these countries, when vaccination rates plummeted in the 1970s and incidence of pertussis infection climbed, a corresponding higher incidence of infantile complication or death did not occur, as many had predicted it would. In 1984, researchers at London's Epidemiological Research Laboratory concluded, in contrasting twenty-five deaths at an 80 percent vaccination rate in 1974 with twenty-three deaths at a 30 percent vaccination rate in 1977, that "since the decline in pertussis immunization, hospital admission and death rates from whooping cough have fallen unexpectedly."

The A.M.A., however, is not convinced that the European model of optional pertussis vaccination is medically worthy of importation to America.

"The incidence of pertussis is cyclic and the severity could also run in cycles," observes A.M.A.'s Nelson. "It's still a very bad disease, a terrible, tragic disease. The burden is on those who say the disease is not still an extraordinarily bad illness to prove that. I don't think you will find very many physicians willing to say we don't have to worry about pertussis anymore, that its severity has lessened."

Medical authorities contend that the kind of documentation Fisher and Coulter present, culled from interviews with over 100 mothers of presumed vaccine-damaged children, are "anecdotal" and not scientifically admissible.

"Most of the pertussis controversy revolves around observations that are anecdotal and unconfirmed," states Plotkin of the A.A.P. "The value of such anecdotes is very limited. On the basis of the information available, I would think there are only rare reactions to pertussis vaccine."

Extensive studies in the U.S. and Britain, explains Giebink, have shown "quite conclusively that some of the most serious of these nervous system disorders are in fact not caused by the vaccine but are only temporally related with it. We've looked at some of the particular diseases using scientific methods and we have not been able to show a cause-and-effect relationship."

CDC's Orenstein concurs. "These adverse events are so rare that we can't detect them. A lot of the responsibility falls on the parent who has to make the connection and file a report. Some of them may forget in their crisis. Suppose we do get all the adverse events reported? It doesn't mean that any of these events are *caused* by the vaccination."

It is precisely statements like these that have infuriated mothers whose babies have suffered damages "temporally" following DPT injections, whatever the true causality might be. Many mothers say their physicians don't listen to them, caution them against hysteria or making trouble, are complacent or patronizing. Other women contend their doctors lied to them and betrayed their trust. Barbara Fisher excoriates this "cavalier disregard for vaccine toxicity and human life."

"We are so conditioned to the idea that our doctor's word is to be trusted without question," said one mother whose infant died thirty-three hours after a DPT shot. "I am a nurse. I watched my son die that day, and I didn't even know what was happening until it was all over."

Mother-activists like Fisher find something immoral lurking within the risk-benefit equations of medical science, especially in light of the lack of exemption options for parents in many states.

"The epidemiologists look at mass vaccination the way a military general studies a battle. A general knows he must sacrifice men to take a hill. This is how government health officials see mass vaccination. They start getting into the idea that some children are expendable. I cannot think of any other instance in our society where we say it's okay to kill children, to have them brain-damaged, because it's for the greater welfare of society."

As Fisher tersely puts it, "When it happens to your child, the risks are 100 percent."

HOLISTIC IMMUNOLOGY

There might be more reasons than symptomatic contraindications arguing the case against mandatory vaccination. According to a variety of holistic practitioners, including M.D.'s, homeopaths, and naturopaths, the general practice of vaccination may have long-term damaging effects on the vitality of the immune system. One such bold M.D. was the late "People's Doctor," Robert Mendelsohn.

Mendelsohn had very impressive credentials to support his strident criticism of vaccinations. He was a practicing pediatrician for twenty-five years, professor at the University of Illinois Medical School, Chairman of the Medical Licensure Committee for Illinois, author of three popular medical guidebooks, and publisher of a medical newsletter for consumers.

For Mendelsohn, vaccinations were a "medical time bomb," the "most threatening" of which was DPT. "The greatest threat of childhood diseases lies in the dangerous and ineffectual efforts made to prevent them through mass immunization," he said. "Although I administered them myself during my early years of practice, I have become a steadfast opponent of mass inoculation because of the myriad hazards they present."

Vaccinations, said Mendelsohn, are one of the harmful sacraments of the modern religion of medicine. "In the total absence of controlled studies, all vaccines today remain, scientifically speaking, unproven remedies—the polite term for medical quackery. The only proven characteristic of vaccines is their devastating adverse effects." Mendelsohn also suggested there might be a causal link between degenerative diseases and immunizations.

Richard Moskowitz is an M.D., homeopath, and former president of the National Center for Homeopathy, now practicing at The Turning Point clinic in Watertown, Mass. He is one of many holistic practitioners who have corroborated Mendelsohn's early indications. In Moskowitz's view *all* vaccinations may be injurious to the functioning and integrity of the immune system.

Moskowitz argues that vaccination may produce a form of immunosuppression and chronic immune failure. The injected virus, because it has been artificially weakened before injection, no longer initiates "a generalized, acute inflammatory response." Instead, it tricks the body into an antibody response—"an isolated technical feat" and only an aspect of the overall immune ability. Worse, the virus may persist in the blood for prolonged periods, perhaps permanently.

"Far from producing a genuine immunity, vaccines may actually interfere with or suppress the natural immune response," says Moskowitz. "By making it difficult or impossible to mount a vigorous, acute response to infection, artificial immunization substitutes a much weaker *chronic* response with little or no tendency for the body to heal itself spontaneously."

Evidence indicates that the individual vaccinations may each have unique deleterious consequences on the immune system. Tetanus may interfere with the immune reaction. It has been linked with peripheral neuropathy, allergic reactions, and laryngeal paralysis. Rubella has been tentatively associated with arthralgia (joint pain) and arthritis. A 1980 report in *Mutation Research* indicated that children who underwent repeated smallpox vaccinations in Czechoslovakia showed chromosomal aberrations in their white blood cells, indicating a mutagenic effect.

The British journal *Medical Hypothesis* reported in 1988 in a study of 200 patients with chronic Epstein-Barr virus syndrome that the disease was attributable to the live rubella virus found in the vaccine. In 1987 a consultant for the World Health Organization announced in the London *Times* that the prevalence of smallpox vaccinations over a thirteen-year period in seven African nations actually triggered the AIDS virus outbreak in those countries. In 1985 a scientist at Harvard's School of Public Health revealed that STLV-3, an AIDS-type virus, had been found in the green monkey *(Cercopithecus)* whose kidney cells were routinely used to culture oral polio vaccine.

Other anomalous long-term medical trends implicating vaccinations have recently been brought to light. Widespread measles vaccinations seem to be shifting the incidence of the disease into older age groups; 80 percent of cases are now occurring in people aged ten to nineteen and with atypical, often untreatable symptoms. Vaccination immunity is clearly less than complete, as 1988 CDC figures showed that of 795 reported cases of pertussis in infants aged three to six months, 49 percent of them had been fully vaccinated.

While holistic health providers are finding alarming grounds for connecting today's auto-immune anomalies and a weakened immune response with vaccines, Giebink of the A.A.P. states unequivocally, "Those are all groundless speculations." ...

IN SEARCH OF WILLING DOCTORS

All fifty states allow a medical exemption for high-risk children. Generally what is required is a written statement by a licensed M.D. indicating that the proposed vaccination is medically contraindicated, based on a previous adverse reaction, a family history of reactions, or a personal history of convulsions, neurological disorders, severe allergies, prematurity, or recent severe, chronic illness.

While individual state regulations vary slightly in terminology, essentially the intention remains uniform, as this excerpt from the New York state regulation makes clear: "If any physician licensed to practice medicine in this state certifies that such immunization may be detrimental to a student's health, the requirements of this section shall be inapplicable until such immunization is no longer found to be detrimental."

Philip Incao, M.D., is a licensed New York state physician with offices in Harlemville, New York, near Albany. Incao has been signing medical exemptions for most of the fifteen years of his family practice. But Incao, who practices anthroposophic medicine (see "The Promise of Anthroposophical Medicine," July 1988 *EW),* as developed by the Austrian philosopher Rudolf Steiner (1861–1925), makes a broader interpretation of "detrimental."

Anthroposophical medicine states that the struggle with childhood infectious diseases is salutary for the child's personal and spiritual development and they should not be suppressed; homeopathic medicines may be used to ameliorate the process, however. In this model the illness is seen as an acute, inflammatory event which mobilizes the immune system. It enables the child's "Ego" (the Higher Self, in other vocabularies) to remodel the inherited body according to its own blueprint.

None of Incao's medical exemptions have been refused. Beginning in 1986, however, his unconventional practice may have provoked New York state health officials to begin what has been a smoldering form of harassment and informal investigation of his anthroposophical procedures. While the medical exemption is nationally available, it shouldn't be surprising to find that most doctors are reluctant to grant it, even in conditions of obvious contraindications —because it bucks too much against the orthodoxy. *DPT: A Shot in the Dark* is full of harrowing examples of distraught families scouring an entire state in search of a sympathetic M.D. to sign their medical exemption.

On the positive side, Washington state recently licensed naturopaths to give vaccinations, which means they can also grant exemptions. In some states, including Florida, chiropractors are allowed to write medical exemptions. The cracks in the orthodoxy may be gradually widening to allow parents more latitude.

BROADENING RELIGIOUS BELIEFS

An exemption from vaccinations based on religious beliefs is permitted in all states except West Virginia and Mississippi. Recent favorable litigation in New York has expanded the legal interpretation of religious beliefs, thereby granting parents further options.

The New York statute defines the parameters for religious exemptions by stating that mandatory vaccination requirements "Shall not apply to children whose parents are bona fide members of a recognized religious organization whose teachings are contrary to the practices herein required." This exemption works fine if a parent in fact belongs to a recognized religion. But what happens if a family has sincere beliefs but is outside

the folds of any church? In 1984 a family in Clinton, New York, found out. They refused to have their two daughters vaccinated and took the issue to court. And they won.

Robert and Kit Allanson had initially secured a medical exemption for their daughters Naomi and Marika, but the school rejected it. The girls were expelled from school, their return pending on vaccination. Allanson secured the legal services of Attorney James Filenbaum and they immediately filed a suit in federal court, suing the school district, superintendent, and principal for $2 million. They also demanded a religious exemption for their girls.

The only weakness in the Allanson strategy was that they didn't belong to any church and the nearest recognizable label they had for their convictions was macrobiotics. The prosecutor had a field day with this.

At the trial, however, Filenbaum brought in a minister and the chairman of the religious department at nearby Hamilton College to testify on behalf of the religious authenticity of the Allansons' beliefs, however much those beliefs might lack an institutional context. After five-and-a-half months of testimony, charges of child neglect, and, Robert Allanson says, "hand-to-hand combat with the government," the Allansons prevailed as the U.S. district judge ruled in their favor.

The Allanson case was a valuable precedent for everyone, even outside of New York. Since the 1984 ruling, Filenbaum has argued another dozen religious exemption cases (in addition to advising hundreds of other clients) and has won nearly all of them....

PERSONAL BELIEFS

Probably the best compromise all around is now legally available in twenty-two states. This is a harassment- and red-tape-free exemption on the grounds of personal or philosophical belief.

Vermont is a "triple-exemption" state which approved the personal belief exemption in 1981. According to Bob O'Grady, administrator of the Epidemiology Division in the Vermont State Health Department in Burlington, of Vermont's 98,600 students enrolled in public and private schools (kindergarten through twelfth grade), .5 percent (493 children) take the personal belief/religious exemption and .2 percent (197 students) take the medical exemption. Clearly 690 exempt and unvaccinated students representing about .7 percent of the school population is not viewed as a threat to public health.

All that is required to obtain the joint religious/philosophical exemption in Vermont, says O'Grady, is a written statement from the parent indicating that she has "a religious or moral conviction opposed to vaccination." The exemption is automatically granted. One needn't even specify the nature or details of the beliefs. Since Vermont has one of the highest vaccination rates (at 98.9 percent) in the country, the option of offering medical, religious, and philosophical exemptions for a tiny minority is a satisfactory compromise among conflicting demands, says O'Grady. "I would have to judge that most people in Vermont feel it is, too."

California also has the personal belief exemption, mandated in 1961 when polio vaccinations were made legally necessary for school admissions. Here a parent must file a letter with the school stating that vaccination is contrary to his or her beliefs, explains Lauren Dales, M.D., chief of the Immunization Unit, California State Department of Health Services in Berkeley.

However, the health officer has the option to "temporarily exclude" a child from school "during the incubation period" if the child is believed to have been exposed to an infectious disease and is still at risk for developing symptoms. Other than that, the California statute "doesn't leave any grounds for a parent's application not to be accepted," says Dales. In his ten years with the department, he's never heard of a complaint from parents.

In California, of 475,000 new pupils each year, about 3,000 take the philosophical/religious exemption and about 1,000 take the medical. "We don't have a problem with these exemptions," says Dales. "We obviously don't want to see disease outbreaks, but when the exemptions are coming in at the low level they are, we don't think they are epidemiologically critical." ...

WHO DECIDES?

The right of freedom of choice in vaccinations is clearly a difficult one to wrest from the hands of the medical establishment, as Barbara Fisher realizes after six years of strenuous effort.

"We haven't gotten anywhere near as far as we had wanted to. We have tried to be as credible as possible. We did our homework before we went out and criticized vaccines. We're dealing with a very powerful and wealthy pharmaceutical industry, with the government, health agencies, and organized medicine. That's a formidable force we're up against."

The exact nature of this "formidable force" may actually lie below the skin of the vaccination controversy and, as Fisher maintains, it may well touch at the "very heart of what is wrong with American medicine today."

The controversy really comes down to two diametrically opposite medical views. Plotkin of the A.A.P., for instance, does not recognize the right of a parent to subject a child to infectious disease. Anthroposophical physician Incao recognizes the necessity for a child to undergo the maturing struggles of early childhood infectious illnesses whereby "the higher self remodels the body in accordance with spiritual ideals."

This stark contrast raises important questions. Do we have the right to be sick anymore? Have we become overly afraid of being sick? Can illness be legislated out of existence, as something aberrant and unnatural?

The fundamental issue could also be seen as a question of one's rights: Does an individual have the right to oversee his/her own immune system (and his or her children's) and its interaction with the environment and the rest of society?

"We're so afraid of nature," says Incao. "What is the purpose of our life? If this purpose is to allow our individuality to unfold and express itself to the fullest, then this happens through the process of the immune system unfolding and reacting as self meets nonself. We become susceptible to infectious disease when we open ourselves to the world. Then we can become full human beings."

And for that voyage of discovery, concludes Incao, vaccinations are contraindicated.

RESOURCES

DPT (Dissatisfied Parents Together)
128 Branch Road
Vienna; VA 22180
(708) 938-DPT3

DPT: A Shot In the Dark, by Harris L Coulter and Barbara Loe Fisher, Warner Books, 1985.

Dangers of Compulsory Immunization: How to Avoid Them Legally, by Tom Finn, Family Fitness Press (P.O. Box 1658, New Port Richey, FL 34291-1658), 1987.

Immunization: The Reality Behind the Myth, by Walene James

POSTSCRIPT

Should All Children Be Immunized Against Childhood Diseases?

Currently, all 50 states require children to be vaccinated before enrolling in school. However, the safety of various vaccines, particularly the whooping cough (DPT) vaccine, continues to be the subject of debate. Although both the American Academy of Pediatrics and the U.S. Public Health Service continue to endorse the whooping cough vaccine, many parents and health providers feel that the risks are too high. Steven Black, codirector of the Kaiser-Permanente Pediatric Vaccine Study Center in Oakland, California, feels that the DPT vaccine is far from ideal. Newer vaccines, he believes, reduce the risks of injury by a significant percentage (see "The Perils of Pertussis," *American Health*, June 1991). Unlike the current DPT vaccine, which uses whole, killed bacteria cells to trigger the formation of antibodies, the new immunizations contain materials that produce immunity without as many side effects. The new vaccines, currently available in Japan but not yet in the United States, cause a significantly lower percentage of some side effects such as high fever and swelling, but whether or not they will reduce the incidence of brain damage is unclear.

Parents of young children are facing two crises relating to immunizations: First, widespread publicity about the genuine but extremely rare adverse effects of the whooping cough vaccine; and second, drug manufacturers' concerns about producing vaccines without protection from expensive lawsuits brought by parents of injured children. As a result, fewer companies are willing to produce vaccines. This, in turn, will lead to vaccine shortages and higher costs (which will be passed on to the consumer). The following articles discuss cost factors in relation to the low rates of immunizations: "Shots in the Dark," *Reason* (November 1994); "Why Haven't Millions of Youngsters Gotten All Their Shots?" *CQ Researcher* (June 18, 1993); "Cheap Shots," *New Republic* (October 26, 1992); and "Unprotected Children," *Atlantic Monthly* (March 1993).

Vaccines other than the DPT vaccine are also thought to be harmful. A 1980 article in *Mutation Research* indicated that children who had smallpox vaccinations in Czechoslovakia showed harmful changes in their white blood cells. Also, in 1988 the British medical journal *Medical Hypothesis* reported a study of 200 patients with a chronic viral disease, Epstein-Barr syndrome. The article claimed that the disease was caused by a live rubella (German measles) virus that was found in a vaccine that was given to the patients. Other articles discussing the risks of vaccination include "Experts Forum," *Mothering* (Summer 1996); "Immunizations: Do You Know the Risks?" *Dr.*

William Campbell Douglass' Second Opinion (May 1994); "Mean Vaccines: For the Record," *Vegetarian Times* (February 1993); and "A New 'P' in DPT," *Vegetarian Times* (July 1992).

The controversies surrounding vaccination continue. The medical community's endorsement of vaccination is evident in the following: "The War We Thought We Had Won," *Medical Update* (April 1996); "Why Aren't We Protecting Our Children?" *RN* (November 1990); and "Complying With Vaccine Law Will Help Prevent Errors," *Nursing* (August 1990). For a comprehensive update on vaccine safety, see "Update: Vaccine Side Effects, Adverse Reactions, Contraindications, and Precautions," *Morbidity and Mortality Weekly Report* (September 6, 1996).

ISSUE 19

Are Homeopathic Remedies Legitimate?

YES: Nancy Bruning, from "The Mysterious Power of Homeopathy," *Natural Health* (January/February 1995)

NO: Stephen Barrett, from "Homeopathy's Legacy: Phony 'Remedies' and Kindred Delusions," *Priorities* (1994)

ISSUE SUMMARY

YES: Author Nancy Bruning claims that neither skeptics nor believers can exactly explain how homeopathy works, but it can successfully treat a wide range of health problems.

NO: Physician and health consumer advocate Stephen Barrett argues that homeopathic remedies are so dilute that they are useless.

Many Americans, disillusioned with traditional medicine, are seeking alternative health providers such as homeopaths, acupuncturists, and chiropractors. Among the various alternatives, homeopathy has recently surged in popularity. Homeopathy is a 200-year-old therapy that employs minuscule doses of natural substances to treat symptoms and disease. Demand for these remedies has never been greater, and consumer advocates and scientists want the Food and Drug Administration (FDA) to regulate the sale of these products, which they claim are worthless.

In 1994, Americans spent more than $165 million on homeopathic medicines. Overall, sales have climbed 25 percent per year since the late 1980s. This surprises many scientists and physicians because homeopathy has been out of fashion since the turn of the century. Interestingly, homeopathy has never lost its appeal in Europe. In England homeopathic services and remedies are even covered by the national health insurance. It also has remained popular in both France and Germany.

Homeopathy is a medical theory and practice that developed over 200 years ago in response to the harsh procedures, such as bloodletting, used in those days. Samuel Hahnemann, a German doctor disenchanted with harsh treatments, developed a theory based on three principles: the minimum dose, the law of similars, and the single remedy. The word homeopathy comes from the Greek words for "like" and "suffering." With the minimum dose, or law of infinitesimals, Hahnemann believed that a substance's strength and effectiveness heightened the more it was diluted. The dilution makes the drug virtually nonexistent, but the homeopathic belief is that the substance has left its imprint or a spirit-like essence that stimulates the body to heal itself. With the law of similars, Hahnemann theorized that if a large amount of a substance causes certain symptoms in a healthy person, smaller amounts of the same substance can cure those symptoms in an ill person. Hahnemann developed this belief after a strong dose of the malaria treatment, quinine, caused his healthy body to develop symptoms similar to those experienced by malaria patients. Finally, a homeopathic practitioner generally prescribes only a single remedy to cover all symptoms that the patient is experiencing.

Although most homeopaths do not recommend that people abandon conventional treatments for AIDS, cancer, and other serious illnesses, they often advise homeopathic remedies along with traditional medications. In most states it is illegal to practice homeopathy without a license to prescribe drugs, but many people with no formal training claim to be homeopaths. The American Medical Association (AMA) does not accept homeopathy, but it does not totally reject it either. The AMA has recently stated that doctors should be aware of alternative therapies and use them if appropriate.

Do homeopathic remedies work? Supporters often point to an analysis of 107 clinical studies published in the *British Medical Journal* in 1991. The results of 81 of these studies suggested that homeopathic treatment was more effective than a placebo, while the others found no difference. There did appear to be methodological problems, however, with many of the studies. The National Center for Homeopathy, an information clearinghouse, points to research published in the *Lancet* (December 10, 1994). The rigorously conducted study showed that asthma patients improved considerably after undergoing homeopathic treatment, though the researchers were at a loss to explain the results. Dr. Herbert Benson, president of the Mind-Body Institute at Deaconess Hospital in Boston, claims that homeopathy's effects are consistent with the placebo effect. For the placebo effect to work, there must be "belief and expectation" that it will, both on the part of the practitioner and the patient. If homeopathy rests solely on faith and belief, sick persons can recover without homeopathic medications. And why do consumers need to spend millions of dollars a year on homeopathic remedies?

In the following selections, author Nancy Bruning states that although scientists scoff at claims that homeopathy can relieve symptoms and treat disease, many people swear that it can. Retired psychiatrist and consumer advocate Stephen Barrett claims that homeopathic remedies are a fraud. He states that "if the FDA required homeopathic remedies to be proven effective in order to remain on the market... homeopathy would face extinction in the United States."

YES
Nancy Bruning

THE MYSTERIOUS POWER
OF HOMEOPATHY

Forget the skeptics—even practitioners of homeopathy struggle to explain this bizarre but seemingly effective system of healing. This is not surprising given that homeopathy defies the known laws of chemistry, physics, and pharmacology. For starters, homeopathic medicines contain substances known to cause the symptoms you want to eliminate. Imagine taking poison ivy pills to relieve itching.

And if that isn't enough, the homeopathic preparations are made by repeatedly diluting the active ingredient—putting an ounce of the ingredient in ten ounces of water, then an ounce of that dilution in ten ounces of water, and so on—until it's unlikely that even a single molecule of the active ingredient will be present in the dose you take. Moreover, the more dilute the preparation, the more potent it is considered to be. All this combines to throw skeptic and believer alike into a baffling realm of theory and speculation where matter dissolves into pure energy, where small permutations in a system can create large changes, and where wave patterns and electromagnetic messages affect not only the body and mind but even the spirit.

Naturally, most scientists scoff at claims that homeopathy can relieve illness. What they can't do, however, is ignore the many people who swear that it can. My own experience a few years ago landed me in the ranks of the believers. When my yoga instructor recommended a popular homeopathic remedy, Calmes Forté, for my insomnia; I tried it, and it worked. Also, I had no druggy feeling the next day, as I might have had with sleeping pills. Over the next several months it continued to work more often than not. But like most people who use homeopathic medicines, I hadn't a clue as to why.

Two years later, I teamed up with a physician trained in homeopathic medicine—Corey Weinstein—and wrote a book about homeopathy. It was then that I learned that this system has an impressive track record and is supported with increasing frequency by publications in scientific journals.

In fact, homeopathy was the medicine of choice for many nineteenth-century American physicians. In the 1850s, however, the newly formed American Medical Association began to rout homeopathy from the halls of "respected" medicine. At the turn of the century there were 15,000 practicing homeopaths in the United States (15 to 20 percent of the entire medical profession), but by the 1970s fewer than 200 practitioners remained.

Now, homeopathy is on the rebound. A survey published in the *New England Journal of Medicine* found that 2.3 million Americans used homeopathy in 1990, and the National Center for Homeopathy estimates that at least 2,500 practitioners use homeopathy in the United States. Sales of homeopathic medicines in health and drug stores are rising at the rate of 25 percent annually as people use these medicines to treat themselves for a variety of problems.

HOW HOMEOPATHY WORKS

There is a principle of homeopathy called the Law of Similars, which holds that "like cures like." This means that a substance that causes certain symptoms in a healthy person can, when given in infinitesimal doses, cure those same symptoms in a sick person. For example, consider the homeopathic remedy *Coffea*. It's made from coffee, well-known for its ability to cause jumpiness and wakefulness. As a remedy, however, *Coffea* is prescribed to calm your nerves and help you sleep. Similarly, *Allium cepa*, which is made from onions, relieves the symptoms of watery eyes and runny nose.

In homeopathy, symptoms are seen neither as enemies to be squashed nor as the disease itself. "Rather," says Dana Ullman, president of the Foundation for Homeopathic Research in Berkeley, California, "they are signs of the body's effort to deal with infection or stress, to defend and heal. Because our bodies are not always completely effective in healing, giving a substance that mimics the body's defense helps trigger that process."

Homeopaths maintain that while suppressing symptoms outright may help you feel better temporarily, it won't help the healing process. In one of the many analogies that homeopaths use to explain their system, countering symptoms with "anti"-histamines or "anti"-biotics is said to be like smashing a beeping smoke alarm instead of looking for the fire that set it off.

Unlike a smoke alarm, however, symptoms are part of the healing process. For instance, even conventional medicine now recognizes that fever helps the body fight infection and that a runny nose clears the body of mucus and dead pathogens.

Homeopaths believe that although symptoms may be unpleasant, they play an important role in healing, and therefore should be stimulated and supported rather than suppressed. Only then can the body rid itself of disease and return to health; the symptoms will fade away naturally when they are no longer needed. Ullman likens homeopathy to "steering *into* a skid" to regain control of your car, rather than steering against the direction of the skid, which only sends you further out of control.

You can take one of two basic categories of homeopathic remedies: *combination* remedies or *single* remedies. Combination remedies include two or more of the single remedies that are most likely to alleviate specific symptoms, such as a cough, indigestion, or muscle aches. Single homeopathic remedies are specific to an individual's overall pattern of symptoms, which in the case of a cough, for example, may include whether the person feels hot or cold, what time of day the cough is worst, and how dry or wet the cough is. Since people's overall symptom patterns will differ, two people with a cough may require different single remedies. Thus, combination remedies are more likely to contain the remedy you will need. For people without experience in homeopathy, they are much easier to use than single remedies.

Combination remedies are used mainly for acute (sudden onset, short-lived) conditions which have simpler and more consistent symptom patterns than chronic (slower developing, longer-lasting) conditions. Acute conditions include minor injuries and wounds, insect bites, burns and sunburn, and muscle strains and sprains. You can also use combination remedies to treat yourself pre- and post-operatively to help deal with shock and to speed healing. And they are often used successfully to fight flus, colds, coughs, and sore throats; headaches and hangovers; digestive problems such as nausea, vomiting, diarrhea, and constipation; and kids' problems, such as earaches, teething pain, and toothaches. A correct combination remedy can even soothe acute emotional reactions such as fear and anxiety before an exam, performance, or other big event.

Brands of combination remedies vary as to the remedies they contain, and although this "shotgun" approach increases the chance a product will contain the remedy you need, it doesn't guarantee it. So if you don't get relief from one particular combination, you may need to try other brands until you find the one that works. If you still fail to see any benefits, don't give up on homeopathy altogether—the combinations you've tried may not contain the particular remedy you require. For another ailment, or at another time, the same or another prod-

uct may work wonderfully. Also, you may need to find a homeopathic specialist who will help you find the correct single remedy needed for your symptoms.

CONSTITUTIONAL REMEDIES

Single remedies (sometimes called constitutional remedies) are often necessary for chronic conditions that have endured for months, years, or your whole life, and which may be more deep-seated and complicated. Choosing the correct single remedy requires some study and perhaps a little luck on the part of the patient, or the skill and expertise of a professional homeopath.

Constitutional homeopathy can often help cure such chronic conditions as acne, allergies, migraine headaches, asthma, depression, anxiety, fatigue, premenstrual syndrome, arthritis, eczema, and psoriasis. Professionally guided constitutional therapy is also recommended if you want to go beyond self-care and cure the underlying disease that may be at the root of recurring acute symptoms.

While combination remedies tend to be easier to use, some homeopaths, such as Jennifer Jacobs, M.D., a family physician in Seattle, encourage people to at least try self-prescribing single remedies for acute conditions. If chosen correctly, they are more effective than the combinations because they are used in higher potencies and are more specific to the individual. However, you can't just wander into a store and expect to choose the right single remedy off the shelf. The playing field can be confusing to the novice, in part because manufacturers label single remedies with just a few parts of the total symptom profile. . . .

Table 1

Picking the Right Remedy

Conditions	Homeopathic Products								
	Aconite	Apis	Arnica	Arsenicum	Belladonna	Bryonia	Carbo veg.	Chamomilla	Ferrum phos.
Acne				x					
Anxiety	x								
Backache			x						
Bruises, Sprains & Strains			x						
Coughs & Cold	x								x
Depression									x
Eczema				x					
Exhaustion			x				x		
Gas				x			x	x	
Headache	x				x	x			x
Indigestion							x		
Insomnia								x	
Irritability		x							
Neck Stiffness	x					x			
PMS								x	
Sinusitis					x				x
Toothache					x			x	

Conditions	Homeopathic Products								
	Gelsemium	Hepar sulph.	Ipecac	Mercurius	Nux vomica	Phosphorus	Pulsatilla	Rhus tox.	Sulphur
Acne				x				x	x
Anxiety	x				x		x		
Backache					x		x	x	
Bruises, Sprains & Strains					x		x	x	
Coughs & Cold		x					x		
Depression				x			x	x	
Eczema		x						x	x
Exhaustion	x				x				
Gas					x				
Headache									
Indigestion			x		x		x		
Insomnia		x		x			x		
Irritability					x	x	x		
Neck Stiffness					x			x	
PMS					x		x	x	
Sinusitis		x					x		
Toothache				x			x		

Source: Nancy Bruning, *Natural Health,* January/February 1995.

RULES FOR HOMEOPATHY

Homeopathy comes with its own set of rules to follow for taking remedies. Some—such as caveats against touching the remedy or drinking coffee—may seem illogical to the average person. And, admittedly there are differences of opinion within the profession as to how strictly you need to observe these rules. However, the consensus is that to be safe and to give homeopathy the best chance of working, it's advisable to follow these guidelines:

1. The frequency of the dosage depends on the intensity of the symptoms. Severe symptoms that come on suddenly, such as earache, may require a dose every five minutes; a slowly developing flu may need the remedy every three or four hours. As the symptoms improve or disappear, increase the interval between doses or stop the medication. Start again if the same symptoms return. However, if there has been no response to the remedy after six doses, switch to another remedy.
2. Avoid touching the remedy with your hands. Instead, tip the required number of pellets into the container cap and from the cap into your mouth; if the tablets are blister-packed, pop them directly into your mouth. Homeopaths say that touching the remedy could contaminate it or inactivate it.
3. Avoid eating or drinking anything but chlorine-free water for fifteen to thirty minutes before and after taking the remedy. And allow the remedy to dissolve slowly under your tongue so it is absorbed directly into the tiny sublingual capillaries. (Some combination tablets include instructions to chew them.)
4. Store homeopathic remedies in their original containers, away from heat and sunlight. Also, keep them away from strong-smelling substances that might contaminate them, such as perfumes, camphor, and eucalyptus. (These and other aromatic substances are found in items that inhabit the medicine chest.) Some homeopaths also advise against drinking herbal teas or ingesting products containing mint (for instance, toothpaste) within a half-hour of taking remedies.
5. Avoid drinking coffee during treatment. Coffee may counteract the remedy's effect by acting as an antidote or by otherwise slowing the healing process.

Another area of debate among homeopaths is the relationship of homeopathic treatment to other forms of medicine. Some homeopaths feel that all you really need to treat an illness is the right homeopathic remedy. However, most say that other natural healing methods help when used appropriately, and that conventional medicine also has its place. Most homeopaths stress the importance of good health habits such as proper diet, exercise, rest, vacation time, satisfying social relationships, creative living, effective stress management, and spiritual nourishment. Since the goal of homeopathy is to stimulate the body's ability to heal, it makes sense to support the body's efforts with healthy living.

NO
Stephen Barrett

HOMEOPATHY'S LEGACY: PHONY "REMEDIES" AND KINDRED DELUSIONS

Homeopathic "remedies" enjoy a unique status in the health marketplace: they are the only quack products legally marketable as drugs. This situation is the result of two circumstances. First, the 1938 Federal Food, Drug, and Cosmetic Act, which was shepherded through Congress by a homeopathic physician who was also a senator, recognizes as drugs all substances included in the *Homeopathic Phamacopeia of the United States*. Second, the FDA [Food and Drug Administration] has not required proof that homeopathic remedies work.

BASIC MISBELIEFS

Homeopathy dates back to the late 1700s when Samuel Hahnemann (1755–1843), a German physician, began formulating its basic principles. Hahnemann was justifiably distressed about bloodletting, leeching, purging and other medical procedures of his day that did far more harm than good. Thinking that these treatments were intended to "balance the body's 'humors' by opposite effects," he developed his "law of similars"—a notion that symptoms of disease can be cured by substances that produce similar symptoms in healthy people. The word "homeopathy" is derived from the Greek words *homeo* (similar) and *pathos* (suffering or disease).

Hahnemann and his early followers conducted "provings" in which they administered herbs, minerals and other substances to healthy people, including themselves, and kept detailed records of what they observed. Later these records were compiled into lengthy reference books called *materia medica*, which are used to match a patient's symptoms with a "corresponding" drug.

Hahnemann declared that diseases represent a disturbance in the body's ability to heal itself and that only a small stimulus is needed to begin the healing process. At first he used small doses of accepted medications. But later he used enormous dilutions and theorized that the smaller the dose, the more powerful the effect—a principle he called the "law of infinitesimals." That, of course, is just the opposite of what pharmacologists have demonstrated.

From Stephen Barrett, "Homeopathy's Legacy: Phony 'Remedies' and Kindred Delusions," *Priorities*, vol. 6, no. 1 (1994), pp. 13–17. Copyright © 1994 by the American Council on Science and Health. Reprinted by permission of *Priorities*, a publication of the American Council on Science and Health, 1995 Broadway, 2nd Floor, New York, NY 10023-5860.

Moreover, if it were true, every substance encountered by a molecule of water might imprint an "essence" that could exert powerful (and unpredictable) medicinal effects when ingested by a person.

The basis for inclusion in the *Homeopathic Pharmacopeia* is not modern scientific testing, but homeopathic "provings" conducted as long as 150 years ago. The current (ninth) edition describes how more than a thousand substances are prepared for homeopathic use. It does not identify the symptoms or diseases for which homeopathic products should be used; that is determined by the practitioner.

Homeopathic products are made from minerals, botanical substances, zoological substances and several other sources. If the medicinal substance is soluble, one part is diluted with either nine or 99 parts of distilled water and/or alcohol and shaken vigorously; if insoluble, it is finely ground and pulverized in similar proportions with powdered lactose (milk sugar). The process is then repeated until the desired concentration is reached. Dilutions of one to ten are designated by the Roman numeral X (1X = 1/10, 3X = 1/1,000, 6X = 1/1,000,000). Similarly, dilutions of one to 100 are designated by the Roman numeral C (1C = 1/100, 3C = 1/1,000,000 and so on). Most remedies today range from 6X to 30X.

According to the laws of chemistry, there is a limit to the dilution that can be made without losing the original substance altogether. This limit, the reciprocal of Avogadro's number (6.023 × 10^{23}), corresponds to homeopathic potencies of 12C or 24X (one part in 10^{24}). Hahnemann himself realized there is virtually no chance that even one molecule of original substance would remain after extreme dilutions. But he believed that the vigorous shaking or pulverizing with each step of dilution leaves behind a "spirit-like" essence—"no longer perceptible to the senses"—which cures by reviving the body's "vital force." This notion is utter nonsense.

THE DECLINE OF HOMEOPATHY

Because homeopathic remedies were actually less dangerous than those of nineteenth-century medical orthodoxy, many medical practitioners began using them. But as medical science and medical education advanced, homeopathy declined sharply, particularly in America, where its schools have either closed or converted to modern methods.

In 1986, I sent a questionnaire to the deans of all 72 U.S. pharmacy schools. Faculty members from 49 schools responded. Most said their school either didn't mention homeopathy at all or considered it of historical interest only. Hahnemann's "law of similars" did not find a single supporter, and all but one respondent said his "law of infinitesimals" was wrong also. Almost all said that homeopathic remedies were neither potent nor effective, except possibly as placebos for mild, self-limiting ailments. About half felt that homeopathic remedies should be completely removed from the marketplace.

In 1987, *Consumer Reports* stated:

Unless the laws of chemistry have gone awry, most homeopathic remedies are too diluted to have any physiological effect.... Any system of medicine embracing the use of such remedies involves a potential danger to patients whether the prescribers are M.D.s, other licensed practitioners, or outright quacks. Ineffective drugs are dangerous drugs when used to treat serious or life-threatening disease. Moreover ... using them for a serious illness or undiagnosed pain instead of obtaining proper medical attention could prove harmful or even fatal.

HYPE FOR SALE

Homeopathic remedies are available from practitioners, health-food stores and drugstores and manufacturers who sell directly to the public. Products are also sold person-to-person through multilevel marketing companies. Several companies sell home-remedy kits. The size of the homeopathic marketplace is unknown because the largest manufacturers keep their sales figures private. However, *Health Foods Business* estimated that 1992 sales through health-food stores totaled about $160 million.

A 1991 survey by the National Board of Chiropractic Examiners (NBCE) found that 36.9 percent of 4,835 full-time chiropractic practitioners who responded said that they had prescribed homeopathic remedies within the previous two years. The 1993 directory of the National Center for Homeopathy (NCH) in Alexandria, Virginia, lists about 300 licensed practitioners, about half of them physicians and the rest mostly naturopaths, chiropractors, acupuncturists, veterinarians, dentists, nurses or physician's assistants. Although several hundred physicians and naturopaths not listed in the NCH directory practice homeopathy to some extent, they appear to be greatly outnumbered by chiropractors.

PRACTICING HOMEOPATHY

Homeopathic physicians who follow Hahnemann's methods closely take an elaborate history to "fit the remedy to the individual." The history typically includes standard medical questions plus many more about such things as emotions, moods, food preferences and reactions to the weather. A remedy is then selected with the help of a *materia medica* or computer program. Other practitioners, whose approaches have not been systematically tabulated, may spend little time with patients. In the 1992 *Digest of Chiropractic Economics*, for example, a chiropractor who runs a homeopathic manufacturing company described how he had treated a patient with a history of hay fever; allergies to dust, mold and animals; frequent sinusitis, constant postnasal drip; frequent cough; cold hands and feet; skipped heart beats; unhealthy skin; insomnia; abdominal bloating; and slowness in healing skin sores. The bill for eleven visits totaling 107 minutes came to $1,007.24.

A few practitioners who consider themselves homeopaths use "electrodiagnostic" devices to help select the remedies they prescribe. These devices—some of which have been seized by enforcement agencies—are little more than fancy galvanometers that measure electrical resistance of the patient's skin when touched by a probe. But these practitioners claim that the instruments detect disease by measuring disturbances in the body's flow of "electromagnetic energy."

HOMEOPATHIC REMEDIES ARE UNDERREGULATED

Federal laws and regulations require that drugs be safe, effective and properly labeled for their intended use. However, the FDA has not applied this framework to most homeopathic remedies. A recent article in a health-food industry trade publication said: "There is more freedom in selling homeopathy than most other categories." Another article even suggested that "when a customer comes into your store complaining of an earache, fever, flu, sore throat, diarrhea or some other common health problem... one word that should immediately come out of your mouth is 'homeopathy.'" A third article said that, because of an FDA crackdown on several nutritional supplements, "more and more companies were turning to herbs and homeopathy to regain sales." Yet another article stated: "Homeopathy is natural medicine's favorite son in the 1990s. Suddenly the category is appearing everywhere—in newspapers, on radio talk shows, on special television programs.... For natural products retailers, it can be a dream come true."

A few companies encourage health professionals to prescribe their products for serious diseases. In 1983, Biological Homeopathic Industries (BHI) of Albuquerque, New Mexico, sent a 123-page catalog to almost 200,000 physicians nationwide. Among its products were *BHI Anticancer Stimulating, BHI Antivirus, BHI Stroke* and fifty other types of tablets claimed to be effective against serious diseases. In 1984, the FDA forced the company to stop distributing several of the products and to tone down its claims for the rest. However, the company's publishing arm issues the quarterly *Biological Therapy: Journal of Natural Medicine*, which regularly contains articles whose authors make questionable claims. An article in the April 1993 issue, for example, listed "indications" for using BHI and Heel products (distributed by BHI) for more than fifty conditions—including cancer, angina pectoris and paralysis. And the October 1993 issue, devoted to the homeopathic treatment of children, includes an article recommending products for acute bacterial infections of the ear and tonsils. The article is described as selections from Heel seminars given in several cities by a Nevada homeopath who also serves as medical editor of *Biological Therapy*.

HOMEOPATHY IN THE MEDIA

The National Center for Homeopathy keeps close track of homeopathy's portrayal by the media. Its September, October and November 1993 newsletters rated 75 articles and broadcasts and concluded that 57 articles (76 percent) were favorable, 13 articles (17 percent) were unfavorable and five articles (seven percent) were neutral. Most reports simply parrot the claims of homeopathy's promoters.

In the United States, homeopathy's most prolific publicist is probably Dana Ullman, M.P.H., president of the Foundation for Homeopathic Education and Research. At a recent meeting, Ullman informed me that his foundation, despite its name, does not fund research because he does not have sufficient time for fund-raising. Nature's Way, of Springville, Utah, is now marketing over-the-counter products formulated by Ullman. The products include: *Insomnia, Sinusitis, Migraine Headache; Vaginitis, Menopause* (for women), and *Earache* (for children). The company has promised an "aggressive marketing strategy"—with ads in healthcare, women's and parenting magazines—intended to "make homeopathy a household word." Its ads claim that "homeopathic medicine offers a significant advantage over its orthodox counterparts." Other companies have marketed such products as *Arthritis Formula, Bleeding, Kidney Disorders, Flu, Herpes, Exhaustion, Whooping Cough, Gon-*

orrhea, Heart Tonic, Gall-Stones, Prostate Pain, Candida Yeast Infection, Cardio Forte, Thyro Forte, Worms and *Smoking Withdrawal Tablets.*

UNIMPRESSIVE "RESEARCH"

Since many homeopathic remedies contain no detectable amount of active ingredient, it is impossible to test whether they contain what their label says. Unlike most potent drugs, they have not been proven effective against disease by double-blind testing.

In 1990, an article in *Review of Epidemiology* analyzed 40 randomized trials that compared homeopathic treatment with standard treatment, a placebo or no treatment. The authors concluded that all but three of the trials had major flaws in their design and that only one of those three had reported a positive result. The authors concluded that there was no evidence that homeopathic treatment has any more value than a placebo.

Proponents trumpet the few "positive" studies as proof that "homeopathy works." Even if their results can be consistently reproduced (which seems unlikely), the most that the study of a single remedy for a single disease could prove is that the remedy is effective against that disease. It would not validate homeopathy's basic theories or prove that homeopathic treatment is useful for other diseases....

NOT PROVEN EFFECTIVE

Homeopaths are working hard to have their services covered in the new health care reform proposals. They claim to provide care that is safer, gentler, "natural," less expensive than conventional care—and more concerned with prevention. I find the "prevention" claim particularly odious because homeopathic treatments prevent nothing and many homeopathic leaders preach against immunization.

If the FDA required homeopathic remedies to be proven effective in order to remain on the market—the standard it applies to other remedies—homeopathy would face extinction in the United States. However, there is no indication that the agency is considering this. FDA officials regard homeopathy as relatively benign and believe that other problems should get enforcement priority. If the FDA attacks homeopathy too vigorously, its proponents might even persuade Congress to rescue them. Regardless of this risk, the FDA should not permit worthless products to be marketed with claims that they are effective.

POSTSCRIPT

Are Homeopathic Remedies Legitimate?

Why do so many Americans seek out alternative medicine such as homeopathy? In a study published in 1993, researchers at Harvard Medical School found that one out of three patients said they had used some kind of alternative treatment, while seven out of ten said they had not told their doctors. The Harvard study estimated that Americans made 425 million visits to alternative practitioners in 1990, spending over $14 billion. Much of the money was paid directly by the consumers since alternative medicine is usually not covered by health insurance. It may be that consumers are dissatisfied with conventional medical care and short, managed care office visits. Alternative medicine may also appeal to the need for consumers to have both their minds and bodies treated.

Medicine and the research establishment are responding. The National Institutes of Health have created the Office of Alternative Medicine, which has funded two full-scale research projects and given numerous study grants. Currently, more than 25 medical schools teach courses on alternative methods. Could there be a problem with this move toward alternatives such as homeopathy? Maybe. Herbal expert Varro Tyler and physician Stephen Barrett claim that homeopathy is a fraud. See "Why Pharmacists Should Not Sell Homeopathic Remedies," *American Journal of Health-System Pharmacy* (May 1, 1995). Many of the studies supporting homeopathy appear to have methodological flaws. Despite this, many consumers seem to be drawn to unproven remedies. It may be that we have gone too far toward the rational end of health care and consumers are seeking out treatment that seems to work despite lack of valid research.

Are there risks to homeopathy? Generally, it is assumed that the dosage is so diluted that there is little therapeutic effect or risk. The main concern is that patients will abandon conventional therapies in favor of the unproven. Readings that explore homeopathy and alternative medicine include "Flu Symptoms," *U.S. News and World Report* (February 17, 1997); "Homeopathy," *Harvard Women's Health* (January 1997); "Funding Alternative Medicine," *Popular Science* (January 1997); "Challenging the Mainstream," *Time* (Fall 1996); "Homeopathy: Real Medicine or Empty Promise," *FDA Consumer* (December 1996); "Does Homeopathy Work?" *Healthline* (February 1996); "Homeopathy," *Mayo Clinic Newsletter* (February 1996); "Is Less Really More?" *Harvard Health Letter* (May 1995); "Homeopathy: Too Much Ado About Nothing," *Skeptical Briefs* (December 1993); and "Unconventional Medicine in the United States," *The New England Journal of Medicine* (January 12, 1993).

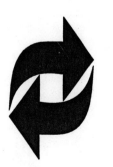

CONTRIBUTORS
TO THIS VOLUME

EDITOR

EILEEN L. DANIEL, a registered dietitian, is an associate professor and chairperson of the Department of Health Science at the State University of New York College at Brockport. She received a B.S. in nutrition and dietetics from the Rochester Institute of Technology in 1977, an M.S. in community health education from SUNY College at Brockport in 1978, and a Ph.D. in health education from the University of Oregon in 1986. A member of the Eta Sigma Gamma National Health Honor Society, the American Dietetics Association, the New York State Dietetics Society, and other professional and community organizations, she is the author or coauthor of over 30 articles on issues of health, nutrition, and health education. Her publications have appeared in professional journals such as the *Journal of Nutrition Education*, the *Journal of School Health*, the *Journal of Health Education*, and the *Journal of the American Dietetics Association*. She is the author of *Jumpstarts with Weblinks: A Guidebook for Fitness/Wellness/Personal Health, 97/98*.

STAFF

David Dean   List Manager
David Brackley   Developmental Editor
Ava Suntoke   Developmental Editor
Tammy Ward   Administrative Assistant
Brenda S. Filley   Production Manager
Juliana Arbo   Typesetting Supervisor
Diane Barker   Proofreader
Lara Johnson   Graphics
Richard Tietjen   Publishing Systems Manager

AUTHORS

BRUCE AMES, a genetic toxicologist, is a professor of biochemistry and molecular biology and the director of the National Institute of Environmental Health Sciences Center at the University of California, Berkeley, where he has been teaching since 1968. He is a member of the National Academy of Sciences and is the recipient of the most prestigious award for cancer research, the General Motors Cancer Research Foundation Prize (1983); the highest award in environmental achievement, the Tyler Prize (1985); and the Gold Medal Award of the American Institute of Chemists (1991). He has been elected to the Royal Swedish Academy of Sciences, Japan Cancer Association, and the Academy of Toxicological Sciences. He is the author or coauthor of 300 scientific publications.

MARCIA ANGELL is a physician, author, and the executive editor of the *New England Journal of Medicine.* She graduated from Boston University School of Medicine and has done postgraduate work in internal medicine as well as in pathology. She frequently writes on ethical issues in medicine and biomedical research and is the author of *Science on Trial: The Clash of Medical Evidence and the Law in the Breast Implant Case* (W. W. Norton, 1996).

STEPHEN BARRETT is a retired psychiatrist and a nationally renowned author, editor, and consumer health advocate. He is a board member of the National Council Against Health Fraud and a scientific and editorial adviser to the American Council on Science and Health. In 1986 he was awarded hororarv life membership in the American Dietetic Association. He has written more than 36 books.

HERBERT BENSON is a physician and associate professor of medicine at Harvard Medical School and the Deaconess Hospital. He is also president and founder of their Mind/Body Institute.

FRANCES M. BERG is a nutritionist and founder, publisher, and editor of *Healthy Weight Journal.* She is an adjunct professor in the Department of Community Medicine and Rural Health of the School of Medicine at the University of North Dakota in Grand Forks, North Dakota. She is the author of eight books and writes the weekly column, *Healthy Living,* published regularly in over 50 newspapers.

DENNIS BERNSTEIN is an associate editor for *Pacific News Service* and a coproducer of KPFA's *Flashpoints* radio show.

DAVID R. BOLDT is a columnist for the *Philadelphia Inquirer.*

NANCY BRUNING is a founding member of Breast Cancer Action. A health and environment writer, she is the author or coauthor of 12 books, including *Breast Implant: Everything You Need to Know* (Hunter House, 1995) and with coauthor Shari Lieberman, *The Real Vitamin and Mineral Book: Going Beyond the RDA for Optimum Health* (Avery, 1990).

DANIEL CALLAHAN, a philosopher, is cofounder and president of the Hastings Center in Briarcliff Manor, New York, where he is also director of International Programs. He received a Ph.D. in philosophy from Harvard University, and he is the author or editor of over 31 publications, including *Ethics in Hard Times* (Plenum Press, 1981); *The Troubled Dream* *of Life: In Search of Peaceful Death* (Simon & Schuster, 1993); and with coauthor Arthur L. Caplan, *Setting Limits: Medical Goals in an Aging Society* (Simon & Schuster, 1987).

SARAH J. CLARK is associated with the Cecil G. Sheps Center for Health Services Research, University of North Carolina at Chapel Hill.

JASON DePARLE is a former editor of the *Washington Monthly*.

EZEKIEL J. EMANUEL is a professor in the Division of Medical Ethics at Harvard Medical School. He is a physician and researcher associated with the Division of Cancer Epidemiology and Control at the Dana Farber Cancer Institute in Boston, Massachusetts. He is the recipient of an American Cancer Society Career Development Award.

LINDA L. EMANUEL is a physician and researcher at the Division of Medical Ethics, Harvard Medical School, Boston, Massachusetts.

KATHLEEN M. FOLEY is a physician in the department of neurology at Memorial Sloan-Kettering Cancer Center in New York City.

GARY L. FREED is a physician with the Division of Community Pediatrics, Department of Health Policy and Administration, Duke University Medical Center, Durham, North Carolina.

MICHAEL FUMENTO is a graduate of the University of Illinois College of Law. A former AIDS analyst and attorney for the U.S. Commission on Civil Rights, Fumento is currently a fellow with Consumer Alert in Washington, D.C. The author of numerous articles on AIDS for publications worldwide, he has written two books, *The Myth of Heterosexual AIDS* (New Republic Books, 1990) and *Science Under Siege: Balancing Technology and the Environment* (William Morrow, 1993). He received the American Council on Science and Health's Distinguished Science Journalist of 1993 Award for *Science Under Siege.*

ROSS GELBSPAN was an editor and reporter at the *Philadelphia Bulletin*, the *Washington Post*, and the *Boston Globe* over a 30-year period. In 1984 he was a corecipient of the Pulitzer Prize for public service reporting.

MARY GORDON is a novelist and short-story writer. She is the author of *Penal Discipline: Female Prisoners* (Gordon Press, 1992), *The Rest of Life: Three Novellas* (Viking Penguin, 1993), and *The Other Side* (Wheeler, 1994).

MARTHA HONEY, a freelance journalist and author, is a research fellow at the Institute for Policy Studies in Washington, D.C.

KEVIN R. HOPKINS is an adjunct senior fellow of the Hudson Institute, a nonprofit research organization, in Indianapolis, Indiana.

DAVID JACOBSEN is a surgeon with Harvard Pilgrim Health Care in Boston.

MICHAEL F. JACOBSON is a microbiologist and the director of the Center for Science in the Public Interest, a health and nutrition consumer advocate group.

WILLIAM B. JOHNSTON is vice president and senior research fellow of the Hudson Institute, a nonprofit policy research organization in Indianapolis, Indiana.

ANDREW G. KADAR is an attending physician at Cedars-Sinai Medical Center in Los Angeles, California, and a clinical instructor in the School of Medicine at the University of California, Los Angeles.

DON B. KATES is a San Francisco civil liberties lawyer and criminologist.

SAMUEL L. KATZ is a physician associated with the division of Pediatric Infectious Diseases, Duke University Medical Center in Durham, North Carolina.

THEA KELLEY is a freelance journalist based in San Francisco.

LESLIE LAURENCE is a health and medical reporter.

RICHARD LEVITON, one of the country's leading health journalists, is a senior writer for *Yoga Journal* in Berkeley, California, a regular contributor to *The Quest,* and was for 7 years a senior writer for *East West,* now named *Natural Health,* in Brookline, Massachusetts. Leviton has written over 150 feature articles. Many of them have been reprinted in the United States and abroad, in Canada, Germany, Switzerland, Israel, and Australia, and some have been republished in topical anthologies.

WILLIAM B. LINDLEY is an associate editor of *Truth Seeker* magazine.

A. KENT MacDOUGALL is a professor emeritus of journalism at the University of California, Berkeley.

ETHAN A. NADELMANN is the director of the Lindesmith Center, a New York drug-policy research institute and an assistant professor of politics and public affairs in the Woodrow Wilson School of Public and International Affairs at Princeton University in Princeton, New Jersey. He was the founding coordinator of the Harvard Study Group on Organized Crime, and he has been a consultant to the Department of State's Bureau of International Narcotics Matters. He is also an assistant editor of the *Journal of Drug Issues* and a contributing editor of the *International Journal on Drug Policy.*

ERIC B. RIMM received a doctorate in epidemiology from the Harvard School of Public Health in 1990 and has since been practicing there as a research associate. He also serves as project director of the Health Professionals Follow-up Study, a prospective epidemiological study designed to investigate the nutritional etiologies of chronic disease among over 50,000 men in the United States. He is a coauthor of over 30 scientific publications, including articles examining associations between alcohol, coffee consumption, and dietary antioxidants (vitamins C, E, and beta-carotene) and risk of cardiovascular disease.

HENRY E. SCHAFFER is a professor of genetics and biomathematics at North Carolina State University in Raleigh.

DAVE SHIFLETT is a writer living in northern Virginia.

S. FRED SINGER is the director of the Washington, D.C.–based Science and Environmental Policy Project (SEPP). He was formerly a professor of environmental sciences at the University of Virginia in Charlottesville and chief scientist for the U.S. Department of Transportation.

MEIR J. STAMPFER is an associate professor of epidemiology at the Harvard University School of Public Health and holds an appointment at Brigham and Women's Hospital. His current research focuses on the influence of diet and exogenous hormones on health. He received a bachelor's degree at Columbia University, an M.D. from New York University School of Medicine, and a Ph.D. in epidemiology from Harvard University. He has published over 140 scientific papers and has a major interest in the influence of diet and exogenous hormones on health.

MARG STARK is a freelance journalist specializing in medical news and features.

JOSH SUGARMANN is the executive director of the Violence Policy Center, an educational foundation that researches firearm violence and advocates gun control. He is the former communications director of the National Coalition to Ban Handguns.

JACOB SULLUM is a senior editor for *Reason* magazine. He writes on several public policy issues, including freedom of speech, criminal justice, and education. His work has appeared in the *Wall Street Journal*, the *New York Times*, and the *Los Angeles Times*. In 1988 he won the Keystone Award for investigative reporting. He has been a fellow of the Knight Center for Specialized Journalism.

ERIC A. VOTH is chairman of the International Drug Strategy Institute and clinical assistant professor with the Department of Medicine at the University of Kansas School of Medicine. He is also the medical director of Chemical Dependency Services at St. Francis Hospital in Topeka, Kansas. He has testified for the Drug Enforcement Administration in opposition to legalizing marijuana, and he is recognized as an international authority on drug abuse.

DIANA CHAPMAN WALSH is a professor in the Department of Health and Social Behavior of the School of Public Health at Harvard University.

JENNIFER WASHBURN is a Brooklyn-based freelance writer.

WILLIAM C. WATERS IV practices medicine in Atlanta.

BETH WEINHOUSE is a health and medical reporter.

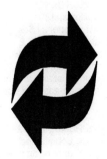

INDEX